Nancy Jacobs, Audiologist
NYC Dept. of Ed. HHVI Reg. 2
3450 E. Tremont Ave, Room 227
Bronx, N.Y. 10465
Tel (718) 794-7422
Fax (718) 794-7435

return to:
Nancy Jacobs
HHVI / Bx Satellite
5500 Broadway, 2nd flr
Bronx, NY 10463

CAPD related classroom observation

- Compensatory strategies -
  Does child know/use any?
  seating close to teacher
  watching teacher speak
  request clarification or repetition.

- Listening environment
  - How many classrooms?
  - background noise
  - reverberation
  - acoustic treatments?
  - ear plugs?
  - medications being taken?

- Teacher Surveys (pre/post FM)
  CHAPS? Fishers? App 6-C

- Lang. processing
  - problems w/ r vs L? p85
  - receptive lang. tests - poor results?
  - expressive lang. ok?

# CENTRAL AUDITORY PROCESSING:
## A Transdisciplinary View

# Central Auditory Processing:
## A Transdisciplinary View

JACK KATZ, Ph.D.
*Professor, Communicative Disorders and Sciences*
*University of Buffalo*
*Buffalo, New York*

NANCY A. STECKER, Ph.D.
*Clinical Assistant Professor*
*Communicative Disorders and Sciences*
*University of Buffalo*
*Buffalo, New York*

DONALD HENDERSON, Ph.D.
*Chairman and Professor*
*Communicative Disorders and Sciences*
*University of Buffalo*
*Buffalo, New York*

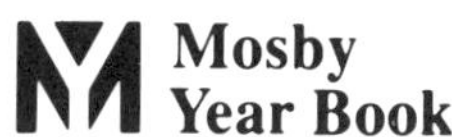


St. Louis Baltimore Boston Chicago London Philadelphia Sydney Toronto

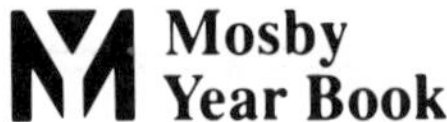

Dedicated to Publishing Excellence

*Sponsoring Editor: David K. Marshall*
*Assistant Editor: Julie Tryboski*
*Assistant Managing Editor, Text and Reference: George Mary Gardner*
*Production Manager: Nancy C. Baker*
*Proofroom Manager: Barbara Kelly*



Mosby–Year Book, Inc.
11830 Westline Industrial Drive
St. Louis, MO 63146



1 2 3 4 5 6 7 8 9 0 CL/MV 96 95 94 93 92

**Library of Congress Cataloging-in-Publication Data**
Central auditory processing: a transdisciplinary view / [edited by]
Jack Katz, Nancy Stecker, Donald Henderson.
p. cm.
Includes bibliographical references and index.
ISBN 1-55664-372-1
1. Word deafness. I. Katz, Jack. II. Stecker, Nancy Austin.
III. Henderson, Donald, 1938-
[DNLM: 1. Auditory Diseases, Central—complications. 2. Auditory
Diseases, Central—diagnosis. 3. Auditory Diseases, Central—
therapy. WV 272 C3973]
RC394.W63C46 1992 92-18767
617.8—dc20 CIP
DNLM/DLC
for Library of Congress

# Contributors

**Susan Ellen Bacon, Ph.D.**
*President, Training Limited*
*Decatur, Illinois*

**Flint A. Boettcher, Ph.D.**
*Research Assistant Professor*
*Hearing Research Lab*
*University of Buffalo*
*Buffalo, New York*

**Steven P. Bornstein, Ph.D.**
*Assistant Professor of Communication Disorders*
*School of Health and Human Sciences*
*University of New Hampshire*
*Durham, New Hampshire*

**Marco Carner, Ph.D.**
*Assistant Professor*
*Department of Otolaryngology*
*University of Verona*
*Verona, Italy*

**Rochelle Cherry, Ed.D.**
*Associate Professor and Head of Audiology*
*Brooklyn College*
*City University of New York*
*New York, New York*

**Laurel Christopherson, M.A.**
*Assistant Professor*
*Department of Communication Disorders*
*Louisiana State University Medical Center*
*New Orleans, Louisiana*

**Carol Cokely, M.A.**
*Research Audiologist*
*Department of Speech and Hearing Sciences*
*Indiana University*
*Bloomington, Indiana*

**Vittorio Colletti, Ph.D.**
*Professor, Department of Otolaryngology*
*University of Verona*
*Verona, Italy*

**Franco G. Fiorino, Ph.D.**
*Assistant Professor*
*Department of Otolaryngology*
*University of Verona*
*Verona, Italy*

**Donald Henderson, Ph.D.**
*Chairman and Professor*
*Communicative Disorders and Sciences*
*University of Buffalo*
*Buffalo, New York*

**Larry Humes, Ph.D.**
*Professor and Director of Audiology*
*Department of Speech and Hearing Sciences*
*Indiana University*
*Bloomington, Indiana*

**Jack Katz, Ph.D.**
*Professor, Communicative Disorders and Sciences*
*University of Buffalo*
*Buffalo, New York*

**Warren D. Keller, Ph.D.**
*Psychologist, Private Practice*
*East Amherst, New York*

**Raymond D. Kent, Ph.D.**
*Professor, Department of Communicative Disorders*
*University of Wisconsin—Madison*
*Madison, Wisconsin*

**Mary Ellen Tekieli Koay, Ph.D.**
*Professor, Speech Pathology and Audiology*
*West Virginia University*
*Morgantown, West Virginia*

**Lloyd E. Lamb, Ph.D.**
*Professor of Communicative Disorders*
*University of New Mexico*
*Albuquerque, New Mexico*

**Judith L. Lauter, Ph.D.**
*John Keys Speech and Hearing Center*
*University of Oklahoma Health Sciences Center*
*Oklahoma City, Oklahoma*

**Paula Menyuk, D.Ed.**
*Professor, Department of Applied Linguistics and Developmental Studies*
*Boston University*
*Boston, Massachusetts*

**Frank E. Musiek, Ph.D.**
*Professor and Director*
*Otolaryngology and Neurology*
*Dartmouth-Hitchcock Medical Center*
*Hanover, New Hampshire*

**Nicholas L. Powers, Ph.D.**
*Research Assistant Professor*
*Hearing Research Lab*
*University of Buffalo*
*Buffalo, New York*

**Richard J. Salvi, Ph.D.**
*Professor, Communicative Disorders and Sciences*
*University of Buffalo*
*Buffalo, New York*

**Daniel Schneider, M.A.**
*Audiologist*
*Genesee Hearing Services*
*Buffalo, New York*

**Christine Sloan, Ph.D.**
*Speech Pathologist, Private Practice*
*Grandville Ferry, Nova Scotia, Canada*

**Nancy A. Stecker, Ph.D.**
*Clinical Assistant Professor*
*Communicative Disorders and Sciences*
*University of Buffalo*
*Buffalo, New York*

**Giuseppe Verlato, Ph.D.**
*Assistant Professor*
*Department of Otolaryngology*
*University of Verona*
*Verona, Italy*

# Preface

The area of central auditory function and its disorders is of relatively recent interest. However, because of the pervasiveness of the auditory system and its critical role in the learning of speech-language and academic skills, it has risen quickly in importance. Specialists in many fields have a keen interest in various aspects of central auditory processing. However, there is a tendency for these groups to communicate primarily within their own disciplines. Thus the important contributions of each group often are not shared with the others. This reduces both our understanding of this family of problems and our effectiveness in dealing with them. It is the purpose of this book to bring together the ideas of different professional groups that all too often do not work and think together, to profit from one another.

*Central Auditory Processing: A Transdisciplinary View* was planned and edited by a committee made up of Jack Katz, Nancy Stecker, and Donald Henderson, of the University of Buffalo. It was supported by the Faculty of Social Sciences, the University's Conferences in the Disciplines, and the Department of Communicative Disorders and Sciences, with the extensive help of Lori Serafino and Sandy Mundier.

Every effort was made to gather information from different specialty areas, including Audiology, Speech-Language Pathology, Psychology, and Otology, and from somewhat different perspectives. Both clinical and laboratory (Hearing-Speech Science) approaches have been addressed, with some attempt from each side to bridge the gaps.

It is our hope that this book will provide the reader with useful ideas to consider in their work with central auditory processing (CAP) and CAP disorders (CAPD), and useful techniques and approaches for evaluating and remediating CAPD. While it is our hope to resolve some of the current questions the reader may have, as teachers we anticipate that this book also will generate new questions for your consideration.

**Jack Katz**
**Nancy A. Stecker**
**Donald Henderson**

see also: Advance Nov. 18, 1996 Vol 6 #46
p 8 - CAPD - Define + measure
p 10 APD
p 21 classroom strategies.

# Contents

*PART* ***I***

# INTRODUCTION

Chapter 1

# Introduction to Central Auditory Processing

**Jack Katz, Ph.D.**
**Nancy A. Stecker, Ph.D.**
**Donald Henderson, Ph.D.**

## THE AUDITORY SYSTEM

It is obvious to both clinicians and researchers that the auditory system is extremely complex. Its influence begins when the pinna shapes the airborne messages that are directed to the outer ear canal. Mechanical transmission through the middle ear provides further filtering and amplification. In fact, for most mammalian ears, including human ears, the shape of the audiogram is a consequence primarily of the acoustic transformation through the external and middle ears. When sound is delivered to the inner ear the mechanical properties of the inner ear provide a detailed analysis of the stimulus. The wide range of frequencies, intensities, and durations of the auditory signals are encoded by the hair cells–eighth nerve complex into neural language, which then is relayed tonotopically to higher levels of the auditory system.

The first station of the brain stem, the cochlear nucleus, is said to recode the auditory signal and transfers much of the message to the opposite side via three major pathways. In addition, information from the cochlear nucleus passes ipsilaterally along the lateral lemniscus. A variety of functions are associated with the brain stem, including localization of sound, squelching background noise, memory, auditory-ocular interaction, and the acoustic reflex, as well as the regulation that is carried out by the olivocochlear bundle. In addition, the auditory brain stem interacts with the reticular activating system and the cerebellum.

On entering the thalamus of the brain, auditory information takes two pathways to the temporal lobe. Primary auditory reception occurs in Heschl's gyri in either hemisphere of the brain. Somewhat different but complementary functions are carried out by the right and left hemispheres. These include auditory-linguistic processing in Wernicke's area and the insular cortex, primarily on the left, and the processing of nonlinguistic information that takes place primarily on the right side. Pathways from each hemisphere course to the opposite side, stimulating, inhibiting, or transferring information.

In the past, research dealing with the auditory system has focused primarily on the peripheral portion. Only in recent years has attention been extended to clarify the contributions of the central auditory nervous system (CANS). This book details the importance of the CANS for effective listening, what factors tend to adversely affect it, how these factors may be measured, and what steps may be taken to minimize the limitations imposed by central auditory processing disorder (CAPD).

## IS THERE CENTRAL AUDITORY PROCESSING?

Presently there is both great interest and great confusion about central auditory processing (CAP) and CAPD. This is not surprising given the size and complexity of the auditory system and the varied functions that it carries out. This section will consider whether there is such a thing as CAP and later sections will consider what CAP does for us and what happens if it fails to function properly.

Many readers may be surprised that there is some question that CAP exists. Logic would have it that if other senses must be processed to be understood, that speech and other auditory signals must be processed as well in order to be perceived. Furthermore, when one comes to appreciate the extensive auditory system that has evolved, it seems reasonable to assume that it must play a critically important role in human communication.

There are those who have suggested that there is little, if any, need for auditory processing.[13, 14] It has been claimed that "very little can be gleaned from the acoustical signal . . . the fuzzy and uninformative acoustic signal."[3] Rather, they believe that we anticipate what is said using our knowledge of the world and our understanding of language. This "top-down" argument suggests that we understand speech using our higher cognitive functions and depend little or not at all on the auditory signal for understanding the spoken word.

We must recognize the vital importance of top-down processing, for without our understanding of language and the world, words and verbal concepts would be meaningless. There should be little argument that the rules of language help us to understand quickly what has been said and that we use these same skills to figure out that which is not clearly heard. Furthermore, to depend on hearing every sound to understand what has been said would be too slow a process and one that would be severely impaired by minor articulatory infractions or the presence of background noise. On the other hand, to indicate a complete dependence upon higher cognitive functions exclusive of the auditory signal would suggest that deafness would be but a minor interference. Hearing aids and telephone amplifiers would be of little value to the user. The implications of an exclusively top-down system for our profession would be drastic considering our interest in speech acoustics and the anatomy and physiology of the speech and hearing mechanism, as well as our current efforts to improve articulation, stuttering, and language disorders.

It is just as important to recognize that without hearing and auditorily processing speech signals we would not develop our top-down skills. In addition, without benefit of the spoken word we would be as handicapped as a person listening to a group of foreign speakers or as a person watching television with the volume turned off. Thus, to view the system as exclusively top-down or bottom-up is not defensible. Although there may be disagreement regarding the details of CAP and who may be most capable to evaluate and remediate CAP problems, we hope that there is no doubt in the reader's mind that the auditory signal and CAP exist and have vital importance for our education and our ability to communicate.

## WHAT IS CENTRAL AUDITORY PROCESSING?

### Terminology

**Central Auditory Processing.**—The term "central auditory processing" is used in this book to refer to the use we make of the auditory signal. Although there are other appropriate terms for this process, CAP is the most commonly used term at this time, and it is the one used by most journals and for book and conference titles. Furthermore, it is useful because it focuses attention on the most obvious aspect of the phenomenon, the role played by the CANS.

**Auditory Processing.**—The term "auditory processing" is used to refer to much the same process as CAP; however, omitting the word "central" implies that auditory processing involves more than the central system. This is indeed the case. The pinna and external auditory meatus resonate to middle and high frequencies that are critical for understanding speech, the middle ear muscles moderate transmission to the cochlea thus avoiding distortion, and the outer hair cells appear to be important in properly tuning the basilar membrane. Without the proper functioning of these peripheral mechanisms, there would be a heavy burden added to the task of the CANS.

**Auditory Perception.**—The term "auditory perception" is favored by many, but used by relatively few people at this time. The term is readily understood by the public and professionals alike. Although the term implies an appreciation at a high level in the central nervous system (CNS), it does not negate the influence of lower levels of the auditory system. The term "auditory perception" has two other benefits: it can be used as a parallel to the term *visual perception,* and it is easily distinguished from hearing sensitivity, presumably a lower-level function.

### Defining Central Auditory Processing

The lack of a widely accepted definition of CAP contributes to the confusion that some may have regarding this topic; however, it is not surprising that this recently identified, highly complex system is not better understood nor its definition agreed upon by professionals. To get a general fix on this topic, it is safe to say that CAP is "what we do with what we hear"—that is, the use we make of what has been heard. If the entire signal is not capable of being heard (e.g., because of a high-frequency hearing loss), then we may need to reduce our expectations because all of the desirable clues may not be available to the auditory system. On the other hand, limitations in dealing with auditory signals above and beyond that of the hearing loss may be labeled CAPD.

For purposes of this book we will use a broad definition of CAP that can accommodate the various professions and orientations represented in the following chapters. It is not meant to be all-inclusive, but rather to provide a common basis for discussion and understanding of the management and application of the heard signal that courses through the auditory system.

The auditory system is involved in a number of sensory and cognitive behaviors. At a sensory-experience level the auditory system not only detects sounds but sorts them in terms of frequency, intensity, and complexity. The code for these primary attributes is probably established at the level of the cochlea. The CANS encodes the localization of sound. This process involves the comparison of signals from each ear and is probably carried out in the olivary complex of the medulla-pons. Also at this level of the brain stem, the auditory system works in concert with the trigeminal and facial nerves to control sound transmission through the middle ear by contraction of the tensor tympani and stapedius muscles. At a higher level of the CNS, the system decodes complex patterns of sound and attributes meaning to sound stimuli. It should be recognized that these are complementary and often simultaneous functions that require parallel processing in the CNS. Although virtually all of the neurons of the eighth nerve entering the cochlear nucleus share common physiological and anatomical characteristics, the second-order neurons leaving the cochlear nucleus fall into five or six different categories. The presumption is that the various cell types leaving the cochlear nucleus are the precursors of the parallel processing that is required for the multiple functions of the auditory system.

Central auditory processing incorporates both serial processing, from one level to the next, as well as parallel processing, simultaneous transmission within a single hemisphere or on both sides. For example, various parts of the auditory signal may be processed in different parts of the auditory nerve at the same time and sequentially, depending on frequency and intensity characteristics. At the level of the cochlear nucleus information is carried up both sides of the brain stem pathway. Effective auditory processing requires the use of both afferent and efferent systems and calls upon sensory, association, and commissural fibers at the level of the brain.

Auditory processing involves attention, detection, and identification of the signal. To be dealt with properly, the information must be selected from among all of the other sensory images for special consideration. This selection process must be carried out at various levels of the auditory system under the control of higher functions.

At the cortical level, auditory processing involves the decoding of the neural message. For this purpose we use many skills from our basic understanding of speech sounds up to our linguistic and world knowledge to determine what was said and meant. Storage of auditory-related information is carried out consciously and unconsciously, for long or brief periods of retention, at various levels of the CANS. Retrieval from these memory stores is also critical to the effective use of what has been heard. In addition to the above, our auditory functions would be in disarray if we were not able to sequence and organize what was heard.

Clearly, a significant breakdown in any of these functions could lead to impairment in the proper use of auditory information. The next section will address these issues.

## SCOPE OF CAPD

Central auditory processing disorder has not been under study for a very long time; nevertheless, a variety of learning and communicative problems have become associated with it. The list of difficulties that are common in those with CAPD is rather long and involves many important functions. When the fundamental characteristics of CAPD are considered (see Chapter 10) it is not difficult to see how these problems may be related. This of course does not imply that there is a causal relationship between CAPD and the associated disabilities. For example, they may be correlated problems but not functionally dependent (e.g., both may result from some third dysfunction); the associated problem simply may be intensified because of the concomitant CAPD; or indeed, the problem might be caused by the auditory processing difficulty.

The most common problem area associated with CAPD is that of learning disabilities (LDs).[9] This association was clearly noted from the early days of studying learning disabilities[8] and even before.[12] Among the many LDs, a weakness in reading was the one first noticed and the one that has been most often related to auditory perceptual difficulties.[10, 11] For example, Monroe[10] in 1932 found a large percentage of poor readers could not auditorily synthesize a few speech sounds into a word. Early studies also reported on the relationship between speech articulation problems and auditory processing difficulties that might underlie them.[18, 19] A recent article also suggests that CAPD may be more common in those with certain voice disorders.[15] Language disorders, especially receptive skills, have been associated with auditory perceptual deficits.[2, 17] However, it is interesting that expressive problems, pragmatic disorders, and more general language disabilities also may be related to CAPD.[20, 21] The influence of otitis media on CAP and other functions has been intensively studied.[4, 7, 16]

A variety of other problems have been associated with CAPD; for example, attention deficit hyperactive disorder often overlaps with CAPD problems, as discussed in Chapter 9. In addition, Green and colleagues[5, 6] and others[1, 22] have discussed auditory processing problems in those with schizophrenia and other psychiatric disorders.

It is our observation that CAPD is a widespread problem that calls for the assistance of many professionals. When the problem is ignored or missed by the professional, it leads to further frustration, failure, and self-doubt on the part of the patient, the family, and teachers. The work with those who have auditory perceptual disorders is especially rewarding and important because when CAPD is understood by the professionals, it can be identified easily by a variety of procedures and appropriate management strategies can be instituted.

## ABOUT THIS BOOK

This book is composed of 17 chapters divided into five major sections. The chapters were contributed by qualified professionals in the areas of speech-language pathology, audiology, and psychology, as well as speech and hearing sciences. Although all of the chapters have clinical relevance, the first 8 deal with more basic issues. Thus, nearly half of the book deals with basic and theoretical information. The importance that we place on these basic areas underscores our belief that in order to have a good understanding of CAP, it is necessary to be grounded in the structure, function, basic science knowledge, and theory of the system under study. The remaining 9 chapters have direct clinical applications. These chapters are divided into aspects that are particularly associated with the work of audiologists and those that are generally carried out by speech-language pathologists. Some of these chapters could have been placed into either section. In fact, we recommend that regardless of the reader's clinical discipline both sections be read to get a broad and more complete picture. In this first chapter, which provides an overview of CAP and CAPD, it is our purpose to show a panoramic view that includes a glimpse of all aspects of the book.

The first major section deals with anatomy and physiology of normal and disordered systems. This section contains four chapters that lay the physical groundwork for understanding auditory processing. Chapter 2 discusses anatomy of the auditory brain stem and cerebrum as well as the normal physiology of this mechanism (based on animal data when human data were unavailable). Chapter 3 discusses the apparent contribution that the acoustic reflex makes to CAP based on both auditory brain stem response (ABR) and speech discrimination findings. Chapter 4 deals with animal studies that demonstrate the influence peripheral hearing disorders have on central functions. These materials provide further support to the notion that the auditory system is highly interdependent and that auditory perception is more than a central phenomenon. The final chapter in this section, chapter 5, discusses the various imaging techniques that are presently available for studying CAP and CAPD. They reveal anatomical and physiological information about the auditory system including the brain stem, thalamus, reception region, and association areas.

The second section contains three chapters that combine theoretical, experimental, and clinical perspectives, applying knowledge from the fields of audiology, speech-language science, and psychology. The first of these chapters, chapter 6, provides a classification system that can be used by various professional fields in dividing the CAPD population into meaningful subgroups. This information relates anatomy, physiology, test results, and behavior and academic performance into a unified taxonomy. Chapter 7 reviews the contemporary research and theories dealing with speech perception and word recognition. The author supports a particle, field, and wave approach in order to appreciate the way speech is perceived. The last chapter in this section, chapter 8, helps to elucidate the professional confusion between CAPD and attention deficit disorder (ADD). Information about each of the disorders is presented, as well as criteria that may be used to separate CAPD from ADD.

The third section of this book contains five chapters dealing with audiological concerns regarding CAP and CAPD. Chapter 9 provides information about behavioral diagnostic procedures and approaches. The chapter emphasizes the importance of assessing all levels of the auditory system, peripheral and central, in order to determine the best management strategies. Chapter 10 is specifically geared to the evaluation of young children. It is obvious that early identification and remediation should be our goal and therefore these activities deserve careful consideration. Chapter 11 deals with the fastest-growing group in this country, the elderly. It is the purpose of this chapter to discuss whether the communication breakdown in the elderly can be shown to be due in part to CAPD exclusive of hearing loss. Chapter 12 is concerned with later brain potentials in evaluating central auditory disorders. This important approach in studying both brain lesion and CAP cases is reviewed. The final chapter in this section is devoted to audiological management of CAPD. In this chapter both classroom strategies, (e.g., assistive listening devices) and direct therapeutic intervention are discussed.

The final section of this book is devoted to approaches and questions dealing mainly with speech-language pathology. The first chapter in this section concerns itself with the relationship of speech problems to CAPD. This chapter provides a classification of available speech and hearing tests that evaluate a continuum of auditory skills. Chapter 15 deals with language impairment and CAPD. A broad language approach is recommended. Chapter 16 discusses the influence of otitis media on disorders of communication. It reviews the literature relating to the controversy concerning the importance of this relationship. The final chapter in this section provides a basis for remediating speech and language problems that are associated with CAPD. This chapter suggests that a gestalt approach be used that goes beyond specific receptive language skills and focuses on the whole child in different settings.

The area of CAP is rapidly evolving in a variety of avenues, both from clinical and research vantage points. It is a field that challenges the talents of many professions, among them those concerned with communicative disorders and psychology, which are the focus of this volume. We believe that this book provides a broad view of both the problems and solutions currently under study and underlines the great potential for future work in this area. It is our hope that the interest and enthusiasm for further study of CAP will come from many professional areas and approaches, because we are convinced that such study will provide the most complete understanding of this process.

## REFERENCES


1. Bruder GE: Cerebral laterality and psychopathology: Dichotic listening studies in schizophrenia and affective disorders. *Schizophr Bull* 1983; 9:134–151.
2. Butler KG: Language processing: Selective attention and mnemonic strategies, in Lasky EZ, Katz J (eds): *Central Auditory Processing Disorders: Problems of Speech, Language and Learning.* Baltimore, University Park Press, 1983, pp 297–315.
3. Duchan JF, Katz J: Language and auditory processing, in Lasky EZ, Katz J (eds): *Central Auditory Processing Disorders: Problems of Speech, Language and Learning.* Baltimore, University Park Press, 1983, pp 31–45.
4. Gottlieb MI, Zinkus PW, Thompson A: Chronic middle ear disease and auditory perceptual deficits. *Clin Pediatr* 1979; 18:725–732.
5. Green P, Hallett S, Hunter M: Abnormal interhemispheric integration in schizophrenics and high risk children, in Flor-Henry P, Gruzelier J (eds): *Laterality and Psychopathology.* Amsterdam, Elsevier, 1983, pp 443–469.
6. Green P, Kotenko V: Superior speech comprehension in schizophrenics under monaural versus binaural listening conditions. *J Abnorm Psychol* 1980; 89:339–408.
7. Holm VA, Kunze LH: Effects of chronic otitis media on language and speech development. *Pediatrics* 1969; 43:833–839.
8. Kass C, Myklebust H: Learning disability: An educational definition. *J Learn Disabil* 1969; 2:38–40.
9. Katz J, Illmer R: Auditory perception in children with learning disabilities, in Katz J (ed): *Handbook of Clinical Audiology.* Baltimore, Williams & Wilkins, 1972, pp 540–563.
10. Monroe M: *Children Who Cannot Read.* Chicago, University of Chicago Press, 1932.
11. Mulder RL, Curtin J: Vocal phonic ability and silent reading achievement. *Elementary Sch J* 1955; 56:121–123.
12. Orton ST: *Reading, Writing and Speech Problems in Children.* New York, WW Norton & Co, 1937.
13. Rees N: Auditory processing factors in language disorders: The view from Procrustes' bed. *J Speech Hear Disord* 1975; 38:304–315.
14. Rees N: Saying more than we know: Is auditory processing disorder a meaningful concept?, in Keith R (ed): *Central Auditory and Language Disorders in Children.* Houston, College Hill Press, 1981, pp 94–120.
15. Saniga RD, Carlin MF: Auditory dysfunction in voice disordered patients. *Am Auditory Soc Bull* 1991; 16:9–10, 22–23.
16. Silva PA, Chalmers D, Stewart I: Some audiological, psychological, educational and behavioral characteristics of children with bilateral otitis media with effusion: A longitudinal study. *J Learn Disabil* 1986; 19:165–169.
17. Sloan C: Auditory processing disorders and language development, in Levenson P, Sloan C (eds): *Auditory Processing and Language: Clinical and Research Perspectives.* New York, Grune & Stratton, 1980, pp 101–116.
18. Stovall JV, Manning WH, Shaw CK: Auditory assembly of children with mild and severe misarticulations. *Folia Phoniatr* 1977; 29:162–172.
19. Travis LE, Rasmus B: Speech sound discrimination ability of cases with functional disorders of articulation. *Q J Speech* 1931; 17:217–226.
20. Wetherby AM, Koegel RL, Mendel M: Central nervous system dysfunction in echolalic autistic individuals. *J Speech Hear Res* 1981; 24:420–429.
21. Young ML: Neuroscience, pragmatic competence and auditory processing, in Lasky EZ, Katz J (eds): *Central Auditory Processing Disorders: Problems of Speech, Language and Learning.* Baltimore, University Park Press, 1983, pp 141–162.
22. Yozawitz A, Bruder G, Sutton S, et al: Dichotic perception: Evidence for right hemisphere dysfunction in affective psychosis. *Br J Psychiatr* 1979; 135:224–237.

*PART II*

# ANATOMICAL AND PHYSIOLOGICAL CONSIDERATIONS

*Chapter* **2**

# Neuroanatomy and Neurophysiology of Central Auditory Processing

**Frank E. Musiek, Ph.D.**
**Lloyd Lamb, Ph.D.**

Auditory processing involves a complex series of neurophysiological and chemical events that begin in the cochlea and proceed upward, encompassing numerous structures and pathways throughout the brain stem and cerebrum. Descending pathways that run throughout the auditory system enhance processing and, ultimately, the interpretation of auditory information.

This chapter presents an overview of central auditory nervous system (CANS) anatomy and physiology, focusing on some of the known or suspected elements of central auditory processing. Significant strides have been made toward understanding the CANS and we highlight some of the more significant research findings. Most of the neurophysiological data presented here have been derived from animal models. Although much of the animal data can be applied to the human model, there are many inconsistancies. Therefore, information from the human model is presented whenever possible.

## BRAIN STEM

### Cochlear Nuclear Complex

There is general agreement that the CANS begins with the cochlear nuclear complex, bilateral groupings of nuclei located on the posterolateral surface of the brain stem at the junction of the pons and the medulla (Fig 2–1). Often referred to as the cochlear nucleus or nuclei (CN), the cochlear nuclear complex consists of three divisions: the anterior ventral CN, the posterior ventral CN, and the dorsal CN. Fibers of the auditory nerve enter this complex at the junction of the anterior ventral and posterior ventral, with each fiber dividing to send branches to the three individual nuclei (Fig 2–2).[145]

The cochlear nuclei are composed of many cell types including, among others, pyramidal, octopus, stellate, and spherical cells.[127] Each of these cells is capable of modifying incoming neural impulses in a characteristic fashion, thus providing the foundation for coding information by the type of neural activity within the CN. Each poststimulatory histogram shows the average response of a given neural unit to a series of short tones presented at the unit's characteristic frequency.[138] The major response patterns are primary-like (initial spike followed by a steady response until the stimulus stops), chopper (on–off–on–off neural response to the stimulus), onset (initial spike to the stimulus onset only), and pauser (similar to primary, but with a pause after the initial spike).[77] One additional response category is the "build-up" response, which is a gradual increase in cell firing during the presentation of a stimulus.[77, 138] Close, though not exclu-

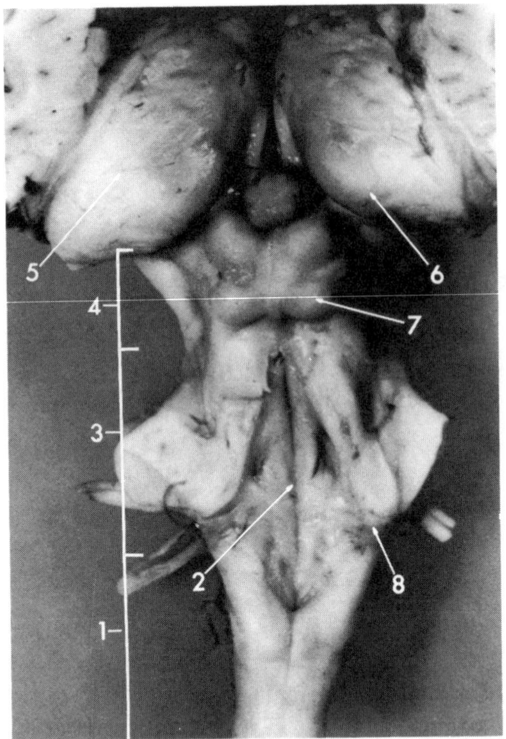


**FIG 2–1.**
Posterior view of human brain stem with cerebrum and cerebellum removed. *1,* Medulla; *2,* fourth ventricle; *3,* pons; *4,* midbrain; *5,* thalamus; *6,* pulvinar; *7,* inferior colliculus; *8,* cochlear nucleus. (From Waddington M: *Atlas of Human Intracranial Anatomy.* Rutland, Vt, Academy Books, 1984. Used by permission.)

sive, agreement has been found between the type of cell and the pattern of response, suggesting important relationships between the anatomy (structure) and physiology (function) of cells within the CN. Thus, it appears that cells within the CN may provide the initial mechanism for central processing and coding of the various properties of an auditory stimulus.

Fibers of the auditory nerve entering the CN are arrayed in systematic fashion in each division of the CN, thus maintaining the frequency arrangement relayed from the cochlea.[144, 164] This tonotopic organization is seen in all three divisions of the CN, with low frequencies being represented ventrolaterally and high frequencies dorsomedially within each nucleus.[144, 164] Tuning curves derived from CN units using tone bursts are similar in shape to those of the auditory nerve.[139] However, some CN fibers yield wider tuning curves than those of auditory nerve fibers,[94] leading one to speculate that CN units may preserve, but not necessarily enhance, frequency resolution of acoustic information coming from the auditory nerve.

The cochlear nuclei lie in the area of the cerebellopontine angle, a lateral recess formed at the juncture of the pons, medulla, and cerebellum. Tumors in this area often affect the CN and may cause central auditory deficits; however, the cerebellopontine angle is sufficiently large to accommodate sizable mass lesions with little compromise of neural function.[107, 112]

The cochlear nuclei are unique among brain stem auditory structures in that their only afferent input is ipsilateral, coming from the cochlea via the auditory nerve. Damage to the CN can result in ipsilateral pure tone deficits[40, 41, 87] and at times may mimic auditory nerve dysfunction.[68] Because the CN is on the posterolateral surface of the brain stem, it often is directly affected by extra-axial tumors such as acoustic neuromas.[40] For this reason, most cerebellopontine angle tumors manifest auditory nerve and brain stem involvement, causing both peripheral and central dysfunction. In cases involving large cerebellopontine angle mass lesions the entire pons may be displaced and compressed, leading to abnormal ipsilateral ear test findings for the auditory brain stem response (ABR) and various monaural central tests.[110, 118]

Within the CN, a fiber pathway called the tuberculoventral tract connects the dorsal and ventral CN. This tract is thought to be primarily inhibitory in nature (D. Ortel, personal communication, 1990). There are three primary neural tracts that project from the cochlear nuclear complex to the superior olivary complex (SOC) and higher levels of the CANS (see Fig 2–2). The dorsal acoustic stria is a large fiber tract that originates in the dorsal and projects contralaterally to the SOC, lateral lemniscus,[166] and inferior colliculus.[77] The intermediate acoustic stria arises from the posterior ventral CN and communicates with the contralateral lateral lemniscus (ventral nucleus) and the central nucleus of the contralateral inferior colliculus.[77] The largest tract, the ventral acoustic stria, emanates from the anterior ventral CN and melds with the trapezoid body as it approaches the midline of the brain stem.[166] The ventral stria projects contralaterally to the SOC and other nuclear groups along the lateral lemnis-

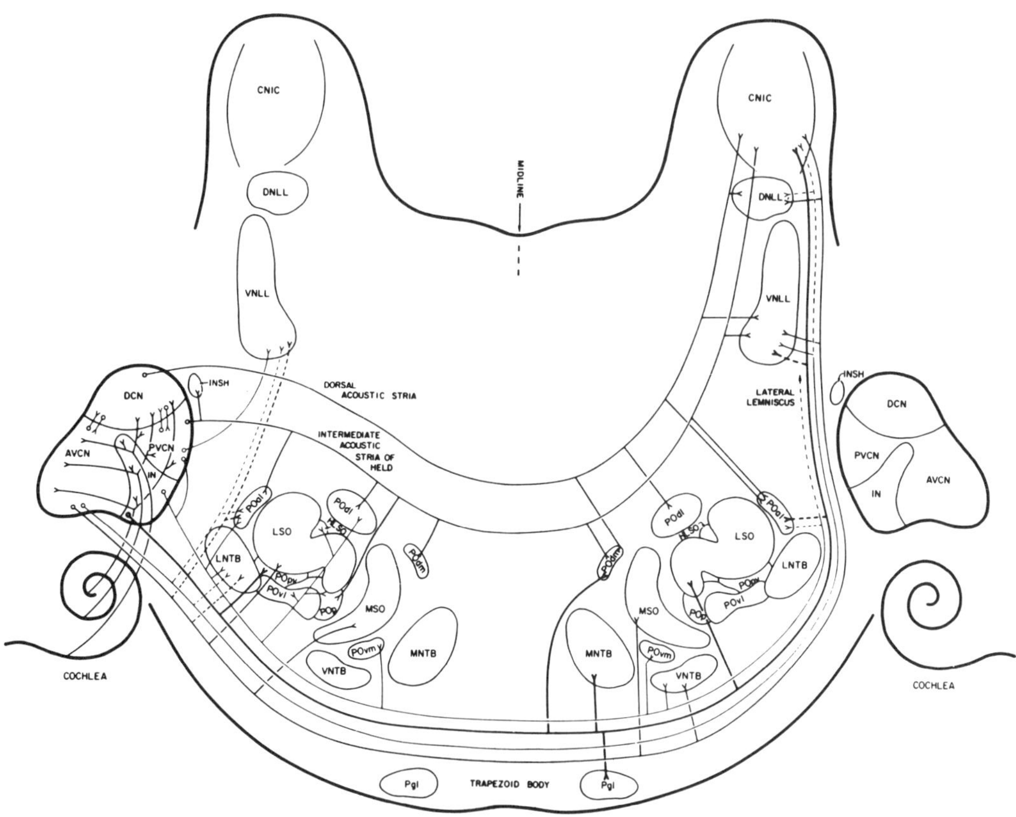


**FIG 2–2.**
Schematic diagram of output pathways of the cochlear nucleus. Solid lines indicate well-documented pathways; dotted lines indicate probable pathways that are not conclusive in their course. *AVCN,* anteroventral cochlear nucleus; *CNIC,* central nucleus of the inferior colliculus; *DCN,* dorsal cochlear nucleus; *DNLL,* dorsal nucleus of the lateral lemniscus; *HLSO,* dorsal hilus of the lateral superior olivary nucleus; *IN,* interstitial nucleus of the cochlear nucleus; *INSH,* interstitial nucleus of the stria of Held; *LNTB,* lateral nucleus of the trapezoid body; *LSO,* lateral superior olivary nucleus; *MNTB,* medial nucleus of the trapezoid body; *MSO,* medial superior olivary nucleus; *Pgi,* lateral paragigantocellular nucleus; *POal,* anterolateral periolivary nucleus; *POdl,* dorsolateral periolivary nucleus; *POdm,* dorsomedial periolivary nucleus; *POp,* posterior periolivary nucleus; *POpv,* posteroventral periolivary nucleus; *POvl,* ventrolateral periolivary nucleus; *POvm,* ventromedial periolivary nucleus; *PVCN,* posteroventral cochlear nucleus; *VNLL,* ventral nucleus of the lateral lemniscus; *VNTB,* ventral nucleus of the trapezoid body. (From Kiang NYS, in Tower DB (ed): *The Nervous System. Human Communication and Its Disorders.* New York, Raven Press, 1975. Used by permission.)

cus. Although these three tracts constitute the primary afferent pathways from the CN, other fibers project ipsilaterally from each division of the CN. Some of these synapse at the SOC and nuclei of the lateral lemniscus within the pons. Others bypass the SOC and nuclei of the lateral lemniscus and synapse at the inferior colliculus only. The dorsal CN also sends a tract of fibers directly to the cerebellum.[166] Although a variety of neural tracts project from the CN to both the ipsilateral and contralateral sides, the contralateral pathways carry the greatest number of fibers (see Figs 2–1 and 2–2).[117]

## Superior Olivary Complex

The SOC is located in the caudal portion of the pons, ventral, and medial to the CN.[117] While there are numerous individual nuclei within the SOC (see Fig 2–2), we will discuss only five. These are the lateral superior olivary nucleus, the medial superior olivary nucleus, the nucleus of the trapezoid body, and two other structures, the lateral and the medial preolivary nuclei. In some animal species the largest and most distinct nucleus is the S-shaped lateral superior olivary nucleus.[97] However, there is evidence suggesting that in humans the medial superior olivary nucleus is the largest of these nuclei.[19]

The lateral superior olivary nucleus is innervated bilaterally,[150] with ipsilateral input coming from the anterior ventral CN, while contralateral innervation arises from both the anterior ventral and posterior ventral CN.[163] The medial superior olivary nucleus also receives both ipsilateral and contralateral input from the anterior ventral CN.[151] Although afferent inputs to the trapezoid body are not completely understood, there appears to be a major contribution from the contralateral CN.[150] Innervation of the lateral and medial preolivary nuclei also is unclear and apparently differs among species, but may come primarily from the ipsilateral anterior ventral CN.[150]

The SOC plays an important role as a relay station in the auditory pathway, and the variety of ipsilateral and contralateral input provides the SOC with the anatomical basis for unique functions in binaural listening.[167] Interaural time[86] and intensity[17] differences reflected in inputs to the SOC are primary determinants of sound localization. Further, the convergence of neural information from each ear assigns the SOC a critical role in listening tasks that require integration and interpretation of binaurally presented signals. For example, audiological tests such as rapidly alternating speech perception and the binaural fusion test are dependent on binaural integration of information by the SOC.[154] These tests often yield abnormal results in cases of SOC pathology or degradation of the signal prior to its reaching the SOC.[88] Measurement of masking level differences (MLDs), one of the more sensitive indices of brain stem integrity, also requires binaural interaction.[85] Temporal cueing at the SOC is critical in MLDs because changing the phase of the stimulus (tones or speech) in the presence of noise results in a change in signal detectability. Several studies have shown MLDs to be affected by low brain stem lesions but not by lesions in the upper brain stem or auditory cortex,[34, 85] further underscoring the role of the SOC in measurement of MLDs.

The SOC also appears to be an important relay station in the reflex arc of the acoustic stapedius muscle reflex.[16] While the neurophysiology of the acoustic reflex is still not completely understood,[59] it is now believed that the reflex involves both direct and indirect neural pathways.[104] The direct reflex arc appears to consist of a three- or four-neuron chain that is activated when either one or both ears are stimulated with sufficiently intense sound. Neural impulses are conducted to the anterior ventral CN via the auditory nerve and from there to the ipsilateral medial superior olivary nucleus and/or facial nerve nucleus. Crossed input appears to come from the anterior ventral CN to the contralateral medial superior olivary nucleus via the trapezoid body. Neurons arising in and around the medial superior olivary nucleus then terminate in the region of the motor nucleus of the facial nerve, from which motor fibers descend to innervate the stapedius muscle. Hence, acoustic stimulation in one ear results in bilateral stapedius muscle contractions.[16]

The existence of an indirect pathway for the acoustic reflex has been postulated for some time. Borg[16] has speculated that the indirect reflex arc is a slower, polysynaptic pathway that may include the extrapyramidal system of the reticular formation.

Despite the lack of complete specification of the neural pathways involved in the reflex arc, there are numerous reports that document the clinical value of acoustic reflex measurements in cases involving brain stem lesions. Hall[59] provides an excellent review of the acoustic reflex and its use in the assessment of brain stem disorders.

As with the CN, tonotopic organization appears to be maintained in all groups of nuclei in the SOC, although the lateral and medial superior olivary nuclei have been studied most extensively. The lateral superior olivary nucleus has a unique tonotopic arrangement, with lower frequencies represented laterally and higher frequencies medially, following the S-shaped structural contour of the nucleus.[156] The lateral superior olivary nucleus also is responsive to a broader range of frequencies than the medial, which largely has low-frequency representation.[117]

The SOC neurons have tuning curves similar to those of the CN.[93] Some SOC tuning curves are wide while others are quite narrow. The discharge patterns seen in post–stimulus-time histograms of SOC neurons are varied but are mainly classified as chopper patterns.[76]

### Lateral Lemniscus

The lateral lemniscus is the primary auditory pathway in the brain stem and comprises both as-

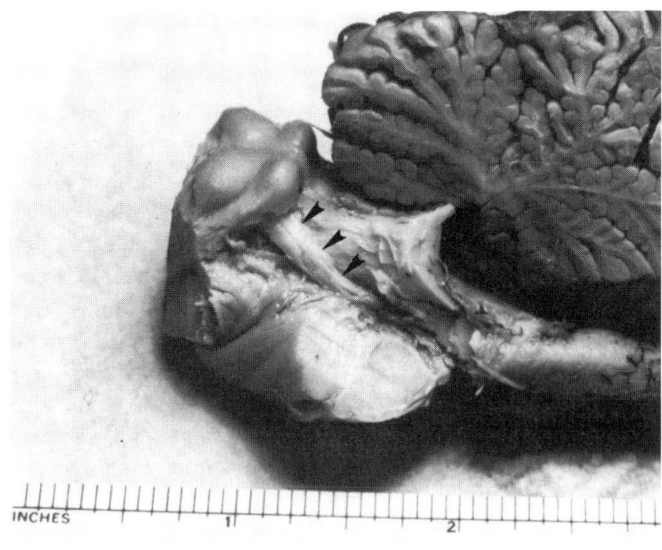


**FIG 2–3.**
Gross dissection showing the lateral lemniscus fiber track coursing rostrally up the lateral pons *(arrows)* and projecting into the inferior colliculus. The superior colliculus is immediately above the inferior colliculus.

cending and descending fibers. The ascending portion extends bilaterally from the CN to the inferior colliculus in the midbrain and contains both crossed and uncrossed fibers of the CN and SOC (Fig 2–3).[55]

Within the lateral lemniscus are two cell groups termed the ventral and dorsal nuclei. These nuclei are located posterolaterally in the upper portion of the pons, near the lateral surface of the brain stem (see Figs 2–2 and 2–3).[45] Afferent input to the nuclei of the lateral lemniscus arises from the dorsal CN on the contralateral side as well as the ventral CN from both sides of the brain stem.[73] Both the ipsilateral and contralateral SOC also provide input to the nuclei.[117] The dorsal lateral lemniscus nuclei from either side of the brain stem are interconnected by a fiber tract called the commissure of Probst.[81] Lemniscal fibers may also cross from one side to the other through the pontine reticular formation.[45] Most of the neurons of the dorsal segment of the lateral lemniscus can be activated binaurally. However, a majority of the neurons from the ventral segment can be activated only by contralateral stimulation.[76] As with the CN and SOC, definite tonotopic organization has been demonstrated for both the dorsal and ventral nuclei of the lateral lemniscus.[19]

## Inferior Colliculus

The inferior colliculus is the largest of the auditory structures of the brain stem[120] and is located on the dorsal surface of the midbrain approximately 3 to 3.5 cm rostral to the pontomedullary junction (see Fig 2–1). From the dorsal aspect of the midbrain, the inferior colliculi are clearly visible as two spherical mounds.[104] Two other rounded projections, the superior colliculi, can also be seen on the dorsal surface of the midbrain, slightly rostral and lateral to the inferior colliculi (see Figs 2–1 and 2–3).[104]

There are two major divisions within the inferior colliculus: the central nucleus or "core," which is composed of purely auditory fibers, and the pericentral nucleus or "belt," which surrounds the central nucleus and consists primarily of somatosensory and auditory fibers.[76]

A majority of the auditory fibers from the lateral lemniscus and lower auditory centers synapse directly or indirectly at the inferior colliculus.[10] Van Noort[157] found that the inferior colliculus receives input from the dorsal and ventral CN, lateral and medial superior olivary nuclei, dorsal and ventral nuclei of the lateral lemniscus, and contralateral inferior colliculus. Other reports[76, 130, 166] suggest that the lower nuclei provide both contralateral and ipsilateral input to the inferior colliculus. There also appears to be a large number of interneurons in the inferior colliculus, suggesting the presence of strong neuronal interconnections (D.K. Morest, personal communication, 1985). The superior colliculi also receive input from the auditory system that apparently is integrated into the reflexes involving the position of the head and eyes.[57]

While the different functions of the inferior colliculus have not been completely defined, many of its functional properties have been described. Like other brain-stem auditory structures, the inferior colliculus has a high degree of tonotopic organization.[91] Moreover, it has a large number of fibers that yield extremely sharp tuning curves, suggesting a high level of frequency resolution.[3] The inferior colliculus contains many time and spatially sensitive neurons,[78, 79, 140] as well as neurons sensitive to binaural stimulation.[11] This suggests a role in sound localization.[104] Finally, in considering its neural connections and its position astride the auditory pathways, the inferior colliculus has been referred to as the "obligatory relay nuclear complex" in transmitting auditory information to higher levels.[117]

Like the lateral lemniscus, the inferior colliculus has a commissure that permits neural communication between its left and right portions.[166] A unique feature of the inferior colliculus is its brachium, a large fiber tract that lies on the dorsolateral surface of the midbrain. This tract projects fibers ipsilaterally to the medial geniculate body (MGB), which is the principal auditory nucleus of the thalamus.

## Medial Geniculate Body

The MGB is located on the inferior dorsolateral surface of the thalamus, just anterior, lateral, and slightly rostral to the inferior colliculus. Although the MGB is in the thalamus and the inferior colliculus in the midbrain, these structures are only approximately 1 cm apart. The MGB contains ventral, dorsal, and medial divisions.[98] Cells in the ventral division respond primarily to acoustic stimuli, while the other divisions contain neurons that respond to both somatosensory and acoustic stimulation.[76, 130] The ventral division appears to be the portion of the MGB that transmits specific auditory discriminative information to the cerebral cortex.[168, 169] The dorsal division projects axons to association areas of the auditory cortex. It has been proposed that this division functions in maintaining and directing auditory attention.[168] The medial division may function as a multisensory arousal system.[168]

Afferent inputs to the MGB are primarily uncrossed, arriving from the inferior colliculus via the brachium. There is conjecture, however, that some input may come from the contralateral inferior colliculus and that some lower nuclei may enter directly on the MGB.[130] In the cat it has been found that there are crossed inputs from the inferior colliculus that connect to the medial division of the MGB (D.K. Morest, personal communication, 1985).

Tonotopic organization has been reported in the ventral segment of the MGB, with low frequencies represented laterally and high frequencies medially.[4] Tuning curves range from broad to sharp, but MGB fibers in general are not as sharply tuned as those of the inferior colliculus.[4] As with the inferior colliculus, the MGB has many neurons that are sensitive to binaural stimulation and interaural intensity differences.[4, 130] Based on long response latencies and after-effects of MGB responses to frequency modulation, Keidel et al[76] have hypothesized that the MGB plays a major role in the processing of natural speech stimuli.

## Reticular Formation

The auditory system like other sensory and motor systems is intricately connected to the reticular formation. The reticular formation could be viewed as having two subsystems: the sensory or ascending reticular activating system (ARAS) and the motor activating system. Our remarks pertain to the ARAS. The reticular formation forms the central core of the brain stem, and is a diffusely organized area with intricately connected nuclei and tracts (W. Mosenthal, personal communication, 1991). The reticular formation is connected to the spinal cord by reticulospinal tracts and to the cerebrum by many (but poorly defined) tracts, such as the medial forebrain bundle, the mammillary peduncle, and the dorsal longitudinal fasciculus. The reticular formation also contains many brain-stem nuclei.

The reticular formation has both ascending and descending tracts on each side of the brain stem, extending from the caudal areas of the spinal cord through the medulla, pons, and midbrain, where diffuse tracts are sent throughout the cerebrum. There are also connections to cerebellum.

It has been shown that when the ARAS is stimulated, the cortex becomes more alert and aware. This increased alertness has been shown by changes in electroencephalogram patterns.[46] Conversely, when the reticular formation is turned off, sleep or coma ensues (W. Mosenthal, personal communication, 1991). The ARAS is a general alarm that responds the same way to any sensory input; its responses prepare the entire brain to act on the incoming stimulus in the appropriate manner.[22] There is some evidence that the ARAS can become sensitive to specific stimuli.[46] This system has a greater reaction to important stimuli than to unimportant ones. This may be one of the mechanisms underlying selective attention and could be related to the ability to hear in noisy surroundings. General listening skills also may be affected by the state of awareness. The profuse connections of sensory structures to the reticular formation and their extensive interactions may make it unnatural to try to separate attention from sensory or cognitive processing of information.

## Vascular Anatomy of the Brain Stem

Many auditory dysfunctions of the brain stem and periphery have a vascular basis. For example, vertebrobasilar disease, "ministrokes," vascular spasms, aneurysms, and vascular loops have all been shown to affect the auditory system.[28, 95, 107]

The major blood supply of the brain stem is the basilar artery, which originates from the left and right vertebral arteries, 1 to 2 mm below the pontomedullary junction on the ventral side of the brain stem. At the low to midpons level the anterior inferior cerebellar artery (AICA) branches from the basilar artery to supply blood to the cochlear nucleus. The CN may also receive an indirect vascular supply from the posterior inferior cerebellar artery.[160] In many instances the AICA will give rise to the internal auditory artery, which supplies the eighth nerve, and then branch into three divisions to supply the cochlear and vestibular periphery. The internal auditory artery sometimes branches directly from the basilar artery.[136]

At the midpons level there are small pontine branches of the basilar artery that, perhaps with some circumferential arteries, indirectly supply the SOC and possibly the lateral lemniscus.[156] There is also a strong possibility that the paramedian branches of the basilar artery supply the SOC and lateral lemniscus. The superior cerebellar arteries are located at the rostral pons or midbrain level; their branches supply the inferior colliculus and in some cases the lateral lemniscus nucleus.[22] At the midbrain level, the basilar artery forms the posterior cerebral arteries. Each posterior cerebral artery has circumferential branches that supply the MGB ipsilaterally (M. Waddington, personal communication, 1985).

A high degree of variability has been shown in the vasculature of the brain stem.[160, 161] Because the vascular pattern varies among specimens, absolute descriptions often are not possible. Also, most brain-stem auditory structures are on the dorsal side of the brain stem and thus may receive secondary and tertiary branches of the key arteries mentioned above.

## Intensity Coding

Auditory fibers in the brain stem fire at a higher rate as sound intensity is increased; however, because the range between the threshold and saturation point of any given fiber is much smaller than the range of intensities audible to the human ear, large intensity increases cannot be encoded by individual nerve fibers.[93]

At high intensities many neurons must interact in order to achieve accurate coding. However the mechanisms of this interaction are poorly understood[59] and most information on intensity coding is based on the study of individual neurons.

Neurons of various brain stem nuclei appear to respond to stimulus intensity in three principal ways.[130, 166] One type of response is referred to as monotonic. This means that as the stimulus intensity increases, the firing rate of the neuron or neurons increases proportionally. The second type of intensity function is monotonic for low intensities, but as stimulus intensity increases the firing rate levels off. In the third type of intensity function the neuronal firing rate reaches a plateau at a relatively low intensity and, in certain cases, actually decreases as intensity increases, resulting in a "rollover" phenomenon. For example, some neurons in the inferior colliculus reach their maximum firing rate 5 dB above their threshold.[166] These three types of intensity coding appear to be common throughout the auditory brain stem, although the extent of each type varies among nuclei groups. From a clinical viewpoint, one might hypothesize that a high-intensity signal would not be appropriately coded when there is damage to brain stem auditory neurons of the first type (monotonic), but not to the latter two types of neurons. This could result in the rollover phenomenon.[69]

### Timing

The latency of brain-stem neuronal responses varies depending on the type of auditory stimulus and the neuron or neuron group being analyzed.[130, 166] Some neurons react quickly to stimulation while others have lengthy latency periods. Some neurons respond only upon termination of the stimulus.

Phase locking is another phenomenon related to timing in the auditory system.[76, 94] Many auditory neurons appear to "lock" onto the stimulus according to phase and will fire only when the stimulus waveform reaches a certain point in its cycle. This is particularly evident with low-frequency sounds. Moreover, at lower frequencies certain neurons will fire on every cycle while at higher frequencies they may fire only at every third or fifth cycle. This phase relationship is especially apparent in lower auditory brain stem neurons and may have considerable relevance to the mechanisms underlying MLDs.[67] Generally, brain-stem auditory neurons have higher firing rates than cortical nerve fibers. How fast a neuron can respond to repeated stimuli depends on its refractory period, defined as the time interval between two successive discharges (depolarization) of a nerve cell. The refractory period is dependent on cell metabolism and dysfunction of metabolic activity will lengthen the period.[153]

### Origins of the Auditory Brain Stem Response

While there is still uncertainty as to the exact origins of some elements of the ABR, recent research[94, 159] has clarified the issue. Moller[94] indicated that wave I of the ABR is generated from the lateral aspect of the auditory nerve, while wave II originates from the medial aspect. Wave III probably has more than one generator, as do other subsequent waves of the ABR; however, it appears that the cochlear nucleus is the principal source of wave III.[94, 159] Wave IV probably has multiple generator sites as well, but it arises predominantly from the SOC with a contralateral influence that may be stronger than the ipsilateral contribution. According to Moller[94] and to Wada and Starr,[159] wave V is generated from the lateral lemniscus. In a simplified view of the ABR origins, it is plausible that the first five ABR waves may be generated entirely within the auditory nerve and pons.

The typical findings of ABR abnormalities on the ear ipsilateral to a brain-stem lesion[25, 106, 119] seem to be inconsistent with known neuroanatomy, which shows a majority of the auditory fibers crossing to the contralateral side on the level of the SOC. One possible explanation for these seemingly contradictory findings may lie in the neural requirements for processing and transmitting different types of stimuli. Relatively simple stimuli, such as clicks and tone pips, may require few auditory fibers for coding and transmission and thus are able to use the smaller but more rapid ipsilateral pathway. Speech, however, is much more complex and apparently needs the longer and more varied contralateral pathway.[108]

Animal studies by Wada and Starr,[159] as well as our own observations with humans, have shown that the first five waves of the ABR are not affected by specific lesions of the inferior colliculus. Unfortunately, the ABR may not be a useful tool in evaluating lesions at or above the inferior colliculus. Powerful clinical tests such as the ABR, MLDs, and acoustic reflexes appear to be restricted to detection of lesions below the midbrain level. In cases where lesions of either the inferior colliculus or the MGB (midbrain and thalamic levels) are suspected, other procedures are necessary to detect and define the abnormality.

## CEREBRUM

### Auditory Cortical Areas

The ascending auditory system continues from the thalamic area to the cerebral cortex through neurons that originate in the medial geniculate bodies and radiate outward to the auditory areas of the brain.

The cerebral cortex (gray matter covering the surface of the brain) is composed of three primary types of nerve cells: pyramidal, stellate, and fusiform. Six cell layers in the cortex can be distinguished by type, density, and arrangement of the nerve cells.[22] The fourth layer is composed of a high proportion of sensory cells, including those that respond to auditory stimulation (M. Marin-Padilla, personal communication, 1986).

Descriptions in the literature vary as to which areas constitute the auditory cortex. Most of this variability results from adapting animal models to the human brain and from disagreement as to whether "association" areas should be included as part of the auditory cortex.[102] We include these association areas because they are critical to understanding the system, although they also contain non–auditory-sensitive fibers.

Heschl's gyrus, sometimes termed the transverse gyrus, is considered to be the primary auditory area of the cortex. This gyrus is located in the sylvian fissure approximately two-thirds posterior on the upper surface of the temporal lobe (supratemporal plane), projecting in a posterior and medial direction. To observe Heschl's gyrus, the temporal lobe must be displaced inferiorly or separated from the brain to expose the supratemporal plane (Fig 2–4). Campain and Minckler[21] analyzed a large number of human brains and found that the configuration of Heschl's gyrus differed on the left and right sides. In some brains double gyri were present on each side, while in others double gyri were present only unilaterally. In a study of 29 human brains, Musiek and Reeves[114] reported that the number of Heschl's gyri ranged from one to three per hemisphere, although there was no significant left-right asymmetry in the number of Heschl's gyri within individual brains. The mean length of Heschl's gyri, however, was found to be greater in the left hemisphere.[114]

The planum temporale is an area on the cortical surface that extends posterior from the most posterior aspect of Heschl's gyrus to the endpoint of the sylvian fissure (see Fig 2–4). Geschwind and Levitsky[52] showed that the planum temporale in the human brain is significantly larger on the left side (3.6 cm) than on the right (2.7 cm). Because the left hemisphere is dominant for speech and the planum temporale is located in the approximate region of Wernicke's area, these investigators reasoned that the planum temporale may be an anatomical correlate to (receptive) language in man. Data from Musiek and Reeves[114] support these earlier findings[52] regarding differences in length of the left and right planum temporale. They suggest, however, that asymmetries in higher-auditory and language function may be due to anatomic differences of the planum temporale as well as Heschl's gyrus.

The supramarginal gyrus curves around the end of the sylvian fissure. This area has been shown to be responsive to acoustic stimulation[23] and is in the approximate region of Wernicke's area, as is the angular gyrus located immediately posterior to the supramarginal gyrus.[52] These are part of a complex association area that appears to integrate auditory, visual, and somesthetic information and therefore is of great importance in the

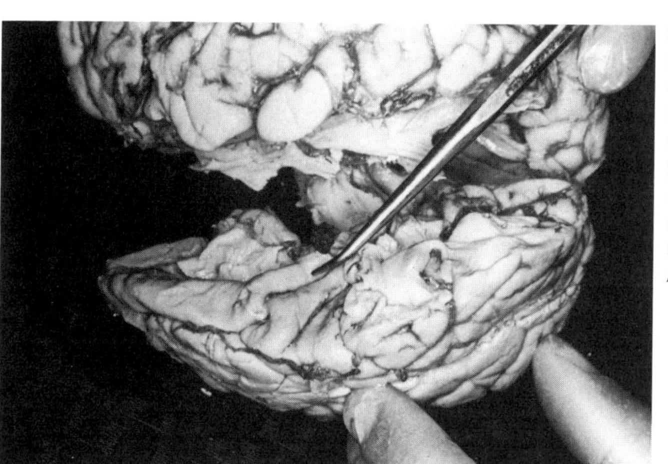

**FIG 2–4.**
Superior temporal plane with probe pointing to two Heschl's gyri. Gyri are divided by Beck's intermedius. Temporal pole is to the extreme left along the superior temporal gyrus. Immediately posterior to the posterior margin of Heschl is the planum temporale, which is just anterior to a transected supramarginal gyrus. (From Musiek FE: *Ear Hear* 1986; 7:283–294. Used by permission.)

visual and somesthetic aspects of language, such as reading and writing.

The sylvian fissure contains the primary auditory area as well as parts of the language area in humans. Rubens[140] reviewed early anatomical work that showed the left sylvian fissure was larger than the right. This finding has been confirmed by others, including Musiek and Reeves,[114] who found that asymmetry of the sylvian fissure was correlated with the greater length of the planum temporale on the left side.

The inferior portion of the parietal lobe and the inferior aspect of the frontal lobe also are responsive to acoustical stimulation.[23, 48] Still another acoustically responsive area is the insula, a portion of the cortex that lies deep within the sylvian fissure medial to the middle segment of the superior temporal gyrus (Fig 2–5). The insular cortex can be observed only if the temporal lobe is removed or displaced inferiorly. In our anatomical observations it appears that the most posterior aspect of the insula is contiguous with Heschl's gyrus.

Within the insula are nerve fibers that are responsive to somatic, visual and gustatory stimulation. The greatest neural activity, however, results from acoustic stimulation.[152] It appears that the posterior aspect of the insula, that portion in closest proximity to Heschl's gyrus, has the most acoustically sensitive fibers.[152] Located just medial to the insula is a narrow strip of gray matter called the claustrum. Little is known about the function of the claustrum, although it seems to be highly responsive to acoustic stimulation.[117, 152]

Anatomical irregularities have been reported in the brains of persons with dyslexia.[49, 74] The planum temporale, normally significantly longer in the left hemisphere, has been found to be bilaterally symmetrical in the brains of patients with dyslexia. Moreover, the brains of dyslexic people contained an unusually high number of cellular abnormalities referred to as cerebrocortical microdysgenesis and defined as nests of ectopic neurons and glia in layer 1 of the cortex. These ectopic areas are often associated with dysplasia of adjacent cortical layers (including focal microgyria) and sometimes with superficial growths known as brain warts. While these focal anomalies may exist in up to 26% of normal brains,[74] they usually are found in small numbers and in the right hemisphere. In patients with developmental dyslexia they occur in much greater numbers, often in the left hemisphere in the area of the perisylvian cortex.[74] These findings suggest possible causes of developmental dyslexia and its relation to central auditory processing (Fig 2–6).

## Brain Prints

Currently, human neuroanatomy can be studied in vivo by computed tomography (CT) scan or by magnetic resonance imaging (MRI). Although these techniques are advanced, they do not always provide quantitative spatial information about brain tissue in fissures or sulci. This is important in estimating asymmetries, lesioned areas, and anatomic regions of the brain. The brain print introduced by Joundet et al[72] can provide a two-di-

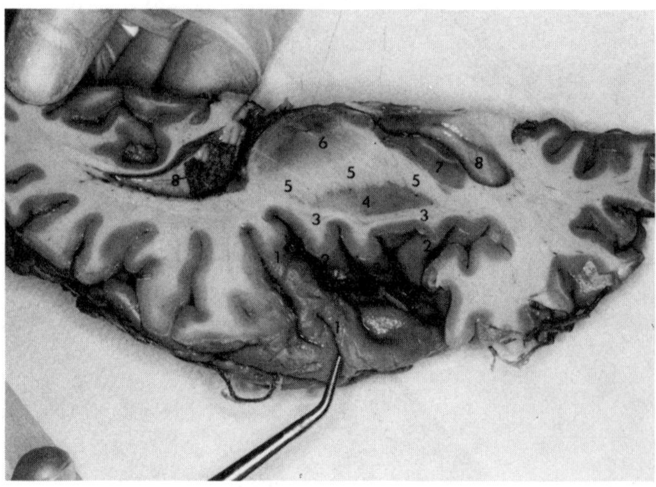


**FIG 2–5.**
Right half of cerebrum, transverse sectioned along the sylvian fissure. *1,* Heschl's gyrus; *2,* insula; *3,* external capsule; *4,* lenticular process; *5,* internal capsule; *6,* thalamus; *7,* caudate; *8,* anterior and posterior lateral ventricle. (From Musiek FE: *Ear Hear* 1986; 7:283–294. Used by permission.)

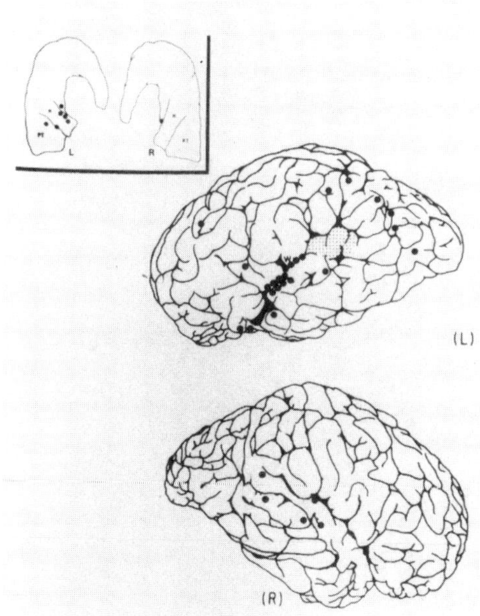


**FIG 2–6.**
Left *(L)* and right *(R)* hemispheres and transverse sections *(upper left)* of Heschl's gyrus *(H)* and planum temporale *(PT)* demonstrating ectopic areas in brain of a learning-disabled (dyslexic) person. (From Galaburda A, et al: *Ann Neurol* 1985; 18:222–235. Used by permission.)

mensional surface map of the unfolded brain allowing views of sulci and area quantification of the cortical surface.

Details of brain-print methodology can be found in Joundet et al.[81] The brain print is dependent on MRI scans performed along the coronal plane with a slice thickness of 3.8 mm. Both $T_1$ and $T_2$ weighted images are obtained to allow optimum sensitivity for various types of pathology. Midsagittal scouts are used to align and mark the section planes on an internalized grid to measure anterior-posterior distances.[155]

The computer reconstruction used to flatten and map the cortical surface involves the following[155]:

1. $T_1$ and $T_2$ weighted images are placed in a photographic enlarger and the images are projected onto paper.
2. The pial surface of each image is traced.
3. Reference points demarcating cortical structures (and lesion areas) are defined and numbered sequentially based on coronal atlases.
4. The tracing is entered into the computer by a digital graphic tablet for straightening, alignment, connection, scaling, and supplemental graphics.
5. Measurements of cortical surface are computed using a digitized planimeter.

Depending on the labeling and computer algorithm used, various maps of cortical surfaces can be generated and studied for anatomical information. The cortical surface can be quantified and various regions of the cortex can be located. In the examples shown (Fig 2–7) the lesions of the cortical surface can be easily measured and quantified. Using these brain prints it was determined in this case that the temporal lobe was larger on the left (176 $cm^2$) than on the right (159 $cm^2$). In regard to lesion effects, the right temporal lobe had 64% of its surface involved vs. only 7% of the left temporal lobe. The lesion involved 100% of both the left and right Heschl's gyri.[155] These are only a sample of the quantitative data that can be obtained using the brain print. Work is underway to use a three-dimensional brain computer reconstruction to provide complementary information to the brain print (W. Loftus, personal communication, 1991).

The brain print provides another way of looking at cortical neuroanatomy. It also can provide critical information as to anatomical correlates to audiologic test results from patients with brain lesions.

## Thalamocortical Connections

Ascending auditory fiber tracts originating in the MGB follow various routes to the cortex and other areas of the brain. One group of fibers provides input to the basal ganglia, the large subcortical gray matter structures composed of the caudate nucleus, putamen, and globus pallidus (see Fig 2–5). The lenticular process, or nucleus, consists of the putamen and globus pallidus and lies between the internal and external capsules (white matter neural pathways) (see Fig 2–5). Animal studies[83] have shown that the MGB sends out fibers that connect to the putamen, the caudate nucleus, and the amygdaloid body, a small almond-shaped expansion located at the tail of the caudate nucleus.

In addition to these connections to the basal ganglia there are two major pathways from the

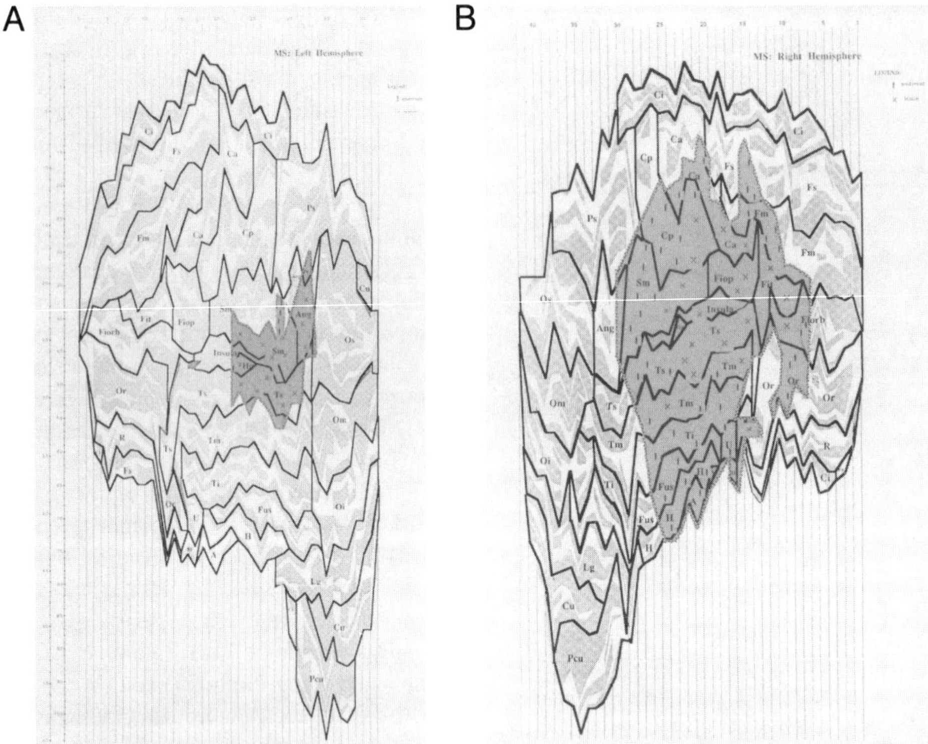


**FIG 2–7.**
Brain prints from left **(A)** and right **(B)** cortical surfaces. Anterior is left for the left hemisphere and right for the right hemisphere. The light areas are gyral crests, dark areas are intrasulcal regions. Lesioned areas (dark gray) are the result of strokes in the middle cerebral artery in both hemispheres. *A*, amygdala; *Ang*, angular gyrus; *BF*, basal forebrain; *Ca*, precentral gyrus; *Ci*, cingulate gyrus; *Cp*, postcentral gyrus; *Cu*, cuneus; *Fiop*, inferior frontal gyrus, pars opercularis; *Fiorb*, inferior frontal gyrus, pars orbitalis; *Fit*, inferior frontal gyrus, pars triangularis; *Fm*, middle frontal gyrus; *Fs*, superior frontal gyrus; *Fus*, fusiform gyrus; *H*, hippocampal region, including the parahippocampal gyrus; *Hg*, transverse gyrus of Heschl; *Lg*, lingual gyrus; *Oi*, inferior lateral occipital gyrus; *Om*, middle lateral occipital gyrus; *Or*, orbitofrontal gyri; *Os*, superior lateral occipital gyrus; *Pc*, precuneus; *Ps*, superior parietal lobule; *R*, rectal gyrus; *Sm*, supramarginal gyrus; *Ti*, interior temporal gyrus; *Tm*, middle temporal gyrus; *TP*, temporal pole; *Ts*, super temporal gyrus; *U*, uncus. (From Tramo M, et al: *J Cog Neurosci* 1990; 2:195–211. Used by permission.)

MGB to the cortex. The first pathway, consisting of all auditory fibers that originate in the ventral MGB, takes a sublenticular course through the internal capsule to the Heschl's gyrus. The second pathway, consisting of auditory, somatic, and possible visual fibers, proceeds from the MGB through the inferior aspect of the internal capsule and ultimately under the putamen to the external capsule. From the external capsule, fibers connect to the insula.[107, 149] There are other connections from the MGB to the auditory cortex that probably overlap the two mentioned here. The pathways described here typify the multiple and complex connections of the thalamocortical auditory anatomy.

### Intrahemispheric Connections of the Auditory Cortex

The primary auditory cortex has both interhemispheric and intrahemispheric connections. Lesions of the primary auditory area in primates have resulted in degeneration of the caudal (posterior) aspect of the superior temporal gyrus and the upper bank of the adjacent superior temporal sulcus.[147] This degeneration pattern suggests the presence of a multisynaptic pathway in the middle and posterior areas of the superior temporal gyrus.[71] The superior temporal gyrus also has fibers that connect to the insula and frontal operculum.

There appear to be few connections of the auditory area to the temporal pole.[117] This finding is interesting in that some audiological studies have attempted to determine the validity of various central auditory tests by using them with patients whose temporal poles have been removed in attempts to control seizure activity.

Auditory cortical areas and other areas of the temporal lobe are connected to areas in the frontal lobe by way of the arcuate fasciculus, one of the "long" association pathways. This large fiber tract travels from the temporal lobe up and around the top of the sylvian fissure and then extends anteriorly to the frontal lobe.[149] Two of the important regions connected through the arcuate fasciculus are Wernicke's area in the temporal lobe and Broca's area in the frontal lobe.[22]

## Interhemispheric Connections

The main connection between the left and right hemispheres is the corpus callosum. The corpus callosum is located at the base of the longitudinal fissure and is the largest fiber tract in the primate brain. The corpus callosum is covered by the cingulate gyri and forms most of the roof of the lateral ventricles.[146] In the adult, the corpus callosum is approximately 6.5 cm long from the anterior genu to the posterior splenium and ranges from approximately 0.5 to 1 cm in thickness.[103] The corpus callosum has great morphological variability but seems to be larger in left-handed people than in right-handed people.[171]

The corpus callosum is composed of long, heavily myelinated axons. The corpus callosum essentially connects the two cortexes and therefore must be considered to span much of the intercortical space above the basal ganglia and lateral ventricles. The corpus callosum is not only a midline structure.[103] It is likely that in many "cortical" lesions some region of the corpus callosum is involved because it encompasses such a large portion of the cerebrum.

The fibers of the corpus callosum are primarily homolateral (connecting to the same locus in each hemisphere), though some fibers are heterolateral (connecting to different loci on each hemisphere).[100] The heterolateral fibers may be more inhibitory than the homolateral fibers. Whether the corpus callosum fibers are inhibitory or excitatory will affect the transcollosal transfer time (TCTT). The TCTT is the latency of an evoked potential recorded from one point on the cortex after stimulation of the homolateral point on the other hemisphere. In the human the TCTT decreases with age, reaching minimum values during the teenage years.[50] This is consistent with increased myelination of the corpus callosum axons, as studies have shown.[173] It has been demonstrated that in primates and humans the TCTT varies greatly, from a minimum of 3 to 6 ms to a maximum in excess of 100 ms.[18, 24, 142] This variability could be viewed as supporting the concept of inhibitory and excitatory neurons in the corpus callosum.

The neural connections of the corpus callosum correspond to various parts of the cortex and its anatomy subserves various regions of the cortex. The most posterior aspect of the corpus callosum is the splenium, which primarily contains visual fibers connecting with the occipital cortex.[123] The trunk makes up the middle portion of the corpus callosum. The posterior half of the trunk is thinner, and this thin area is called the sulcus. It is in this region that most of the auditory fibers from the temporal lobe and insula are found. The frontal and parietal lobes are also represented in the trunk region. The anterior part of the corpus callosum is termed the genu and has olfactory fibers and fibers from the anterior insula.[123]

The auditory areas of the corpus callosum warrant further discussion. The auditory area at midline has been shown to be just anterior to the splenium in the posterior half of the corpus callosum. This information comes from primate research[123] but there are also data on humans that help localize the auditory areas. Baran et al[9] have shown that there is little or no change in dichotic listening or pattern perception (tasks requiring interhemispheric transfer) performance after the sectioning of the anterior half of the corpus callosum; however, persons with complete section of the corpus callosum demonstrate markedly poor performance on these auditory tasks.[111]

Though we have a considerable amount of knowledge of the anatomy of the corpus callosum at midline, little is known about the course of the transcallosal auditory pathway (TCAP). Present information about the TCAP comes from anatomical and clinical studies.[35] The TCAP begins at the auditory cortex, courses posteriorly, runs superiorly around the lateral ventricles, crosses a periventricular area known as the trigone, and then courses medially and inferiorly into the cor-

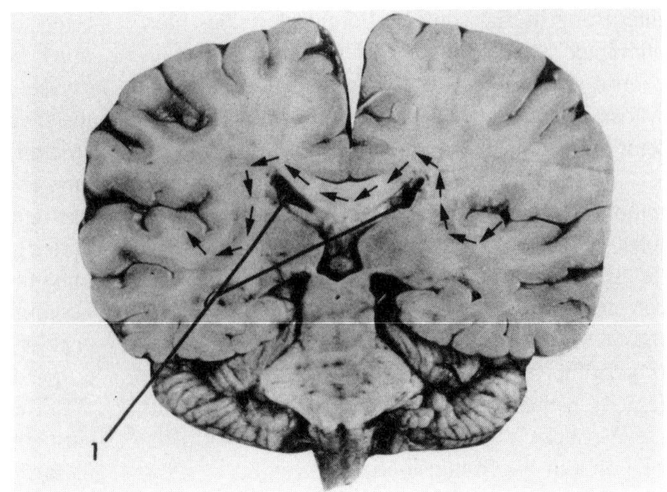


**FIG 2–8.**
Coronal section depicting the transcallosal auditory pathway *(arrows)*. Pathway courses from the primary auditory areas around the lateral ventricles *(1)* and through the mid region of the corpus callosum.

pus callosum proper (Fig 2–8). Any lesions along the TCAP can result in degraded interhemispheric transfer.

A recent study demonstrates size differences in the corpus callosum between children with attention-deficit disorders and matched controls. The corpora of the experimental group were smaller in the auditory area and in the genu as compared with those of the control group.[66]

The vascular anatomy of the corpus callosum is rather simple. The posterior fifth (splenium) is supplied by branches of the posterior cerebral artery.[22] The remaining segment is supplied by the pericallosal artery, which is a branch of the anterior cerebral artery.[22]

### Tonotopic Organization

As in the brain stem, there is distinct tonotopic organization in the auditory cortex. Tonotopic organization has been demonstrated in the primary auditory cortex of the primate, with low frequencies being represented rostrolaterally and high frequencies caudomedially.[90] Using positron emission tomography (PET) to measure changes in cerebral blood flow, Lauter et al[82] demonstrated a similar pattern in the human brain. Tones of 500 Hz evoked increased activity in the lateral part of Heschl's gyrus, while 4,000-Hz tones resulted in increased activity in the medial position. Most tonotopic information on the insular cortex has been obtained from studies in the cat.[172] In the cat insula, the high-frequency neurons appear to be in the superior portion with the low-frequency neurons in the inferior segment.[172]

In the primary auditory area where cells are sharply tuned, highly definable tonotopic organization and isofrequency strips (contours) can be found.[132] Despite many attempts to show a relationship between columnar organization and tonotopicity, no frequency-specific columns have been located. However, there does seem to be a spatial component to frequency representation in the auditory cortex; it requires approximately 2 mm to encompass the frequency range of one octave. For extremely high frequencies, less space is needed to represent an octave range.[99]

Some types of tuning curves obtained from the auditory cortex are unique. Broad and sharp as well as multipeaked tuning curves have been recorded from cortical neurons.[132] The multipeaked tuning curves may be observed primarily from cortical recordings. Neurons in the primary auditory cortex appear to receive a narrow frequency-tuned excitatory input from the contralateral ear. This frequency-intensity "response area" may be flanked by inhibitory inputs that originate from adjacent cochlear sites.[129] Cortical neurons may respond briskly to brief acoustic events but show poorer spike discharge rates to sustained, steady-state acoustic signals.[171]

### Intensity Coding

The discharge or firing rate of cortical neurons in primates varies as a function of intensity and takes two forms—monotonic and nonmonotonic.[128] Most of the neurons in the primary auditory cortex display rate-intensity functions similar to that of the auditory nerve; that is, the firing rate is monotonic for increments of roughly 10 to 40 dB. Higher intensities do not result in increased firing rates. Many of the neurons in the auditory cortex are sharply nonmonotonic. In some cases, the firing rate may be reduced to a spontaneous level with a 10-dB increase above the optimum intensity.[130, 132]

Phillips[129] reported similar results with cats, identifying both monotonic and nonmonotonic profiles. For some nonmonotonic neurons, firing rates decreased precipitously, often to zero, at stimulus levels above the best sound pressure level. Phillips also found that the introduction of wide-band noise raised the threshold level of the cortical neurons. However, once threshold sensitivity was achieved in noise, the firing rate increased in a manner similar to the nonmasked condition, with the intensity profile remaining basically unchanged. With successive increments in the level of the masking noise, the tonal intensity profile is displaced toward progressively higher SPLs.

Animal studies have shown some cortical neurons to be intensity selective; that is, certain cells respond only within a given intensity range, but collectively the neurons cover a wide range of intensities. For example, cortical cells may respond maximally, minimally, or not at all at a given intensity. When the intensity is changed, different cells may respond at a maximum level, and the previous neurons may respond minimally or not at all.[90]

### Timing

Like the brain stem, the auditory cortex responds in various ways to the onset, presence, and cessation of acoustic stimuli. Abeles and Goldstein[1] found four types of responses of cortical neurons to a 100 ms tone. One type of neuron sustained a response for the duration of the stimulus, although the firing rate was considerably less at the cessation of the tone. "On" neurons responded only to the onset, and "off" neurons responded only after the tone was terminated. The fourth type responded to both the onset and termination of the tone, but did not sustain a response during the tone.

Additional information on timing a temporal processing in the auditory cortex can be found in the work of Goldstein et al.[56] These investigators studied cells in the primary auditory area of rats and found four categories of response to clicks presented at different rates. Approximately 40% of the cells responded to each click at rates of 10 to 1,000/sec, whereas 25% cells did not respond at all. A third group of cells showed varying response patterns as the click rate changed, and the fourth group of cells responded only to low click rates.

Timing within the auditory cortex plays a critical role in localization abilities. Many neurons in the primary auditory cortex are sensitive to the interaural phase as well as to intensity differences.[12] There is general agreement that in a sound field more cortical units fire to sound stimuli from a contralateral source than from an ipsilateral source.[42, 43] This finding provided the basis for the initial clinical work on sound localization. As early as 1958, Sanchez-Longo and Forster[143] reported that patients with temporal lobe damage had difficulty locating sound sources in the sound field contralateral to the damaged hemisphere. Recently, Moore et al[96] studied the abilities of both normal and brain-damaged subjects to track a fused auditory image as it moved through auditory space. The perceived location of the auditory image, which varies according to the temporal relationship of paired clicks presented (one each, from matched speakers) is referred to as the precedence effect. While normal subjects were able to track the fused auditory image accurately, two subjects with unilateral temporal lobe lesions (one in the right hemisphere and one in the left) exhibited auditory field deficits opposite the damaged hemispheres. Results of these investigations[9, 111] are consistent with other localization and lateralization studies that have shown contralateral ear effects.[84, 135]

### Electrical Stimulation of Auditory Cortex

Penfield and associates[125, 126] conducted several auditory stimulation experiments during neurosurgical procedures performed on humans. These investigators electrically stimulated areas along the margin of the sylvian fissure while the patient, under local anesthesia, reported what he or she heard. Many of Penfield's patients did not report any auditory experience or sensation during electrical stimulation; however, some reported hearing buzzing, ringing, chirping, knocking, humming, and rushing sounds during stimulation of the superior gyrus of the temporal lobe. These sounds were generally referred to the contralateral ear and to a lesser extent to both ears.

During electrical stimulation of the auditory areas of the brain, patients often reported the impression of hearing loss, yet they heard and understood words spoken to them. Patients also claimed that the voice of the surgeon changed in pitch and loudness during electrical stimulation.

In 1963, Penfield and Pernot[124] reported cases in which electrical stimulation of the left posterior-superior temporal gyrus and Heschl's gyrus resulted in the patient's hearing voices, people shouting, and other similar acoustic phenomena. When the right auditory cortex was stimulated, most patients who responded heard music and singing.

## Lateralization of Function in Auditory Cortex

One of the key principles in central auditory assessment using behavioral tests is related to lateralization of the deficit. It is well known that behavioral tests typically indicate deficiencies in the ear contralateral to the damaged hemisphere. This contralateral ear deficit may relate to the fact that each ear provides more contralateral than ipsilateral input to the cortex. This view has strong physiological support. Mountcastle[99] reported that the threshold for activation of cortical neurons by contralateral stimulation is generally 5 to 20 dB lower than for ipsilateral stimulation. Celesia[23] has shown that near-field evoked potentials recorded from the auditory cortex in humans during neurosurgery are of greater amplitude for contralateral than ipsilateral ear stimulation.

Similar findings showing a stronger contralateral representation have also been reported in cats.[39] Late auditory evoked potentials recorded with electrodes over the temporal-parietal areas of the human scalp also have revealed differences between contralateral and ipsilateral stimulation. Generally, the auditory evoked potentials recorded from contralateral stimulation are earlier and of greater amplitude than those recorded ipsilaterally[20]; however, this is not always the case and controversy surrounds these findings for far-field evoked potentials.[39]

## Behavioral Ablation Studies

Measuring the effects of partial or total ablation of the auditory cortex in animals by monitoring their auditory behavior has been of great value in localization of function. Ablation experiments have served as the basis for development of several auditory tests. Kryter and Ades[80] in one of the first studies involving ablation of the cat auditory cortex found little or no effect on absolute thresholds or differential thresholds for intensity. These findings are consistent with data subsequently obtained from humans with brain damage or surgically removed auditory cortices.[13, 64]

However, several other investigators[61, 62, 129] have reported that bilateral ablations of the primate auditory cortex results in severe hearing loss for pure tones. Bilaterally ablated animals demonstrated gradual recovery, but many retained some permanent pure-tone sensitivity loss, especially in the midfrequencies.[61] Unilateral cortical ablations resulted in hearing loss in the ear contralateral to the lesion with normal hearing in the ipsilateral ear.[62] Permanent residual hearing loss has also been reported in humans with bilateral cortical lesions.[8, 70, 174] Differences among animal species are shown in findings with opossums[137] and ferrets[137] in which auditory threshold recovery is almost complete following bilateral lesions of the auditory cortex.

The effects of auditory cortex ablation on frequency discrimination remains unclear, even after many areas of research. Some early studies[5, 92] reported that frequency discrimination was lost after ablation of the auditory cortex, while later studies[32] contradicted these early findings. These discrepancies may be related to the difficulty of the discrimination tasks, as each study employed a different test paradigm to measure pitch perception. The complexity of the tasks, and not the differences in frequency discrimination, is probably responsible for the discrepant findings.[130]

Since ablation of the auditory cortex has little or no effect on absolute or differential thresholds for intensity or frequency, more complex tasks were sought to examine the results of cortical ablation. Diamond and Neff,[38] using patterned acoustic stimuli, examined the ability of cats to detect differences in frequency patterns after various bilateral cortical ablations. Following ablation of primary and association auditory cortices the cats could no longer discriminate different acoustic patterns, and despite extensive retraining they could not relearn the pattern task. Based on subsequent studies, Neff[115] reported that auditory cortex ablations primarily affected temporal sequencing and not pattern detection or frequency discrimination of the tones composing the patterns. Colavita[26, 27] demonstrated in cats that ablation of only the insular-temporal region resulted in the inability to discriminate temporal patterns. The early research of Diamond and Neff influenced Pinheiro in her development of the frequency (pitch) pattern test, which has proved to be a valuable clinical central auditory test with humans.[101, 113, 134] Another pattern perception test, duration patterns, has emerged recently as a potentially valuable clinical tool.[105] Based on these studies, it appears that temporal ordering is a critical part of pattern perception, which in turn is affected by lesions of the auditory cortex.

Other studies have also shown that the temporal dimension of hearing is linked to the integrity of the auditory cortex. Gershuni et al.[51] demonstrated that a unilateral lesion of dog's auditory cortex resulted in decreased pure tone sensitivity for short but not long tones for the ear contralateral to the lesion.

In contrast, Cranford[31] showed that cortical lesions had no effect on brief-tone thresholds in cats. However, Cranford[33] also demonstrated that auditory cortex lesions in cats markedly affected the frequency difference limen for short- but not long-duration tones presented to the contralateral ear. Following the animal study, Cranford examined brief tone frequency difference limens in seven human subjects with unilateral temporal lobe lesions.[33] Findings with human subjects were essentially the same as those with animals. Brief-tone thresholds for subjects with temporal lobe lesions were the same as those of a normal control group, but the brief-tone frequency difference limen was markedly poorer for subjects with lesions. The frequency difference limen was poorer for the contralateral ear for stimulus durations under 200 msec.

## Vascular Anatomy in the Auditory Cortex

The primary artery that supplies blood to the auditory cortex is the middle cerebral artery.[160] The middle cerebral artery branches directly from the internal carotid artery at the base of the brain. While its route varies considerably among specimens, it courses primarily within the sylvian fissure in an anterior-to-posterior direction.[160] The artery varies in length and may be only 2 cm long before its branching becomes diffuse.[51] However, in some cases it may run almost the entire length of the sylvian fissure before it becomes the angular artery, which courses posteriorly and laterally on the brain surface.

In viewing the anterior aspect of the middle cerebral artery, the first major branch that supplies an auditory region is the fronto-opercular artery. This artery takes a superior course, supplying the anterior portion of the insula. The central sulcus artery just posterior to the fronto-opercular artery supplies the posterior insula and the anterior parietal lobe. Branching inferiorly from the middle cerebral artery are three arteries that course over the middle and posterior part of the temporal lobe.[160] These three arteries (anterior, middle and posterior temporal) supply the middle and superior temporal gyri. A combination of the middle cerebral artery and angular artery probably supplies the primary auditory area as well as the angular gyrus and part of the supramarginal gyrus. The other part of the supramarginal gyrus is supplied by the posterior parietal artery.

Vascular insults involving the middle cerebral artery can result in considerable tissue damage to gray and white matter in the temporal-parietal regions of the brain. These lesions, among the most common anomalies affecting the auditory cortex, are devastating not only to the morphology of the auditory cortex but also to its function.

## Efferent Auditory System

Although the efferent auditory system likely functions as one unit, the pathways are divided into two sections. There has been a great deal of recent work on the caudalmost part of the system (the olivocochlear bundle), but little is known about the more rostral system. The rostral efferent pathway starts at the auditory cortex and descends to the medial geniculate and midbrain regions, including the inferior colliculus. There appears to be a "loop" system between the cortex and these structures. There are also fibers that descend from the cortex to motor neurons in the brain stem.

The inferior colliculus also receives efferents from the medial geniculate.[131] It is possible that efferent fibers may give rise to other efferent fibers along the entire length of the pathway. This would provide a complete efferent connection from the cortex to the periphery.[60] Although there is some evidence for this complete pathway, the definitive anatomy is not known.

It has been shown that electrical stimulation of the cortex results in excitation or inhibition of single units in the lower auditory system.[141] There has also been physiologic evidence for a descending train of impulses that eventually reach the cochlea from the cortex.[36]

The olivocochlear bundle is the best known circuitry of the efferent system. There are two main tracts of the olivocochlear bundle, the lateral and the medial.[162] The lateral tract originates from cells near the lateral superior olive and is mostly composed of uncrossed, unmyelinated fibers that terminate on the (ipsilateral) dendrites beneath the inner hair cells. The medial tract is composed of myelinated fibers that originate in the area around the medial superior olive. Most fibers cross to the opposite cochlea where they connect directly to the outer hair cells (Fig 2–9). The lateral and medial olivocochlear bundle also connect to various divisions of the CN before they course along the vestibular nerves in the internal auditory meatus.[131, 162]

Some early physiologic studies have shown that stimulation of the crossed olivocochlear bundle fibers resulted in reduced neural response from the cochlea and auditory nerve[47]; however, stimulation of the lateral aspect of the SOC has lowered the threshold of fibers in the CN.[29] Hence, it appears that the olivocochlear bundle has the potential for modulating the activity coming from the cochlea in either an excitatory or inhibitory manner.

Pickles and Comis[133] showed that application of atropine (a cholinergic blocker) in the region of the olivocochlear bundle resulted in poorer hearing in noise. Several other studies have shown that the bundle plays an important role for hearing in noise.[37, 116] The mechanism underlying this facilitation for hearing in noise may be related to the medial olivocochlear bundle potential ability to trigger outer-hair-cell expansion and contraction, thereby enhancing or damping basilar-membrane activity. An important part of this function of the olivocochlear bundle has to do with its neurotransmitters. It appears that the olivocochlear bundle is a central mechanism that has some control over the periphery.

## AUDITORY NEUROCHEMISTRY

Recently there has been increased interest and study of the neurotransmitters of the auditory system. There are many reasons for this interest but perhaps the main one is very basic. Information obtained by the periphery must be transmitted to the brain and this process of neurotransmission requires neurotransmitters. These neurochemical substances provide for the synapse between two

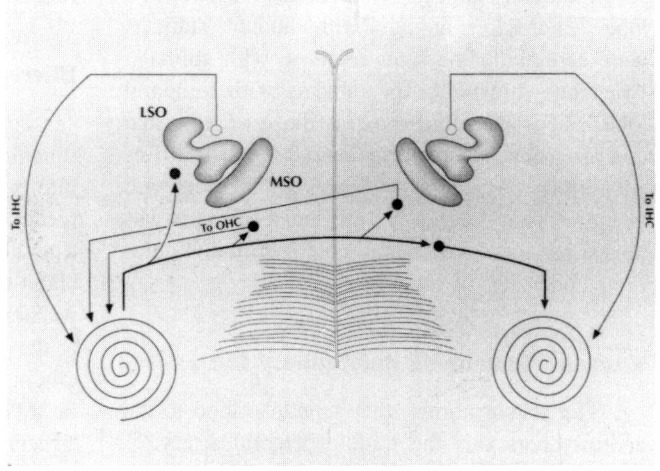


**FIG 2–9.**
Anatomy of the olivocochlear bundle showing the afferent systems (*arrows* pointing towards the lateral *[LSO]* and medial superior olivary *[MSO]* nuclei) and efferent systems (*arrows* pointing towards the cochlea). The olivocochlear bundle fibers originating from the area around the MSO are mostly crossed. Fibers originating from around the LSO are mostly uncrossed. (From Musiek FE, Hoffman D: *Ear Hear* 1990; 11:395–402. Used by permission.)

nerve cells to take place. Therefore the characteristics of the synapse as well as the neurotransmitter may determine many of the characteristics of auditory function or processing. Certainly without synaptic activity auditory function as we know it would not take place. Since many of the known neurotransmitters are associated with the central auditory system, it is appropriate to review the neurochemistry as part of a discussion of neuroanatomy and physiology. In addition, much of the research on auditory neurotransmitters has profound clinical implications.

### Structure of Neurotransmission

The main structure in neurotransmission is the synapse. It is the connecting link between nerve cells and involves the synaptic button of the axon, which communicates neurochemically with the dendrites or soma of another nerve cell (Figs 2–10 and 2–11). The neurotransmitters are released by vesicles and diffuse across the synaptic region to bind to receptors, which are proteins embedded in the adjacent cell membrane (Fig 2–12). The binding of a neurotransmitter can cause several events to occur. One such event is the change in ion flow across the cell membrane, which can result in a change in the receptor potential (postsynaptic cell). After a number of transmitter-receptor interactions in a restricted time period, the postsynaptic cell will depolarize and fire its own impulse or action potential. This action is associated with an excitatory neurotransmitter[109]; an inhibitory neurotransmitter can cause hyperpolarization of the postsynaptic cell membrane, which makes the cell difficult to excite (fire an impulse).[109] There are many other biochemical actions of the cell that can influence the nature of the synapse, but they are beyond the scope of this review.

In present-day medicine, many therapeutic drugs are used to affect the synaptic activity. Some drugs may mimic natural neurotransmitters by binding to and activating the postsynaptic receptor; these are termed agonists. An antagonist causes an opposite effect; it can bind to the receptor but not activate it. By binding to the receptor it also blocks the natural neurotransmitter function.

### Auditory Neurotransmission (Afferent)

If neurotransmitters can control synaptic activity, then it seems possible to control the functions that are based on these synaptic interactions. The neurotransmitters must first be identified and localized. Strict criteria must be met before a chemical can be considered a neurotransmitter[109]; however, once these neurotransmitters are identified, treatments with agonists and antagonists may provide new information on function and dysfunction of a system.

It is not known which neurotransmitter operates between the hair cells and the auditory nerve in the cochlea, but glutamate is thought to be a possibility.[14] Glutamate or aspartate are also thought to be involved in auditory nerve-to-cochlear nucleus transmission.[14, 58] The cochlear nucleus probably has several excitatory neurotransmitters, including aspartate, glutamate, and

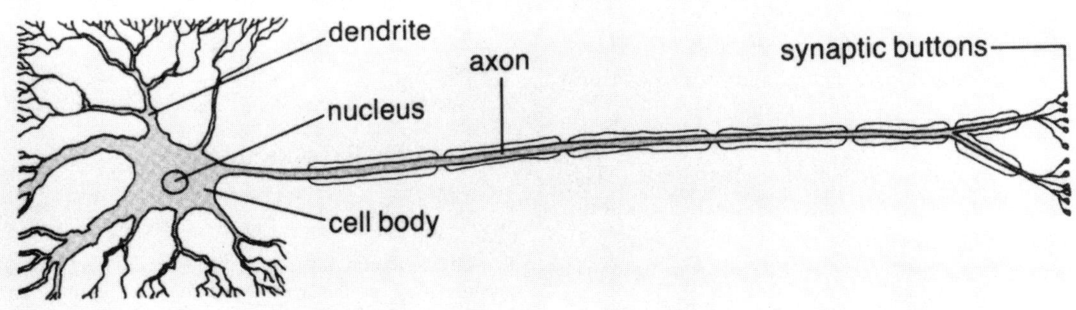


**FIG 2–10.**
Typical nerve cell. (From Ornstein R, Thompson R, Macaulay D: *The Amazing Brain,* Boston, 1984, Houghton-Mifflin. Used by permission.)

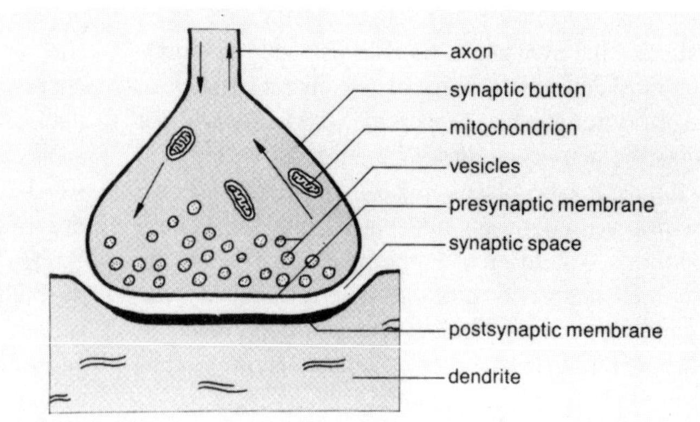


**FIG 2–11.**
Anatomy of a synapse. (From Ornstein R, Thompson R, Macaulay D: *The Amazing Brain,* Boston, 1984, Houghton-Mifflin. Used by permission.)

acetylcholine (ACh).[6, 54, 121] Gamma-aminobutyric acid (GABA) and glycine are inhibitory amino acids found at high levels in the cochlear nucleus.[53] Both GABA and glycine are also found in the SOC.[63, 165] Excitatory amino acids, such as quisqualate, glutamate, and *N*-methyl-D-aspartate (NMDA), have been localized in the SOC.[122] Adams and Wenthold[2] suggested that glycine and glutamate are found in the inferior colliculus. Both NMDA and aspartate have been shown to increase activity at the level of the inferior colliculus.[44]

There are few data on auditory cortex neurotransmitters. There is some evidence that ACh and some of the opiate drugs have effects on auditory cortex activity or evoked potentials; however, more research is necessary to understand the neurochemistry in this brain region.[89, 158]

## Auditory Neurotransmission (Efferent)

More information is available on efferent rather than afferent neurotransmitters. Specifically, the neurotransmission of the olivocochlear bundle has been heavily studied (see Fig 2–9). The olivocochlear bundle system can be viewed as two systems. One is lateral and originates from the area around the lateral superior olive; the other is medial and rises from the region of the medial olive. Both systems are cholinergic.[7] The lateral system also has enkephalin and dynorphin, which are opioid peptides (Fig 2–13).[65] These efferent neurotransmitters can be found in the perilymph of the cochlea. Applying ACh to the olivocochlear bundle mimics effects of electrical stimulation of the bundle.[15]

## Auditory Function

A number of studies have examined neurotransmitter effects on auditory function, measured either electrophysiologically or behaviorally. For example, auditory nerve activity during sound stimulation was reduced when glutamatergic blockers were profused through the cochleas of guinea pigs.[30] An increase in spontaneous and

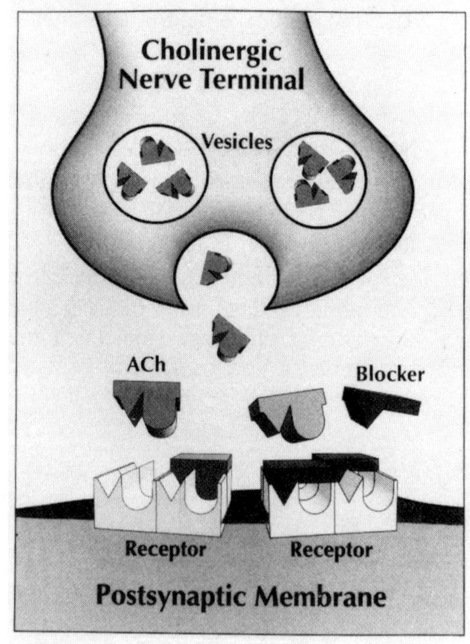


**FIG 2–12.**
Neurotransmission (across a synapse) showing acetylcholine *(ACh)* as the neurotransmitter (an agonist) and an example of a blocker (an antagonist) for ACh. (From Musiek FE, Hoffman D: *Ear Hear* 1990; 11:395–402. Used by permission.)

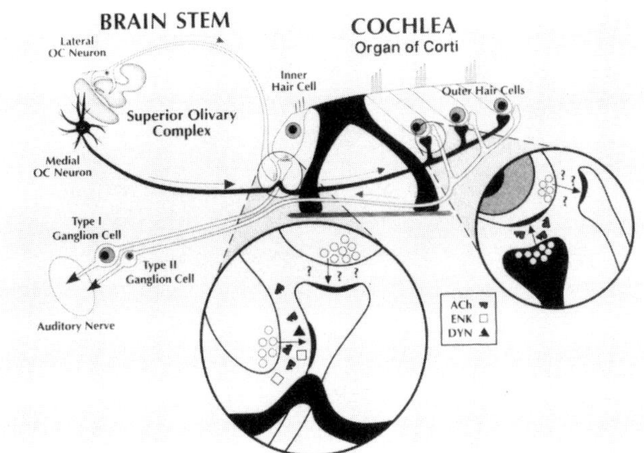


**FIG 2–13.**
Lateral and medial olivocochlear connections to inner (efferent neurons) and outer hair cells of the cochlea. Also shown are efferent neurotransmitters that interact at these sites. (From Musiek FE, Hoffman D: *Ear Hear* 1990; 11:395–402. Used by permission.)

acoustically stimulated firing rates of CN fibers was noted with the application of the excitatory amino acid aspartate. This effect was reversed when an antagonist drug was administered. A similar study using agonists (glutamate, aspartate, NMDA) and antagonists at the level of the inferior colliculus showed similar neural modulating results.[44]

In humans, the late auditory evoked potential (P2) showed an increase in amplitude when naloxone (an opioid antagonist) was administered. In the same study an opioid agonist (fentanyl) reduced the P2 amplitude.[158]

Auditory function of the olivocochlear bundle and neurotransmission have been studied. As mentioned earlier, it appears that the olivocochlear bundle plays a role in enhancing hearing in noise.[133, 170] It is also thought that this mechanism is mediated by the chemical interaction of the olivocochlear bundle and the hair cells of the cochlea. The fact that outer hair cells can expand and contract may be intimately related to the olivocochlear bundle, because neurotransmitters may control this hair cell function. This in turn may allow olivocochlear bundle modulation of incoming impulses via the outer hair cells by regulating their motor activity.

Recent studies done on chinchillas have shown that the auditory nerve action potential can be significantly enhanced by injecting pentazocine, an opioid agonist.[148] This effect is noted only at intensity levels near threshold and clearly involves the olivocochlear bundle system since opioids are found in the (lateral) system.

The studies on auditory function and neurotransmission may eventually provide a manner in which hearing can be enhanced therapeutically. Research that has been done in this area emphasizes neurochemistry's intimate role in auditory physiology.

## SUMMARY

This chapter has presented an overview of topics in neuroanatomy and neurophysiology that are relevant to central auditory processing. We have selected topics and subtopics to provide important background information and current data on structure and function of the central auditory system. New information on neurochemistry, brain prints and brain morphology in learning-disabled people will become more and more important aspects not only of neuroanatomy and neurophysiology but also of clinical management of those with central auditory dysfunction. It is also hoped that this commentary will encourage those interested in central auditory assessment and management to become serious students of brain anatomy and physiology, for without a thorough understanding of structure and function, test findings mean little.

### Acknowledgment

We thank Alicia Green for editorial assistance in the preparation of this manuscript.

## REFERENCES


1. Abeles M, Goldstein M: Responses of a single unit in the primary auditory cortex of the cat to tones and to tone pairs. *Brain Res* 1972; 42:337–352.
2. Adams J, Wenthold R: Immunostaining of GABA-ergic and glycinergic inputs to the anteroventral cochlear nucleus. *Neurosci Abstr* 1987; 13:1259.
3. Aitken LM, Webster WR, Veale JL, et al: Inferior colliculus. I. Comparison of response properties of neurons in central, pericentral, and external nuclei of adult cat. *J Neurophysiol* 1975; 38:1196–1207.
4. Aitkin LM, Webster WR: Medial geniculate body of the cat: Organization and response to tonal stimuli of neurons in the ventral division. *J Neurophysiol* 1972; 35:365–380.
5. Allen W: Effect of destroying three localized cerebral cortical areas for sound on correct conditioned differential responses of the dog's foreleg. *Am J Physiol* 1945; 144:415–428.
6. Altschuler R, Wenthold R, Schwartz A, et al: Immunocytochemical localization of glutaminase-like immunoreactivity in the auditory nerve. *Brain Res* 1984; 29:173–178.
7. Altschuler RA, Fex J: Efferent neurotransmitters, in Altschuler RA, Hoffman DW, Bobbin RP (eds): *Neurobiology of Hearing: The Cochlea.* New York, Raven Press, 1986, pp 383–396.
8. Auerbach S, Allard T, Naeser M, et al: Pure word deafness. Analysis of a case with bilateral lesions and a defect at the prephonemic level. *Brain* 1982; 105:271–300.
9. Baran JA, Musiek FE, Reeves AG: Central auditory function following anterior sectioning of the corpus callosum. *Ear Hear* 1986; 7:359–362.
10. Barnes W, Magoon H, Ranson S: The ascending auditory pathway in the brain stem of the monkey. *J Comp Neurol* 1943; 79:129–152.
11. Benerento L, Coleman P: Responses of single cells in cat inferior colliculus to binaural click stimuli: Combinations of intensity levels, time differences, and intensity differences. *Brain Res* 1970; 17:387–405.
12. Benson D, Teas D: Single unit study of binaural interaction in the auditory cortex of the chinchilla. *Brain Res* 1976; 103:313–338.
13. Berlin C, Lowe-Bell S, Janetta P et al: Central auditory deficits after temporal lobectomy. *Arch Otolaryngol* 1972; 96:4–10.
14. Bledsoe S, Bobbin R, Puel J: Neurotransmission in the inner ear, in Jahn A, Santo-Sacchi J (eds): *Physiology of the Ear*. New York, Raven Press, 1988, pp 385–406.
15. Bobbin RP, Konishi T: Acetylcholine mimics crossed olivocochlear bundle stimulation. *Nature* 1971; 231:222–224.
16. Borg E: On the organization of the acoustic middle ear reflex. A physiologic and anatomic study. *Brain Res* 1973; 49:101–123.
17. Boudreau JC, Tsuchitani C: Cat superior olive S-segment cell discharge to tonal stimulation, in Neff WD (ed): *Contributions to Sensory Physiology,* vol 4. New York, Academic Press, 1970, pp 143–213.
18. Bremer F, Brihaye J, Andre-Balisaux G: Physiologie et pathologie du corps calleux. *Schweiz Arch Neurol Psychiatr* 1956; 78:31–32.
19. Brugge IF, Geisler CE: Auditory mechanisms of the lower brain stem. *Am Rev Neurosci* 1978; 1:363–394.
20. Butler R, Keidel W, Spreng M: An investigation of the human cortical evoked potential under conditions of monaural and binaural stimulation. *Acta Otolaryngol* 1969; 68:317–326.
21. Campain R, Minckler J: A note in gross configurations of the human auditory cortex. *Brain Lang* 1976; 3:318–323.
22. Carpenter M, Sutin J: *Human Neuroanatomy.* Baltimore, Williams and Wilkins, 1983.
23. Celesia G: Organization of auditory cortical areas in man. *Brain* 1976; 99:403–414.
24. Chang H-T: Cortical response to activity of callosal neurons. *J Neurophysiol* 1953; 16:117–131.
25. Chiappa K: *Evoked Potentials in Clinical Medicine.* New York, Raven Press, 1983.
26. Colavita F: Auditory cortical lesions and visual patterns discrimination in cats. *Brain Res* 1972; 39:437–447.
27. Colavita F: Insular-temporal lesions and vibrotactile temporal pattern discrimination in cats. *Psychol Behav* 1974; 12:215–218.
28. Colclasure J, Graham S: Intracranial aneurysm occurring as a sensorineural hearing loss. *Otolaryngol Head Neck Surg* 1981; 89:283–287.
29. Comis S, Whitfield I: Influence of centrifugal pathways on unit activity in the cochlear nucleus. *J Neurophysiol* 1968; 31:62–68.
30. Cousillas H, Cole KS, Johnstone BM: Effect of spider venom on cochlear nerve activity consistent with glutamatergic transmission at hair cell-afferent dendrite synapse. *Hear Res* 1988; 36:213–220.
31. Cranford J: Detection vs. discrimination of brief tones by cats with auditory cortex lesions. *J Acoust Soc Am* 1979; 65:1573–1575.

32. Cranford J, Igarashi M, Stramler J: Effect of auditory neocortical ablation on pitch perception in the cat. *J Neurophysiol* 1976; 39:143–152.
33. Cranford J, Stream R, Rye C, et al: Detection vs. discrimination of brief duration tones: Findings in patients with temporal lobe damage. *Arch Otolaryngol* 1982; 108:350–356.
34. Cullen J, Thompson C: Masking release for speech in subjects with temporal lobe resections. *Arch Otolaryngol* 1974; 100:113–116.
35. Damasio H, Damasio A: Paradoxic ear extension in dichotic listening: Possible anatomic significance. *Neurology* 1979; 25:644–653.
36. Desmedt J: Physiological studies of the efferent recurrent auditory system, in Keidel W, Neff W (eds): *Handbook of Sensory Physiology,* vol 2. Berlin, Springer-Verlag, 1975, pp 219–246.
37. Dewson J: Efferent olivocochlear bundle: Some relationships to stimulus discrimination in noise. *J Neurophysiol* 1968; 31:122–130.
38. Diamond I, Neff W: Ablation of temporal cortex and discrimination of auditory patterns. *J Neurophysiol* 1957; 20:300–315.
39. Donchin E, Kutas M, McCarthy G: Electrocortical indices of hemispheric utilization, in Harnad S, et al (eds): *Lateralization in the Nervous System*. New York, Academic Press, 1976.
40. Dublin W: *Fundamentals of Sensorineural Auditory Pathology*. Springfield, Ill, Charles C Thomas, 1976.
41. Dublin W: The cochlear nuclei—pathology. *Otolaryngol Head Neck Surg* 1985; 93:448–463.
42. Eisenmann L: Neurocoding of sound localization: An electrophysiological study in auditory cortex of the cat using free field stimuli. *Brain Res* 1974; 75:203–214.
43. Evans E, Cortical representation, in de Reuck A, Knight J (eds): *Hearing Mechanisms in Vertebrates*. London, Churchill Livingstone, 1968, pp 277–287.
44. Faingold CL, Hoffmann WE, Caspary DM: Effects of excitant amino acids on acoustic responses of inferior colliculus neurons. *Hear Res* 1989; 40:127–136.
45. Ferraro J, Minckler J: The human lateral lemniscus and its nuclei. The human auditory pathways. A quantitative study. *Brain Lang* 1977; 4:277–294.
46. French J: The reticular formation. *Sci Am* 1957; 66:1–8.
47. Galambos R: Suppression of auditory nerve activity by stimulation of efferent fibers to cochlea. *J Neurophysiol* 1956; 19:424–437.
48. Galaburda A, Sanides F: Cytoarchitectonic organization of the human auditory cortex. *J Comp Neurol* 1980; 190:597–610.
49. Galaburda A, Sherman G, Rosen G, et al: Developmental dyslexia: Four consecutive patients with cortical anomalies. *Ann Neurol* 1985; 18:222–235.
50. Gazzaniga M, Sperry R: Some functional effects of sectioning the cerebral commissure in man. *Proc Natl Acad Sci USA* 1962; 48:1765–1769.
51. Gershuni J, Baru A, Karaseva T: Role of auditory cortex and discrimination of acoustic stimuli. *Neurol Sci Trans* 1967; 1:370–372.
52. Geschwind N, Levitsky W: Human brain: Left-right asymmetries in temporal speech region. *Science* 1968; 161:186–187.
53. Godfrey D, Carter J, Berger S, et al: Quantitative histochemical mapping of candidate transmitter amino acids in the cat cochlear nucleus. *J Histochem Cytochem* 1977; 25:417–431.
54. Godfrey D, Park J, Dunn J, et al: Cholinergic neurotransmission in the cochlear nucleus, in Drecher D (ed): *Auditory Neurochemistry*. Springfield, Ill, Charles C Thomas, 1985, pp 163–183.
55. Goldberg JM, Moore RY: Ascending projections of the lateral lemniscus in the cat and the monkey. *J Comp Neurol* 1967; 129:143–155.
56. Goldstein M, DeRibaupierre R, Yeni-Komshian G: Cortical coding of periodicity pitch, in Sachs M (ed): *Physiology of the Auditory System*. Baltimore, National Education Consultants, Inc, 1971.
57. Gordon B: The inferior colliculus of the brain. *Sci Am* 1972; 227:72–82.
58. Guth P, Melamed B: Neurotransmission in the auditory system: A primer for pharmacologists. *Ann Rev Pharm Toxicol* 1982; 22:383–412.
59. Hall JW III: The acoustic reflex in central auditory dysfunction, in Pinheiro ML, Musiek FE (eds): *Assessment of Central Auditory Dysfunction: Foundations and Clinical Correlates*. Baltimore, Williams and Wilkins, 1985, pp 103–130.
60. Harrison J, Howe M: Anatomy of the descending auditory system (mammalian), in Keidel W, Neff W (eds): *Handbook of Sensory Physiology,* vol 1. Berlin, Springer-Verlag, 1974.
61. Heffner H, Heffner R: Hearing loss in Japanese Macaques following bilateral auditory cortex lesions. *J Neurophysiol* 1986; 55:256–271.
62. Heffner H, Heffner R, Porter W: Effects of auditory cortex lesion on absolute thresholds in Macaques. Proceedings, Society for Neuroscience Annual Meeting, Dallas, October 20, 1985.

63. Helfert R, Altschuler R, Wenthold R: GABA and glycine immunoreactivity in the guinea pig superior olivary complex. *Neurosci Abstr* 1987; 13:544.
64. Hodgson W: Audiological report of a patient with left hemispherectomy. *J Speech Hear Disord* 1967; 32:39–45.
65. Hoffman DW: Opioid mechanisms in the inner ear, in Altschuler RA, Hoffman DW, Bobbin RP (eds): *Neurobiology of Hearing: The Cochlea.* New York, Raven Press, 1986, pp 371–382.
66. Hynd GW, Semrud-Clikeman M, Lorys AR, et al: Corpus callosum morphology in attention deficit-hyperactivity disorder: Morphometric analysis of MRI. *J Learn Disord* 1991; 24:141–146.
67. Jeffress L, McFadden D: Differences of interaural phase and level of detection and lateralization. *J Acoust Soc Am* 1971; 49:1169–1179.
68. Jerger J, Jerger S: Auditory findings in brain stem disorders. *Arch Otolaryngol* 1974; 99:342–350.
69. Jerger J, Jerger S: Diagnostic significance of PB word functions. *Arch Otolaryngol* 1971; 93:573–580.
70. Jerger J, Weikers N, Sharbrough F, et al: Bilateral lesions of the temporal lobe: A case study. *Acta Otolaryngol (Suppl)* 1969; 258:1–51.
71. Jones E, Powell T: An anatomical study of converging sensory pathways within the cerebral cortex of the monkey. *Brain* 1970; 93:793–820.
72. Jouandet M, Tramo M, Herron D, et al: Brainprints: Computer generated two dimensional maps of the human cerebral cortex in vivo. *J Cog Neurosci* 1989; 1:88–117.
73. Jungert S: Auditory pathways in the brain stem. A neurophysiologic study. *Acta Otolaryngol (Suppl)* 1958; 138.
74. Kaufman W, Galaburda A: Cerebrocortical microdysgenesis in neurologically normal subjects: A histopathological study. *Neurology* 1989; 39:238–243.
75. Kavanagh G, Kelly J: Hearing in the ferret *(Mustela putorius):* Effects of primary auditory cortical lesions on thresholds for pure tone detection. *J Neurophysiol* 1988; 60:879–888.
76. Keidel W, Kallert S, Korth M, et al: *The Physiological Basis of Hearing.* New York, Thieme-Stratton, 1983.
77. Kiang NYS: Stimulus representation in the discharge patterns of auditory neurons, in Tower DB (ed): *The Nervous System. Human Communication and Its Disorders,* vol 3. New York, Raven Press, 1975, pp 81–96.
78. Knudson EI, Konishi M: Monaural occlusion shifts receptive-field locations of auditory midbrain units in the owl. *J Neurophysiol* 1980; 44:687–695.
79. Knudson EI, Konishi M: Space and frequency are represented separately in auditory midbrain of the owl. *Neurophysiology* 1978; 41:870–884.
80. Kryter K, Ades H: Studies on the function of the higher acoustic centers in the cat. *Am J Psychol* 1943; 56:501–536.
81. Kudo M: Projections of the nuclei of the lateral lemniscus in the cat. An autoradiographic study. *Brain Res* 1981; 221:57–69.
82. Lauter J, Herscovitch P, Formby C, et al: Tonatopic organization of human auditory cortex revealed by positron emission tomography. *Hear Res* 1985; 20:199–205.
83. LeDoux J, Sakaguchi A, Reis D: Subcortical efferent projections of the medial geniculate nucleus mediate emotional responses conditioned to acoustic stimuli. *J Neurosci* 1983; 4:683–698.
84. Liden G, Rosenthal V: New developments in diagnostic auditory neurological problems, in Paparella M, Meyerhoff W (eds): *Sensorineural Hearing Loss, Vertigo and Tinnitus.* Baltimore, Williams and Wilkins, 1981.
85. Lynn G, Gilroy J, Taylow P, et al: Binaural masking level differences in neurological disorders. *Arch Otolaryngol* 1981; 107:357–362.
86. Masterson B, Thompson GC, Bechtold JK, et al: Neuroanatomical basis of binaural phase difference analysis for sound localization: A comparative study. *J Comp Physiol Psychol* 1975; 89:379–386.
87. Matkin N, Carhart R: Auditory profiles associated with Rh incompatibility. *Arch Otolaryngol* 1966; 84:502–513.
88. Matzker J: Two new methods for the assessment of central auditory functions in cases of brain disease. *Ann Otol Rhinol Laryngol* 1959; 68:1188–1197.
89. McKenna T, Ashe J, Hui G, et al: Muscarinic agonists modulate spontaneous and evoked unit discharge in auditory cortex of the cat. *Synapse* 1988; 2:54–68.
90. Merzenich M, Brugge J: Representation of the cochlear partition on the superior temporal plane of the Macaque monkey. *Brain Res* 1973; 50:275–296.
91. Merzenich MM, Reid MD: Representation of the cochlea within the inferior colliculus of the cat. *Brain Res* 1974; 77:397–415.
92. Meyer D, Woolsey C: Effects of localized cortical destruction on auditory discriminative conditioning in the cat. *J Neurophysiol* 1952; 15:149–162.

93. Møller A: *Auditory Physiology*. New York, Academic Press, 1983.
94. Møller AR: Physiology of the ascending auditory pathway with special reference to the auditory brain stem response (ABR), in Pinheiro ML, Musiek FE (eds): *Assessment of Central Auditory Dysfunction: Foundations and Clinical Correlates*. Baltimore, Williams and Wilkins, 1985, pp 23–41.
95. Møller M, Møller A: Auditory brain stem evoked responses (ABR) in diagnosis of eighth nerve and brain stem lesions, in Pinheiro ML, Musiek FE (eds): *Assessment of Central Auditory Dysfunction: Foundations and Clinical Correlates*. Baltimore, Williams and Wilkins, 1985, pp 43–65.
96. Moore C, Cranford J, Rahn A: Tracking for a "moving" fused auditory image under conditions that elicit the precedence effect. *J Speech Hear Res* 1990; 33:141–148.
97. Moore JK: The human auditory brain stem: A comparative view. *Hear Res* 1987; 29:1–32.
98. Morest DK: The neuronal architecture of medial geniculate body of the cat. *J Anat* 1964; 98:611–630.
99. Mountcastle V: Central neural mechanisms in hearing, in Mountcastle V (ed): *Medical Physiology*, vol 2. St Louis, Mosby–Year Book, 1968.
100. Mountcastle V: *Interhemispheric Relations and Cerebral Dominance*. Baltimore, Johns Hopkins Press, 1962.
101. Musiek FE: Application of central auditory tests: An overview, in Katz J (ed): *Handbook of Clinical Audiology*. Baltimore, Williams and Wilkins, 1985.
102. Musiek FE: Neuroanatomy, neurophysiology and central auditory assessment. II. The cerebrum. *Ear Hear* 1986; 7:283–294.
103. Musiek FE: Neuroanatomy, neurophysiology, and central auditory assessment. III. Corpus callosum and efferent pathways. *Ear Hear* 1986; 7:349–358.
104. Musiek FE, Baran JA: Neuroanatomy, neurophysiology, and central auditory assessment. I. Brain stem. *Ear Hear* 1986; 7:207–219.
105. Musiek F, Baran J, Pinheiro M: Duration pattern recognition in normal subjects and patients with cerebral and cochlear lesions. *Audiology* 1990; 29:304–313.
106. Musiek FE, Geurkink N: Auditory brain stem response and central auditory test findings for patients with brain stem lesions. *Laryngoscope* 1982; 92:891–900.
107. Musiek FE, Gollegly KM: ABR in eighth nerve and low brain stem lesions, in Jacobson JT (ed): *The Auditory Brain Stem Response*. San Diego, College-Hill Press, 1985, pp 181–202.
108. Musiek FE, Gollegly K, Kibbe K, et al: Current concepts on the use of ABR and auditory psychophysical tests in the evaluation of brain stem lesions. *Am J Otol (Suppl)* 1988; 9:25–35.
109. Musiek F, Hoffman D: An introduction to the functional neurochemistry of the auditory system. *Ear Hear* 1990; 11:395–402.
110. Musiek FE, Kibbe-Michael K: The ABR wave IV–V abnormalities from the ear opposite large CPE tumors. *Am J Otol* 1986; 7:253–257.
111. Musiek FE, Kibbe K, Baran J: Neuroaudiological results from split-brain patients. *Semin Hear* 1984; 5:219–229.
112. Musiek FE, Kibbe-Michael K, Geurkink N, et al: ABR results in patients with posterior fossa tumors and normal pure tone hearing. *Otolaryngol Head Neck Surg* 1986; 94:568–573.
113. Musiek FE, Pinheiro M: Frequency patterns in cochlear, brain stem, and cerebral lesions. *Audiology* 1987; 26:79–88.
114. Musiek FE, Reeves AG: Asymmetries of the auditory areas of the cerebrum. *J Am Acad Audiol* 1990; 1:240–245.
115. Neff W: Neuromechanisms of auditory discrimination, in Rosenblith W (ed): *Sensory Communication*. New York, Wiley and Sons, 1961.
116. Nieder P, Nieder I: Antimasking effect of crossed olivocochlear bundle stimulation with loud clicks in guinea pig. *Exp Neurol* 1970; 28: 179–188.
117. Noback CR: Neuroanatomical correlates of central auditory function, in Pinheiro ML, Musiek FE (eds): *Assessment of Central Auditory Dysfunction: Foundations and Clinical Correlates*. Baltimore, Williams and Wilkins, 1985, pp 7–21.
118. Nodar R, Kinney S: The contralateral effects of large tumors on brain stem auditory evoked potentials. *Laryngoscope* 1980; 90:1762–1768.
119. Oh S, Kuba T, Soyer A, et al: Lateralization of brain stem lesions by brain stem auditory evoked potentials. *Neurology* 1981; 31:14–18.
120. Oliver DL, Morest DK: The central nucleus of the inferior colliculus in the cat. *J Comp Neurol* 1984; 222:237–264.
121. Oliver D, Potashner S, Jones D, et al: Selective labeling of spiroganglion and granule cells with D-aspartate in the auditory system of the cat and guinea pig. *J Neurosci* 1983; 3:455–472.
122. Otterson O, Storm-Mathison J: Glutamate- and GABA-containing neurons in the mouse and rat brain, as demonstrated with a new immunocy-

tochemical technique. *J Comp Neurol* 1984; 229:374–392.

123. Pandya D, Seltzer B: The topography of commissural fibers, in Lepore F, Pitito M, Jasper H (eds): *Two Hemispheres—One Brain: Functions of the Corpus Callosum*. New York, Alan R Liss, Inc, 1986.
124. Penfield W, Perot P: The brain's record of auditory and visual experience: A final summary and discussion. *Brain* 1963; 86:596–695.
125. Penfield W, Rasmussen T: *The Cerebral Cortex of Man*. New York, Macmillan and Co, 1950.
126. Penfield W, Roberts L: *Speech and Brain Mechanisms*. Princeton, NJ, Princeton University Press, 1959.
127. Pfeiffer RR: Classification of response patterns of spike discharges for units in the cochlear nucleus. Tone burst stimulation. *Exp Brain Res* 1966; 1:220–235.
128. Pfingst B, O'Conner T: Characteristics of neurons in auditory cortex of monkeys performing a simple auditory task. *J Neurophysiol* 1981; 45:16–34.
129. Phillips D: Neural representation of sound amplitude in the auditory cortex: Effects of noise masking. *Behav Brain Res* 1990; 37:197–214.
130. Pickles J: *An Introduction to the Physiology of Hearing*, ed 1. New York, Academic Press, 1982.
131. Pickles JO: *An Introduction to the Physiology of Hearing*, ed 2. New York, Academic Press, 1988, p 246.
132. Pickles J: Physiology of the cerebral auditory system, in Pinheiro ML, Musiek FE (eds): *Assessment of Central Auditory Dysfunction: Foundations and Clinical Correlates*. Baltimore, Williams and Wilkins, 1985.
133. Pickles JO, Comis SD: Role of centrifugal pathways to cochlear nucleus in detection of signals in noise. *J Neurophysiol* 1973; 29:1131–1137.
134. Pinheiro M, Musiek F: Sequencing and temporal ordering in the auditory system, in Pinheiro M, Musiek FE (eds): *Assessment of Central Auditory Dysfunction: Foundations and Clinical Correlates*. Baltimore, Williams and Wilkins, 1985, pp 219–238.
135. Pinheiro M, Tobin H: Interaural intensity differences for intracranial lateralization. *J Acoust Soc Am* 1969; 40:1482–1487.
136. Portman M, Sterkers J, Charachon R, et al: *The Internal Auditory Meatus: Anatomy, Pathology, and Surgery*. New York, Churchill Livingstone, 1975.
137. Ravizza R, Masterton R: Contribution of neocortex to sound localization in opossum *(Didelphis virginiana)*. *J Neurophysiol* 1972; 35:344–356.
138. Rhode W: The use of intracellular techniques in the study of the cochlear nucleus. *J Acoust Soc Am* 1985; 78:320–327.
139. Rose JE, Galambos R, Hughes JR: Microelectrode studies of the cochlear nuclei of the cat. *Johns Hopkins Hosp Bull* 1959; 211–251.
140. Rubens A: Anatomical asymmetries of the human cerebral cortex, in Harnad S et al (eds): *Lateralization in the Nervous System*. New York, Academic Press, 1986.
141. Ryugo D, Weinberger N: Corticofugal modulation of the medial geniculate body. *Exp Neurol* 1976; 51:377–391.
142. Salamy A: Commissural transmission: Maturational changes in humans. *Science* 1978; 200:1409–1410.
143. Sanchez-Longo L, Forster F: Clinical significance of impairment of sound localization. *Neurology* 1958; 8:118–125.
144. Sando I: The anatomical interrelationships of the cochlear nerve fibers. *Acta Otolaryngol* 1965; 59:417–436.
145. Schuknecht HT: *Pathology of the Ear*. Cambridge, Mass, Harvard University Press, 1974.
146. Selnes OA: The corpus callosum: Some anatomical and functional considerations with special reference to language. *Brain Lang* 1974; 1:111–139.
147. Seltzer B, Pandya D: Afferent cortical connections and archetectonics of the superior temporal sulcus and surrounding cortex in Rhesus monkey. *Brain Res* 1978; 149:1–24.
148. Staley T, Kalish R, Musiek F, et al: Effects of opiate drugs on auditory evoked potentials in the chinchilla. *Hear Res,* in press.
149. Streitfeld B: The fiber connections of the temporal lobe with emphasis on the Rhesus monkey. *Int J Neurosci* 1980; 11:51–71.
150. Strominger NL, Hurwitz JL: Anatomical aspects of the superior olivary complex. *J Comp Neurol* 1976; 170:485–497.
151. Strominger NL, Strominger AL: Ascending brain stem projections of the anteroventral cochlear nucleus in the rhesus monkey. *J Comp Neurol* 1971; 143:217–232.
152. Sudakov K, MacLean P, Reeves A, et al: Unit study of exteroceptive inputs to the claustrocortex in the awake sitting squirrel monkey. *Brain Res* 1971; 28:19–34.
153. Tasaki I: Nerve impulses in individual auditory nerve fibers of the guinea pig. *J Neurophysiol* 1954; 17:97–122.
154. Tobin H: Binaural interaction tasks, in Pinheiro

ML, Musiek FE (eds): *Assessment of Central Auditory Dysfunction: Foundations and Clinical Correlates*. Baltimore, Williams & Wilkins, 1985, pp 151–171.

155. Tramo M, Bharucha J, Musiek F: Music perception in cognition following bilateral lesions of auditory cortex. *J Cognitive Neurosci* 1990; 2:195–211.
156. Tsuchitani C, Boudreau JC: Single unit analysis of cat superior olive S-segment with tonal stimuli. *J Neurophysiol* 1966; 29:684–697.
157. Van Noort J: *The Structure and Connections of the Inferior Colliculus: An Investigation of the Lower Auditory System*. Leiden, Van Corcum, 1969.
158. Velasco M, Velasco F, Castaneda R, et al: Effect of fentanyl and naloxone on human somatic and auditory-evoked potential components. *Neuropharmacol* 1984; 23:359–366.
159. Wada S, Starr A: Generation of auditory brain stem responses. III. Effects of lesions of the superior olive, lateral lemniscus and inferior colliculus on the ABR in guinea pig. *Electroencephalogr Clin Neurophysiol* 1983; 56:352–366.
160. Waddington M: *Atlas of Cerebral Angiography With Anatomic Correlation*. Boston, Little, Brown and Co, 1974.
161. Waddington M: *Atlas of Human Intracranial Anatomy*. Rutland, Vt, Academy Books, 1984.
162. Warr WB: Efferent components of the auditory system. *Ann Otol Rhinol Laryngol* 1980; 89:114–120.
163. Warr WB: Fiber degeneration following lesions in the anterior ventral cochlear nucleus of the cat. *Exp Neurol* 1966; 14:453–474.
164. Webster DB: Projection of the cochlea to cochlear nuclei in Merriam's kangaroo rat. *J Comp Neurol* 1971; 143:323–340.
165. Wenthold R, Huie D, Altschuler R, et al: Glycine immunoreactivity localized in the cochlear nucleus and superior olivary complex. *Neuroscience* 1987; 22:897–912.
166. Whitfield IC: *The Auditory Pathway*. Baltimore, Williams and Wilkins, 1967.
167. Willeford JA, Burleigh JM: *Handbook of Central Auditory Processing Disorders in Children*. Orlando, Grune and Stratton, 1985.
168. Winer JA: The human medial geniculate body. *Hear Res* 1984; 15:225–247.
169. Winer JA: The medial geniculate body of the cat. *Adv Anat Embryol Cell Biol* 1985; 86:1–98.
170. Winslow R, Sachs M: Effect of electrical stimulation of the crossed olivocochlear bundle on auditory nerve responses to tones in noise. *J Neurophysiol* 1987; 57:1002–1021.
171. Witelson S: Wires of the mind: Anatomical variation in the corpus callosum in relation to hemispheric specialization and integration, in Lepore F, Ptito M, Jasper H (eds): *Two Hemispheres—One Brain: Functions of the Corpus Callosum*. New York, Alan R Liss, Inc, 1986.
172. Woolsey C: Organization of cortical auditory system: A review and synthesis, in Rasmussen G, Windell W (eds): *Neuromechanics of the Auditory and Visibility Systems*. Springfield, Ill, Charles C Thomas, 1960.
173. Yakovlev P, LeCours A: Myelogenetic cycles of regional maturation of the brain, in Minkowski A (ed): *Regional Development of the Brain in Early Life*. Philadelphia, FA Davis, 1967.
174. Yaqub B, Gascon G, Al-Nosha M, et al: Pure word deafness (acquired verbal auditory agnosia) in an Arabic-speaking patient. *Brain* 1988; 111:457–466.

*Chapter* 3

# Acoustic Reflex in Frequency Selectivity: Brain Stem Auditory Evoked Response and Speech Discrimination

**Vittorio Colletti, M.D.**
**Franco G. Fiorino, M.D.**
**Giuseppa Verlato, M.D.**
**Marco Carner, M.D.**

## CLINICAL APPLICATION OF ACOUSTIC REFLEX

By definition the central auditory system begins at the termination of the eighth nerve in the cochlear nucleus. As is discussed in the chapters by Musiek and Salvi et al., the cochlear nucleus of the brain stem is quite complex and its outputs are involved in both afferent and efferent functions. The brain stem contains the nuclei of the primary auditory feedback systems; i.e., the olivocochlear system, which influences the operation of hair cells and the acoustic reflex (AR), which influences the transmission of sound through the middle ear. The following discussion highlights AR—a particularly important diagnostic tool in audiology and neuro-otology—and how the AR influences suprathreshold processing of sounds.

The afferent and efferent pathways of the reflex can be involved in a variety of neurological, inflammatory, degenerative, and neoplastic diseases. For example, in sensorineural hearing loss the amount of reflex decay during stimulation, as well as the relationship between hearing level and the reflex threshold, allow the differentiation of cochlear from eighth nerve pathologies.[1, 25, 30, 38]

The efferent limb of the reflex is explored in the diagnosis of ossicular chain disorders, such as otosclerosis and discontinuity,[35, 39] and in facial nerve palsy, where it can assume a prognostic value.[24] Abnormal reflexes are also recorded when stapedial muscle function is altered by myopathic diseases such as myasthenia gravis and hyperthyroidism.[27]

Since the early 1970s the investigations of Colletti,[11, 12] Bosatra et al,[9] Jerger and Jerger[26] and others have shown the acoustic reflex to be a valuable diagnostic tool in the diagnosis of brainstem lesions, such as in multiple sclerosis,[12] syringobulbia,[9] tumors,[21, 23] vertebrobasilar insufficiency,[9, 14] Friedreich's ataxia, and glue-sniffing polyneuropathy.[14] Furthermore, the diagnostic power of the AR in brain stem disorders has been improved by a more detailed and refined analysis of the reflex time course.[6, 11] For example, the temporal dispersion of reflex transmission through a diseased brain stem appears as an increase in latency and rise time,[10, 12] while bilateral comparison of crossed and uncrossed reflexes gives important indications as to the site of the lesion.[26]

## TONIC INFLUENCES OF HIGHER CNS STRUCTURES ON ACOUSTIC REFLEX

It must be stressed that the AR may be altered by pathological conditions that affect the ascending auditory pathway or its activity may be modulated by higher subcortical and cortical structures.

Both the AR[2] and the olivocochlear efferent system[22] are under the tonic facilitory influences from higher centers. In humans, however, the AR is not affected by vascular, traumatic, or tumoral damage to cortical structures that impairs auditory perceptual behavior.[20] This apparent discrepancy between clinical and experimental data could be explained by the observation that decerebration or bilateral ablation of auditory cortical area is necessary to inhibit the acoustic reflex in unanesthetized cats, while unilateral removal of this area or extensive cortical lesions sparing the auditory cortical area are ineffective.[2]

The existence of a tonic central inhibition on the AR has also been proposed[29] based on the observation that the reflex threshold improves with low blood-ethanol concentrations[36] and in brain-injured patients.[18] The assumption is that the brain injury or ethanol releases the AR from tonic inhibition. However, it should be noted in the former study the threshold shift was very small, amounting to 0.5 dB, while in the latter study a limited number of patients (three) was examined. Nevertheless, it is conceivable that localized brain damage could enhance the AR via selective withdrawal of inhibitory influences on the olivocochlear bundles.[5]

## PHASIC INFLUENCES OF HIGHER CNS STRUCTURES ON ACOUSTIC REFLEX

In the conscious cat, the middle ear muscles contract spontaneously during attention and desynchronized sleep thereby increasing the threshold of auditory arousal.[3] After bilateral ablation of auditory cortical area, the AR is no longer affected by wakefulness or sleep and gradually disappears during repetitive stimulation.[2]

In humans the amplitude of phasic AR decreases during attention.[17] In contrast, the AR is activated before and during vocalization.[8] We also recently evidenced a depression of phasic AR at the onset of dynamic exercise, which we attributed to cortical and/or brain stem involvement.[13]

## INFLUENCES OF ACOUSTIC REFLEX ON AUDITORY PROCESSING

Several studies exist on AR activity modulation of the central nervous system, but it is still unclear whether the reflex can modify central auditory processing. It is well known that the AR affects peripheral sound transmission primarily by the attenuation of acoustic input, mainly in the low frequency range.[4] As a consequence, the masking effect of low frequency tones on high ones is partially prevented[41] and the dynamic range from auditory threshold to discomfort level is increased.

The effect of attenuation of low frequencies on central auditory processing is not well known. It has been reported that absence of the AR in subjects having undergone stapedectomy with stapedius tendon section or suffering from Bell's palsy causes a deterioration in speech discrimination.[7, 28] However, it is not clear whether this effect results from the lack of AR activity or from the drop in speech discrimination owing to the hearing loss that can occur in such diseases.

A more thorough study of the AR effect on normal psychoacoustic and electrophysiologic phenomena could contribute to the elucidation of the influence of AR activity on sound processing.

## Experimental Studies

The present investigation analyzes the AR influence on three different levels of auditory processing. Psychoacoustic tuning curves were evaluated to study peripheral frequency analysis, whereas evoked potential input-output responses were assessed as an index of intensity encoding in the brain stem. Finally, speech discrimination and speech perception tests investigated more complex auditory function involving the cortex.

Subjects who had undergone stapedectomy with stapedius tendon section (STS) or with tendon preservation (STP), along with normally hearing volunteers, served as subjects in the research. Stapedectomized patients provide the best human model available for evaluating auditory tasks in the presence and absence of the acoustic reflex. It has been demonstrated that when surgery has been successful and bone conduction is well preserved, stapedectomy exerts little if any trauma to the inner ear, in contrast to total stapedectomy.[15, 37]

### *Experiment 1—Frequency Selectivity in Subjects With STS and STP*

Frequency selectivity was estimated from measurements of psychophysical tuning curves (PTC).[42] Psychophysical tuning curves are obtained by plotting the minimum intensity of a continuous tone over a range of frequencies required to mask an intermittent test tone. They furnish a picture of the frequency selectivity of the auditory system, providing information on the capacity of the ear to discriminate a sound in the presence of another tone; the sharper the curve, the greater the selectivity.

**Methods.**—Psychophysical tuning curves were examined in 10 subjects with STP and in 10 with STS at test frequencies of 500 and 4,000 Hz. Psychophysical tuning curves from a third group of 10 normally hearing volunteers were also investigated. Data were reported in each experiment as means and standard error of the means (SEM). The mean age for the STP group was 39 (SEM = 7), for the STS group 38.1 (SEM = 6.5), and for the control group 39 (SEM = 8.3).

The air-bone gap was less than 10 dB in all subjects and hearing level (HL) was within 30 dB at all the audiometric frequencies tested. The mean hearing level was 15 dB HL in the normal subjects, 20 dB HL in the STS group, and 21 dB HL in the STP group.

Subjects listened to a continuous masking tone and an interrupted pure tone of 500 or 4,000 Hz (duty cycle of 50%) at 10 and 30 dB (sensation level; relative to auditory threshold) for 2 seconds. Masker frequencies were spaced above and below the pure-tone probe frequency. The result of masking was the typical V-shaped tuning curve. Frequency selectivity was estimated by measuring the bandwidth 10 dB above PTC and the steepness of the low- and high-frequency tails was considered.

**Results.**—Figure 3–1 shows the average 500 and 4,000 Hz PTCs obtained with the test tone at 10 dB SL. All three groups have similar shapes at the tip and the steepness of the tails is similar in the normal and STP groups; however, the low-frequency tail is clearly lower in STS patients ($P < .05$). At 4,000 Hz, the trends between groups were essentially the same. However, the STS group had a significantly shallower low frequency tail. At the higher level, 30 dB SL, there is a trend for all three groups to have shallower PTS, with the STS group having significantly shallower low frequency tails (Fig 3–2).

**Discussion.**—The normal frequency or auditory selectivity retained at PTC tip frequencies in STP and STS subjects confirms that stapedectomy is a functionally conservative surgery that exerts little if any trauma to the inner ear. Total stapedectomy instead results in a widening of the PTC tip along with a slight deterioration of auditory threshold at high frequencies (Colletti et al, unpublished observations).

The steepness of PTC low-frequency tails decreases as a function of the test-tone intensity.[19] This, however, cannot explain the shallower low-frequency tails observed in STS subjects in the present research; the hearing level of this group was only slightly worse than that of normal subjects and quite similar to the hearing level of STP patients. A reasonable alternate explanation is that the stapedius muscle contraction improves frequency selectivity through attenuation of low frequencies, thereby reducing the upward spread of masking.

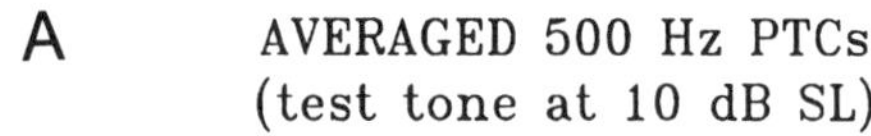


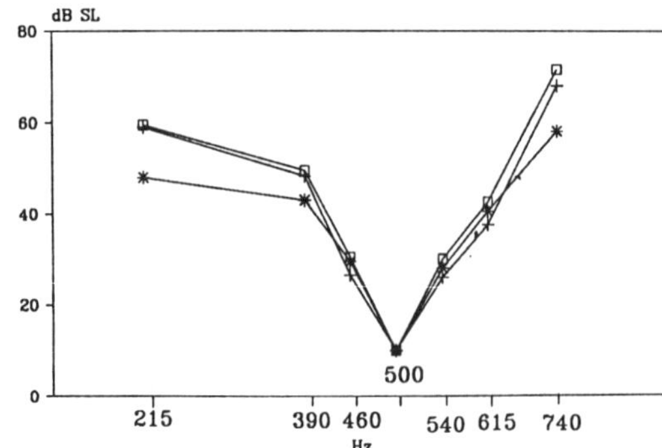


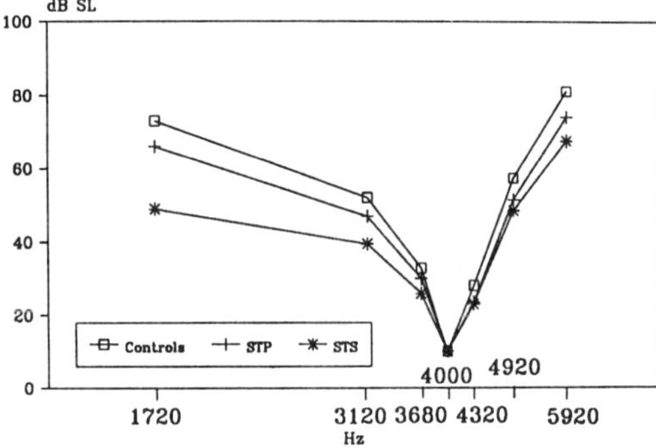


**FIG 3–1.**
Averaged 500 Hz and 4,000 Hz psychoacoustical tuning curves (PTC) in stapedotomy with stapedius tendon preservation (STP), stapedotomy with tendon section (STS), and controls. Test tone at 10 dB SL (re: auditory threshold).

### *Experiment 2—Auditory Brain Stem Response in Subjects With STS and STP*

The acoustic reflex plays a role in the encoding of intensity by modulating the passage of sound through the middle ear. This experiment assessed the effect of STP and STS on the encoding of loudness by measuring the latency and amplitude of the ABR.

**Methods.**—Five patients with STP and five with STS were examined. The mean ages were 37 years (SEM = 6) and 37.8 years (SEM = 6.5), respectively. As in experiment 1, hearing levels were within 30 dB HL in every subject and the air-bone gap was less than 10 dB.

The stimuli were clicks (0.1 msec duration) with alternating polarity presented at intensities of 80, 100, and 120 dB SPL p.e. and at a rate of 21 stimuli per second. The EEG activity was recorded using a commercial averager and silver/silver chloride electrodes. The positive (active) electrode was connected to the vertex, the negative electrode (reference) to an earlobe, and the ground to the forehead. Electrode impedance was kept below 3,000 Ω. ABR signals were fed through a filter passing the 30–2,500 Hz band.

Latencies of waves I, III, and V were evaluated in the two groups.

**Results.**—The STP and STS groups presented very similar latencies with respect to all waves studied (Fig 3–3). In the absence of the AR, wave V latency was slightly reduced at the highest intensity, although not significantly. Nev-

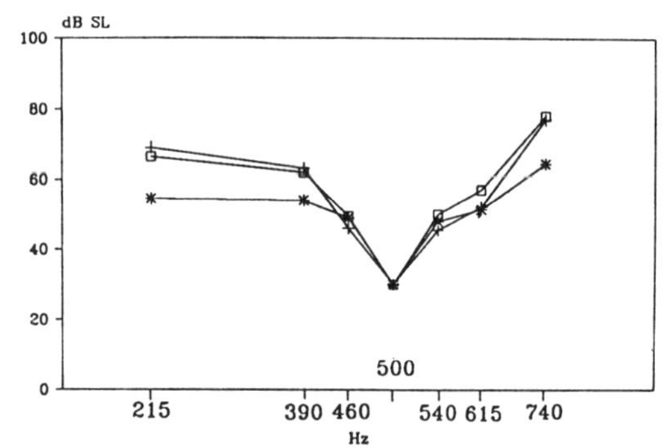


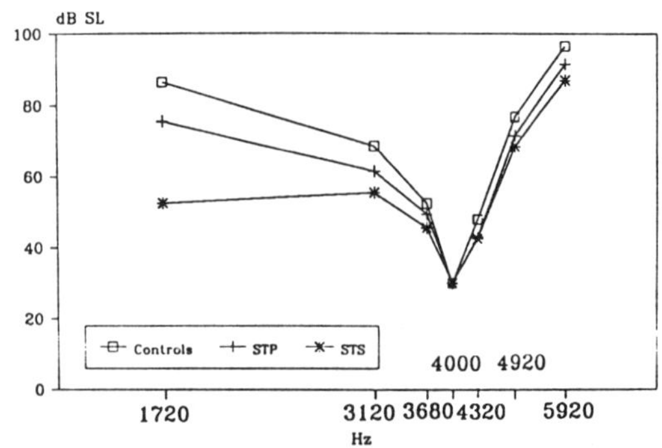


**FIG 3–2.**
Averaged 500 Hz and 4,000 Hz psychoacoustical tuning curves (PTC) in stapedotomy with tendon preservation (STP), stapedotomy with tendon section (STS), and controls. Test tone at 30 dB SL (re: auditory threshold).

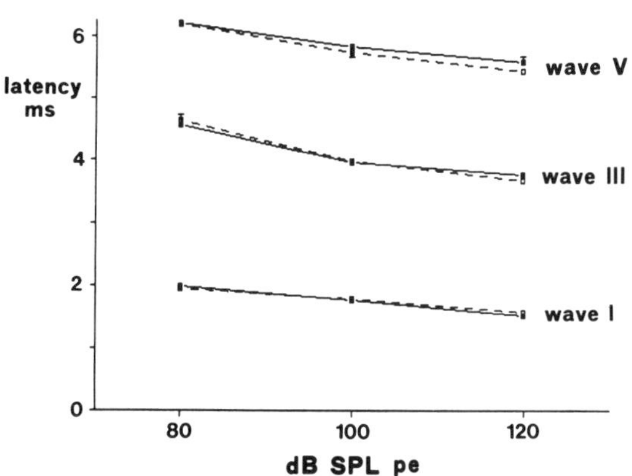


**FIG 3–3.**
Latency of waves I, III, and V as a function of stimulus intensity (alternated clicks, 21/sec) in stapedotomy patients with tendon section *(dashed line)* and those with tendon preservation *(continuous line)*.

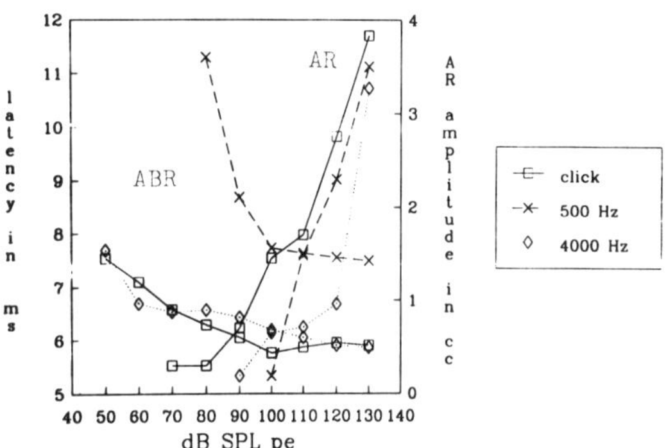


**FIG 3–4.**
Wave V latency *(descending curves)* and acoustic reflex (AR) amplitude *(ascending curves)* as a function of the intensity of eliciting stimuli in a representative subject.

ertheless, it is not possible to rule out an effect of the AR on ABR waves since the number of subjects examined was rather small.

### *Experiment 3—Auditory Brain Stem Response in Normally Hearing Subjects*

**Methods.**—Because the AR mainly attenuates low-frequency tones, ABRs evoked with stimuli of different frequencies were compared in eight normally hearing volunteers, aged 27.7 ± 2 years.

Alternated tone bursts (logons) of 500 and 4,000 Hz were utilized at a repetition rate of 21 stimuli per second; the intensity was increased from 50 to 130 dB SPL in 10-dB steps.

The input-output function of wave V latency was related to the amplitude/intensity function of the AR, elicited with the same stimuli utilized for the ABR recordings. Because of technical limitations, the contralateral reflex was used.

**Results.**—Figure 3–4 describes a representative case. Wave V latencies are displayed with the descending curves and the AR amplitudes for the same stimuli are represented by the ascending curves.

A gradual decrease in latency was observed when using clicks and 4,000-Hz logons, while the latency-intensity function at 500 Hz presented an abrupt change in slope approximately when the contralateral AR was activated (i.e., 100 dB SPL).

To determine the deflection points of the curves, data were fitted with two different lines, below and above saturation, and the best fit was selected[16] (Fig 3–5). A close correspondence was found between the calculated deflection points and the contralateral AR threshold at 500 Hz, while at 4,000 Hz the deflection point preceded AR threshold by 16 dB (Fig 3–6). Since the ipsilateral reflex threshold occurs approximately 10 dB below the contralateral one,[32] it can be assumed that the wave-V latency input-output function reached saturation simultaneously with the AR development at 500 Hz, while the saturation was independent from the AR at 4,000 Hz.

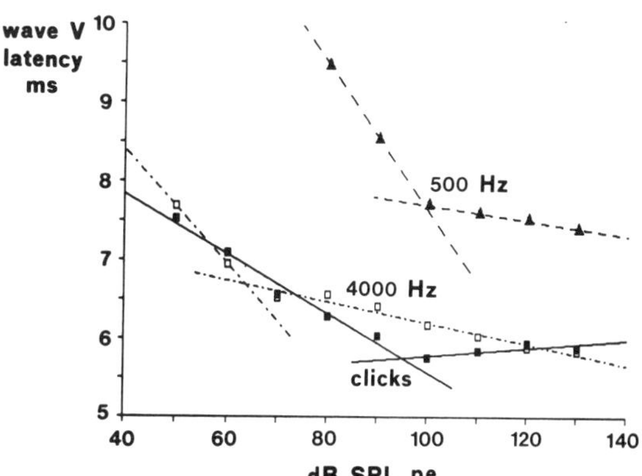


**FIG 3–5.**
Deflection points of wave V latency-intensity functions obtained by fitting experimental data according to Conconi (1988) to same representative subject as in Figure 3–4.

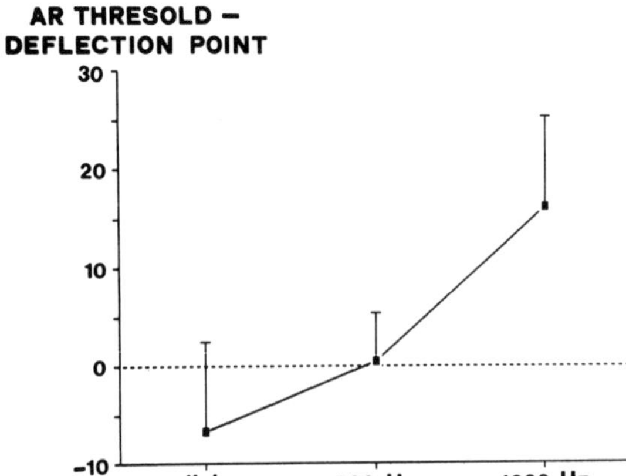


**FIG 3–6.**
Acoustic reflex threshold minus the intensity corresponding to the deflection point of wave V latency input-output function. Values given as mean ± SD.

**Discussion.**—The outcomes of experiments 2 and 3 do not allow us to conclude that the AR clearly affects ABR-wave latencies. However, it seems reasonable to suggest that the AR is partly involved in the faster saturation of the wave V latency input-output function, observed with 500 Hz stimulation and not with 4,000 Hz stimulation (see Figs 3–4 and 3–5).

### *Experiment 4—Speech Audiometry in STS and STP Subjects*

The previous experiments have shown how the AR can refine the systems frequency selectivity and influence the intensity coding of low frequencies. A more practical question is whether the AR influences subjects' speech discrimination, especially in the presence of background noise.

**Methods.**—STP (n = 10) and STS (n = 10) subjects were tested using speech audiometry with ipsilateral masking. Recall that both groups had an air-bone gap of less than 10 dB and air conduction auditory thresholds within 30 dB at all audiometric frequencies. STP and STS subjects had a mean age, respectively, of 36 ± 5.5 and 37.5 ± 7.8 years, which did not differ significantly from a third group of 10 normally hearing volunteers used as controls (36.5 ± 7.2 years).

The performance-intensity function for Italian disyllabic phonetically balanced words (PB) was plotted, using verbal repetition as the response method. The level at which subjects reached maximum discrimination (PB maximum) was determined. The experiment consisted of administering the words at 20 and again at 50 dB SL with respect to PB maximum, in the presence of ipsilateral masking with speech noise at signal-to-noise ratios of +10, 0, and −10.

**Results.**—Discrimination scores diminished as a function of ipsilateral masking intensity in all groups (Fig 3–7); however, the best scores were attained in normal and STP subjects, while speech discrimination in the STS group was significantly worse ($P < .01$) both at 20 and at 50 dB SL. For signal-to-noise ratios of +10, 0, and −10 dB average scores at 20 dB SL were 92%, 66%, and 7% correct, respectively, for the STP subjects and 82%, 52%, and 2% correct for the STS subjects.

The results of this experiment indicate that the AR improves speech discrimination in the presence of ipsilateral masking. At a signal-to-noise (S/N) ratio of 0 dB the difference in percent correct between the STS and STP group was 14% and 20%, respectively, for presentation levels of 10 and 30 dB SL.

This phenomenon can be attributed to the attenuation of sound energy in the low-frequency range provided by the AR. Upward spread of masking to high-frequency speech sounds is thus limited, resulting in an improvement of speech intelligibility.

It must be considered, however, that a hearing impairment at high frequencies owing to surgical trauma to the inner ear could be the cause of speech discrimination problems after surgery for otosclerosis. And indeed this phenomenon frequently occurs after total stapedectomy and has been reported in the findings of different authors, such as Smyth and Hassard,[37] McCandless and Goering,[28] and Colletti and co-workers.[15] Our groups of subjects had excellent hearing levels and discrimination scores that always reached the value of 100% when tested in quiet surroundings. However, ipsilateral masking had a differential effect on speech discrimination that decreased significantly in the group with severed stapedius tendons.

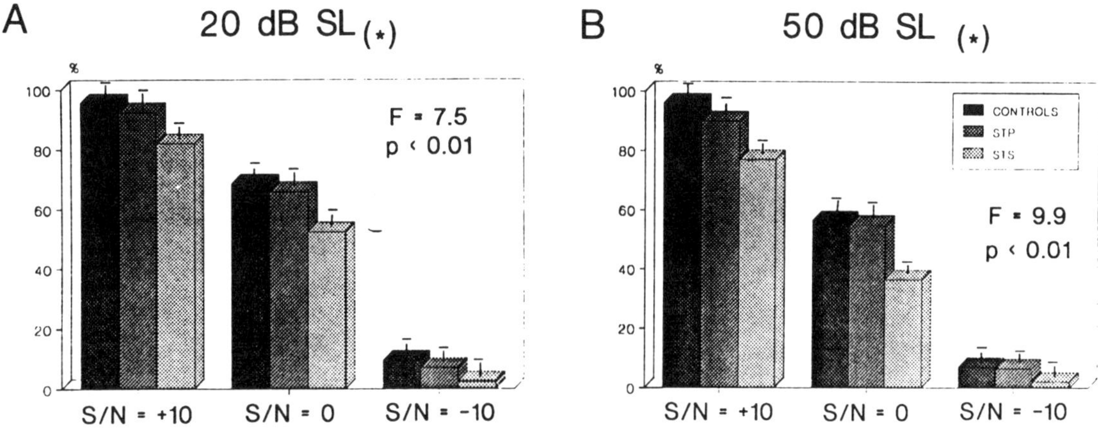


**FIG 3–7.**
Discrimination score at 20 dB SL and at 50 dB SL (re: threshold of maximum discrimination) at different signal-to-noise ratios.

## CONCLUSIONS

The outcomes of the present investigation indeed suggest that the AR affects auditory processing; frequency selectivity and speech discrimination are impaired in the absence of AR activity in stapedectomized patients. However, when intensity encoding is evaluated with ABR, the effects are seen only at low frequencies. Specifically, the results indirectly suggest that the AR could be involved in the rapid saturation of wave V latency input-output function, observed in the AR range with low-frequency tones in normal subjects (see Figs 3–4 and 3–5). Interestingly, in the literature the attenuation of the wave V latency-intensity function has not been correlated directly with the AR, but both phenomena have been linked to the same factor, the loudness discomfort level.[34, 40]

Another electrophysiologic event that might reflect an AR influence is the well-known adaptation of the ABR to an increase in stimulation rate.[33] As stimulation rates increase there is a delay of wave latencies and a decrease in wave amplitudes. Such variations could be partially accounted for by the temporal summation of the AR, which effectively attenuates sound transmission through the middle ear.[31] Further studies are thus warranted to elucidate AR influences on ABR waves; however, the current results show the importance of the AR in frequency selectivity and speech discrimination in noise.

## REFERENCES

1. Anderson H, Barr B, Wedenberg E: Intra-aural reflexes in retrocochlear lesions, in Hamberger C, Wersall J (eds): *Nobel Symposium 10: Disorders of the Skull Base Region.* Stockholm, Almquist and Wiskell, 1969, pp 49–55.
2. Baust W, Berlucchi G: Reflex response to clicks of cat's tensor tympani during sleep and wakefulness and the influence thereon of the auditory cortex. *Arch Ital Biol* 1964; 102:686–712.
3. Baust W, Berlucchi G, Moruzzi G: The auditory input during sleep and wakefulness. *Pflugers Arch* 1964; 280:S89–S91.
4. Borg E: A quantitative study of the effect of the acoustic stapedius reflex on sound transmission through the middle ear of man. *Acta Otolaryngol* 1968; 66:461–472.
5. Borg E: Efferent inhibition of afferent acoustic activity in the unanesthetized rabbit. *Exp Neurol* 1971; 31:301.
6. Borg E: Dynamic characteristics of the intra-aural muscle reflex, in Feldman AS, Wilber LA (eds): *Acoustic Impedance and Admittance: The Measurement of Middle Ear Function.* Baltimore, Williams and Wilkins, 1976, pp 236–299.
7. Borg E, Zakrisson JE: Stapedius reflex and speech features. *J Acoust Soc Am* 1973; 54:525–527.
8. Borg E, Zakrisson JE: The activity of the stapedius muscle in man during vocalization. *Acta Otolaryngol* 1975; 79:325–333.
9. Bosatra A, Russolo M, Poli P: Modifications of the stapedius muscle reflex under spontaneous and

experimental brain-stem impairment. *Acta Otolaryngol* 1975; 80:61–66.

10. Bosatra A, Russolo M, Poli P: Oscilloscopic analysis of the stapedius muscle reflex in brain stem lesions. *Arch Otolaryngol* 1976; 102:284–285.
11. Colletti V: Biometric aspects of the stapedius reflex. *Acta Otorhinolaryngol Belg* 1974; 28:545–552.
12. Colletti V: Stapedius reflex abnormalities in multiple sclerosis. *Audiology* 1975; 14:63–71.
13. Colletti V, Fiorino FG, Verlato G, et al: Physical exercise and active protection from temporary threshold shift. *Acta Otolaryngol* 1991; 111:234–239.
14. Colletti V, Sittoni V: Diagnostic application of stapedial reflex and ABR in neurological disorders. *Adv Audiol* 1985; 3:198–209.
15. Colletti V, Sittoni V, Fiorino FG: Stapedotomy with and without stapedius tendon preservation versus stapedectomy. Long-term results. *Am J Otol* 1988; 9:136–141.
16. Conconi F, Ballarin E, Borsetto C, et al: Use of the heart rate deflection point to assess the anaerobic threshold (reply to letter). *J Appl Physiol* 1988; 64:1759–1760.
17. Corcoran AL, Cleaver VCG, Stephens SDG: Attention, eye closure and the acoustic reflex. *Audiology* 1980; 19:233–244.
18. Downs DW, Crum MA: The hyperactive acoustic reflex: Four case studies. *Arch Otolaryngol* 1980; 106:401–404.
19. Florentine M, Buus S, Scharf B, et al: Frequency selectivity in normally-hearing and hearing impaired observers. *J Speech Hear Res* 1980; 23:646–669.
20. Gelfand SA, Silman S: Acoustic reflex threshold in brain-damaged patients. *Ear Hear* 1982; 3:93–95.
21. Greisen O, Rasmussen PE: Stapedius muscle reflexes and otoneurological examinations in brainstem tumors. *Acta Otolaryngol* 1970; 70:366–370.
22. Gummer M, Yates GK, Johnstone BM: Modulation transfer function of efferent neurons in the guinea pig cochlea. *Hear Res* 1988; 36:41–52.
23. Hayes D, Jerger J: Patterns of acoustic reflex and auditory brainstem response abnormality. *Acta Otolaryngol* 1981; 92:199–209.
24. Ide M, Morimitsu T, Ushisako Y, et al: The significance of stapedial reflex test in facial nerve paralysis. *Acta Otolaryngol (Stockh) (Suppl)* 1988; 446:57–63.
25. Jerger J, Harford E, Clemis J, et al: The acoustic reflex in eighth nerve disorder. *Arch Otolaryngol* 1974; 99:409–413.
26. Jerger S, Jerger J: Diagnostic value of crossed vs uncrossed acoustic reflexes. *Arch Otolaryngol* 1977; 103:445–453.
27. Laurian N, Laurian L, Sadov R, et al: New clinical applications of the stapedial reflex. *J Laryngol Otol* 1983; 97:1099–1103.
28. McCandless GA, Goering DM: Changes in loudness after stapedectomy. *Arch Otolaryngol* 1974; 100:344–350.
29. Mangham CA: The effect of drugs and systemic disease on the acoustic reflex, in Silman S (ed): *The Acoustic Reflex: Basic Principles and Clinical Applications*. Orlando, Fla, Academic Press, 1984, pp 441–468.
30. Metz O: Threshold of reflex contractions of muscles of middle ear and recruitment of loudness. *Arch Otolaryngol* 1952; 55:536–543.
31. Møller AR: Acoustic reflex in man. *J Acoust Soc Am* 1962; 34:1524–1534.
32. Møller AR: *Auditory Physiology*. New York, Academic Press, 1983.
33. Moore EJ: Effects of stimulus parameters, in Moore EJ (ed): *Bases of Auditory Brain-Stem Evoked Responses*. New York, Grune and Stratton, 1983, pp 221–251.
34. Niemeyer W: Relations between the discomfort level and the reflex threshold of the middle ear muscles. *Audiology* 1971; 10:172–176.
35. Olivier JC, Garcin M, Cagnol C: Interêt de l'impedancemetrie de Madsen dan les otites à tympan ferme et l'otospongiose. *Cah d'ORL* 1970; 5:491–498.
36. Robinette MA, Brey RH: Influence of alcohol on the acoustic reflex and temporary threshold shift. *Arch Otolaryngol* 1978; 1:31–37.
37. Smyth GDL, Hassard TH: Eighteen years experience in stapedectomy: The case for the small fenestra operation. *Ann Otol Rhinol Laryngol* 1978; 87:49–55.
38. Stach BA: The acoustic reflex in diagnostic audiology: From Metz to present. *Ear Hear* 1987; 8:36S–42S.
39. Terkildsen K, Osterhammel P, Bratlau P: Acoustic middle ear muscle reflexes in patients with otosclerosis. *Arch Otolaryngol* 1973; 98:152–155.
40. Thornton ARD, Farrell G, McSporran EL: Clinical methods for the objective estimation of loudness discomfort level (LDL) using auditory brainstem responses in patients. *Scand Audiol* 1989; 18:225–230.
41. Wiggers HC: The functions of the intra-aural muscles. *Am J Physiol* 1937; 120:771–780.
42. Zwicker E, Schorn K: Psychoacoustical tuning curves in audiology. *Audiology* 1978; 17:120–140.

Chapter 4

# Functional Changes in Central Auditory Pathways Resulting From Cochlear Diseases

Richard J. Salvi, Ph.D.
Donald Henderson, Ph.D.
Flint A. Boettcher, Ph.D.
Nicholas L. Powers, Ph.D.

During the past 50 years, researchers have learned a great deal about how the central auditory system functions in normal ears; however, relatively little is known about how the system functions when the inner ear or cochlea is damaged. The purpose of this paper is to review some of the functional changes that occur in the central auditory system of listeners with sensorineural hearing loss. Specifically, how do neurons in the central auditory system respond when the cochlea is compromised or when the peripheral inputs to the system are partially or completely cut off? Research in this area has received relatively little attention because sensorineural hearing loss has been considered a peripheral disorder. That is, the perceptual distortions that are associated with sensorineural hearing loss (e.g., tinnitus, poor speech discrimination, loudness recruitment, abnormal temporal integration) have been attributed to distortion in the neural code originating in the cochlea.[17, 18, 25–27, 32, 34] Although the neurophysiological changes observed in the periphery may account for some of the distortions in hearing, a full understanding of the disorders must ultimately take into account the functional changes that take place in the central auditory system. To appreciate the striking and unexpected changes in the central auditory pathway when the cochlea is damaged, it may be useful to briefly review some of the important anatomical and physiological properties of the system.

## ANATOMY AND PHYSIOLOGY

One of the most remarkable features of the auditory system is the ability to separate highly complex sounds into their constituent frequencies. In the cochlea, a given frequency preferentially excites a specific group of hair cells along the length of the cochlea (Fig 4–1). High frequencies stimulate hair cells near the basal (stapes) end of the cochlea and low frequencies activate hair cells near the apical end of the cochlea. This mapping of frequency to location is referred to as a tonotopic organization. Acoustic information transduced by the hair cells is subsequently conveyed to the central auditory system through approxi-

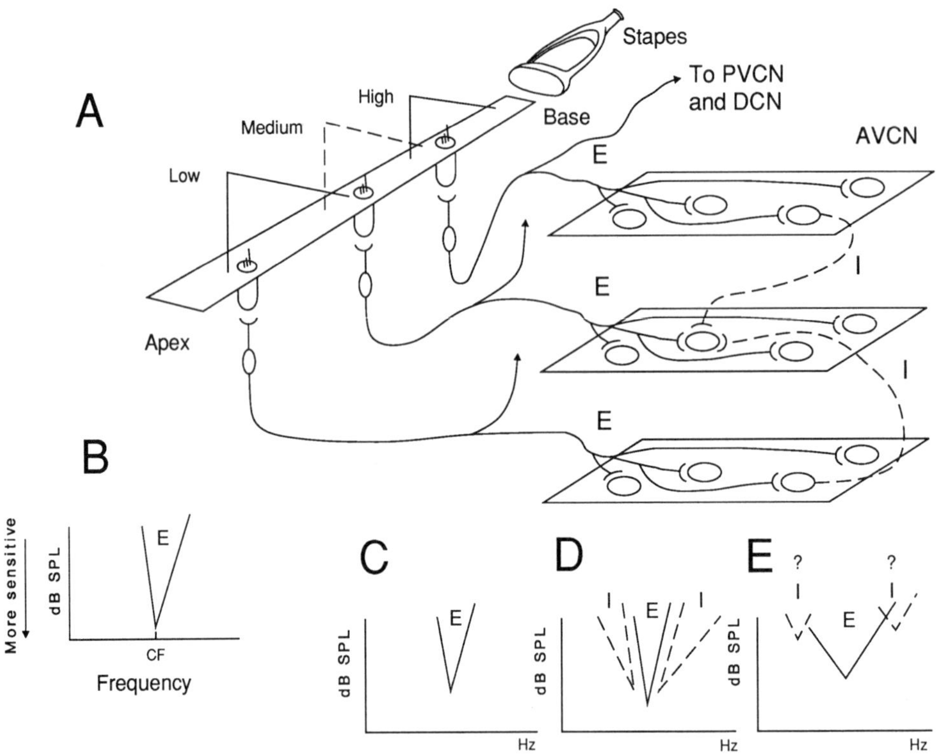


**FIG 4–1.**
**A,** highly simplified schematic illustrating the flow of neural activity out of the cochlea into the cochlear nucleus. Apex and base of the cochlear partition illustrate where low-, medium-, and high-frequency stimuli are transduced. Stimulation of an inner hair cell results in an increase in the discharge rate of an auditory nerve fiber. Each auditory nerve fiber innervates a single inner hair cell. Auditory nerve fiber axons project into the CN complex where they bifurcate; the ascending branches synapse on many neurons in isofrequency sheets in the anteroventral CN (AVCN). Neurons in the top isofrequency sheet in AVCN are excited *(E)* by high frequencies; those in the bottom isofrequency sheet are excited by low frequencies. Neural connections between isofrequency sheets in AVCN *(dashed lines)* are inhibitory *(I)*. **B,** auditory nerve-fiber tuning curve shows the frequency-intensity combinations that cause a just-noticeable increase in the discharge rate; i.e., the tuning curve outlines the excitatory response area. The frequency that excites the neuron with the lowest sound pressure level (the tip of the tuning curve) indicates the characteristic frequency *(CF)* of the neuron. **C,** response area of a cochlear nucleus unit with only an excitatory *(E)* region. **D,** some units in the cochlear nucleus have excitatory *(E)* response areas flanked by inhibitory *(I)* response areas above and below CF *(middle)*. Inhibitory response areas indicate frequency and intensity combinations that inhibit the neuron (decrease in discharge rate). **E,** after presenting a traumatizing stimulus to the inhibitory region above CF, it might be expected that the excitatory response area *(E)* becomes broader and the inhibitory areas *(I)* decrease or are eliminated relative to preexposure measures.

mately 30,000 auditory nerve fibers. Because most (90% to 95%) auditory nerve fibers make synaptic contact with a single inner hair cell,[35] the output of each fiber provides information from a relatively restricted frequency region of the cochlea.

The response properties of auditory nerve fibers are relatively simple and homogeneous across the population of neurons. A common characteristic of an auditory nerve fiber is the production of action potentials in the absence of acoustic stimulation, a behavior known as spontaneous activity. If tone bursts of an appropriate frequency and intensity are presented, the auditory nerve fiber will be excited, resulting in an increase in its discharge rate above its spontaneous discharge rate. A tuning curve, which represents the "audiogram" of a single neuron, shows the frequency-intensity combinations that cause a just-noticeable increase in a neuron's discharge rate (see Fig 4–1,B). Each tuning curve has a low-threshold, narrowly tuned tip and the frequency where threshold is lowest is referred to as the characteristic frequency (CF). Notice that the intensity axis for a tuning curve is reversed relative to a clinical audiogram; that is, the highest sensitivity is indicated by the lowest point in the tuning curve. A behavioral audiogram results from the contribution of many neurons with different CFs that span the entire range of hearing.

After leaving the cochlea, each auditory nerve fiber enters the cochlear nucleus (CN) and branches, with an ascending branch terminating in the anteroventral CN and a descending branch leading to the dorsal CN and the posteroventral CN. The frequency-place (tonotopic) map that projects out of the cochlea is subsequently maintained at each division of the cochlear nucleus as well as higher levels of the auditory pathway. Figure 4–1,A shows a highly simplified schematic of how the inputs from the auditory nerve are transformed into isofrequency sheets containing neurons with relatively complex response properties. Each auditory nerve fiber activates a thin layer or sheet of neurons all tuned to approximately the same frequency (see Fig 4–1,A). The characteristic frequency of these isofrequency sheets increases in an orderly manner resulting in a tonotopic axis.

Most neurons in the central auditory pathway receive input from afferent and efferent nerve fibers. Furthermore, some neurons may receive both excitatory and inhibitory inputs, as shown in Figure 4–1,A. Consequently, the response properties of neurons in the central auditory system are considerably more complex than in the auditory nerve. For example, Figure 4–1,C illustrates the response of a CN neuron receiving only excitatory inputs; the neuron is excited only by acoustic stimulation of the appropriate frequency and intensity. On the other hand, some neurons in the CN have both inhibitory and excitatory inputs. The response of this neuron would show excitatory response areas that are flanked by frequency regions that inhibit the neuron's firing (see Fig 4–1,D). Still others are inhibited by low-intensity sounds in a narrow frequency region and are excited only at high stimulus levels.[7, 42]

The functional characteristics of neurons above the level of the cochlear nucleus become increasingly complex owing in part to more complicated inhibitory, efferent, and binaural influences.[37] Thus, one finds neurons that are sensitive to particular stimulus features such as a difference in intensity and/or difference in time of arrival at the two ears.[4] In addition, some neurons appear to be sensitive to changes in stimulus level[36] and temporal characteristics of the stimulus.[33] This brief review outlining the functional complexity of the central auditory system may provide some insights into the functional changes that occur in the central auditory pathway described below.

## Enhancement of Evoked Potential Amplitude With Peripheral Loss

For a number of years we have been using the auditory evoked response to estimate how much hearing loss chinchillas develop after being exposed to high levels of noise. The basic experimental paradigm is as follows. Chronic recording electrodes are implanted at various locations within the auditory pathway (round window, cochlear nucleus, inferior colliculus) of normal chinchillas that have been made monaural by surgical destruction of one cochlea as described in earlier reports.[11, 27] After a suitable recovery time, the auditory evoked response is measured over a wide range of frequencies and intensities as described previously.[29] The animals are exposed to loud, damaging sounds and the measurements are repeated.

Figure 4–2 shows evoked response data from the inferior colliculus of one animal before and after exposure to a 2-kHz pure tone (105 dB SPL re 20 mPa; 5 days). This exposure consistently produced 20 to 30 dB of permanent threshold shift (PTS) between 2 and 8 kHz (see Fig 4–2,B). Figure 4–2 also shows a preexposure, postexposure pair of evoked response waveforms (see Fig 4–2,A) and amplitude-level functions (amplitude of the evoked response as a function of sound pressure level) obtained at 0.5 kHz (see Fig 4–2,C) and 4 kHz (see Fig 4–2,D) before and after the exposure. After the exposure, higher sound levels were required to elicit the evoked response at 4 kHz caused by the hearing loss; however, once threshold was exceeded the response amplitude increased rapidly and saturated at a maximum amplitude that was similar to the maximum preexposure amplitude. At intermediate sound levels, the amplitude exceeded the preexposure values. By contrast, the traumatizing exposure had no effect on the threshold at 0.5 kHz; however, the postexposure amplitude-level function increased rapidly and saturated at a level that

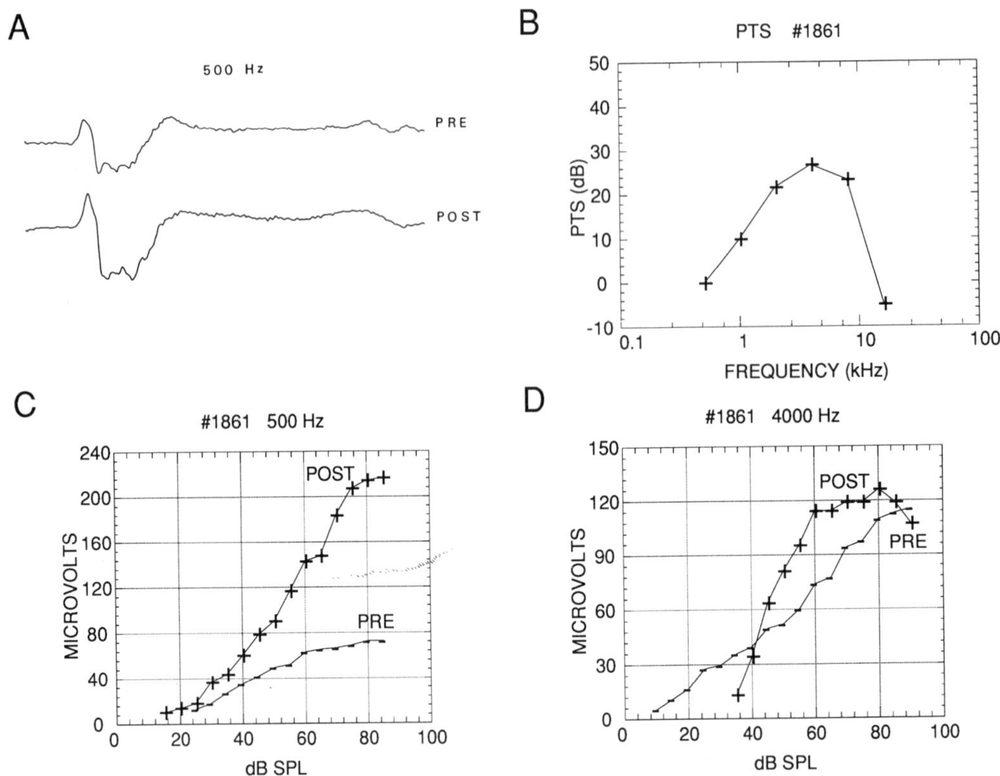


**FIG 4–2.**
**A,** preexposure and postexposure evoked-response waveforms in response to 500-Hz tone bursts. Note that the amplitude of the postexposure waveform is larger than that of the preexposure waveform. **B,** permanent threshold shift (PTS) as a function of frequency. The hearing loss was induced by a 2 kHz tone, 105 dB SPL for 5 days. **C,** evoked response amplitude as a function of sound-pressure level for tone bursts presented at 500 Hz. **D,** evoked response amplitude-level functions in response to 4-kHz tone bursts. (Adapted from Salvi RJ et al: *Hear Res* 1990; 50:245–248. Used by permission.)

was almost three times greater than the maximum preexposure amplitude. In spite of the change in amplitude, there was little or no change in the morphology of the evoked response waveform (see Fig 4–2,A).

In order to illustrate the trends in our data, we divided each value of the postexposure amplitude-level function by the maximum preexposure amplitude for that animal. Thus, a normalized amplitude of 1.5 would mean that the postexposure amplitude was 50% larger than the largest preexposure value; Figure 4–3 shows the normalized amplitude-level functions at the four test frequencies for all 10 subjects. After the exposure, the maximum amplitude of the evoked response was typically depressed (i.e., the maximum normalized amplitude was less than 1) at 4 and 8 kHz. By contrast, the maximum amplitude of the evoked response was typically much larger than normal at 0.5 and 2 kHz. It is important to note the evoked response amplitude is typically enhanced at frequencies associated with the low-frequency edge of the hearing loss (0.5 and 2 kHz), whereas the amplitude is reduced for frequencies of maximum loss.

Does the enhancement of the amplitude of the evoked potential seen in the inferior colliculus originate in the periphery or is it a central auditory phenomenon? To address this issue, a second experiment was done with chronic electrodes stereotaxically implanted in the cochlear nucleus, inferior colliculus, and on the round window of the chinchilla. Afterward, the animals were exposed for 2 hours to a 2.8-kHz tone at 105 dB SPL. Figure 4–4 shows the amplitude-level functions measured on the low-frequency edge of the hearing loss (1 kHz) at three different recording locations in the same animal. The compound action potential (CAP) recorded from the round window of the cochlea showed a slight loss in sensitivity and a significant reduction in amplitude 24 hours after the exposure. By 30

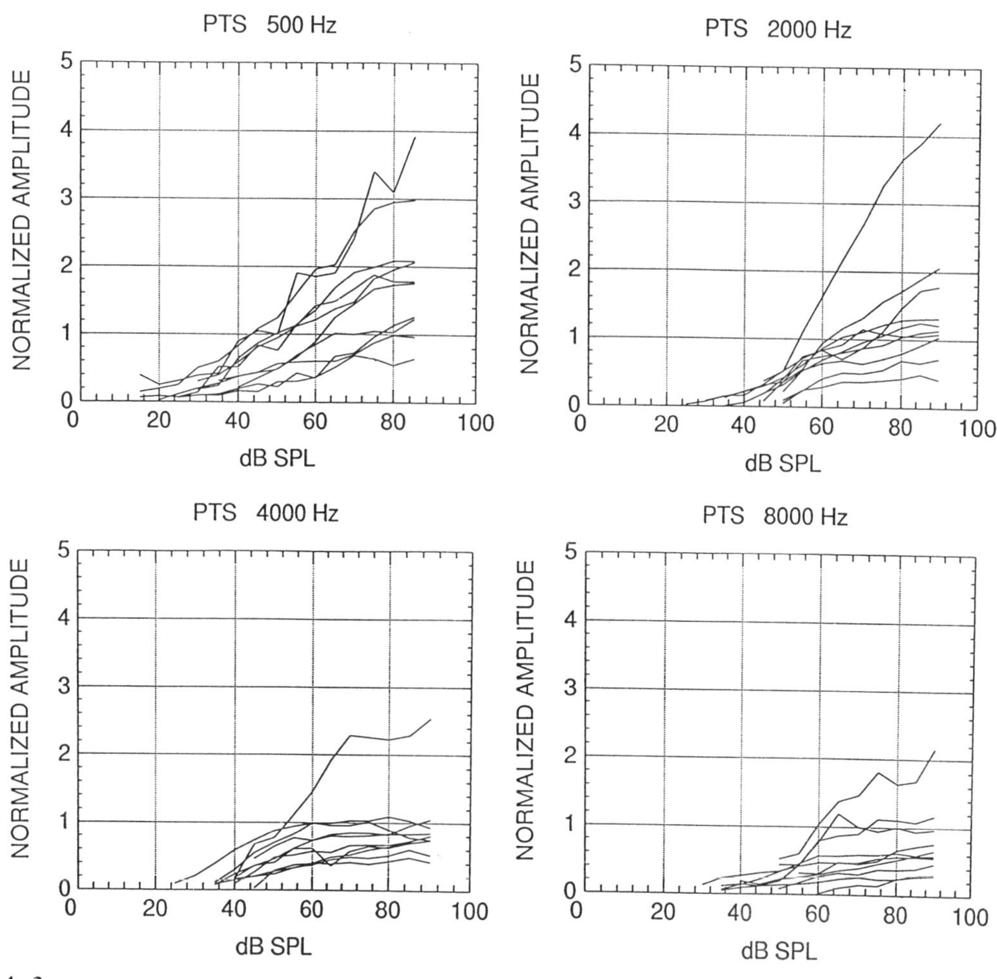


**FIG 4–3.**
Normalized evoked response amplitude as a function of stimulus level recorded from chronic electrodes implanted into the inferior colliculus. Data from 10 chinchillas with permanent threshold shift (PTS) induced by a 2-kHz pure tone. Each postexposure amplitude-level function was normalized to the maximum preexposure amplitude obtained from the same animal at that particular frequency. Normalized values greater than 1.0 indicate that the postexposure value exceeded the maximum preexposure amplitude. (From Salvi RJ et al: *Hear Res* 1990; 50:245–258. Used by permission.)

days postexposure, the amplitude-level function had essentially recovered to normal values. The response from the CN also showed a loss in sensitivity and a significant drop in amplitude 24 hours after the exposure. Some recovery occurred by 30 days postexposure; however, the amplitudes were still significantly depressed at high sound levels. The amplitude-level functions from the inferior colliculus were significantly different from those measured at more peripheral recording sites. The evoked response from the inferior colliculus showed a loss in sensitivity 24 hours after the exposure; however, the function increased steeply once threshold was exceeded and the maximum amplitude was substantially larger than normal. The evoked response amplitude was still much larger than normal 30 days after the exposure even though the threshold was normal.

To summarize, the amplitude of the evoked response from the inferior colliculus is often larger than normal after acoustic trauma whereas the amplitude of the evoked responses are generally smaller than normal in the CN and auditory nerve. This suggests that the enhancement phenomenon originates in the central auditory pathway; however, its exact origins are not yet known.

One question that may be important for understanding the underlying mechanisms responsible for the enhancement phenomenon is how long

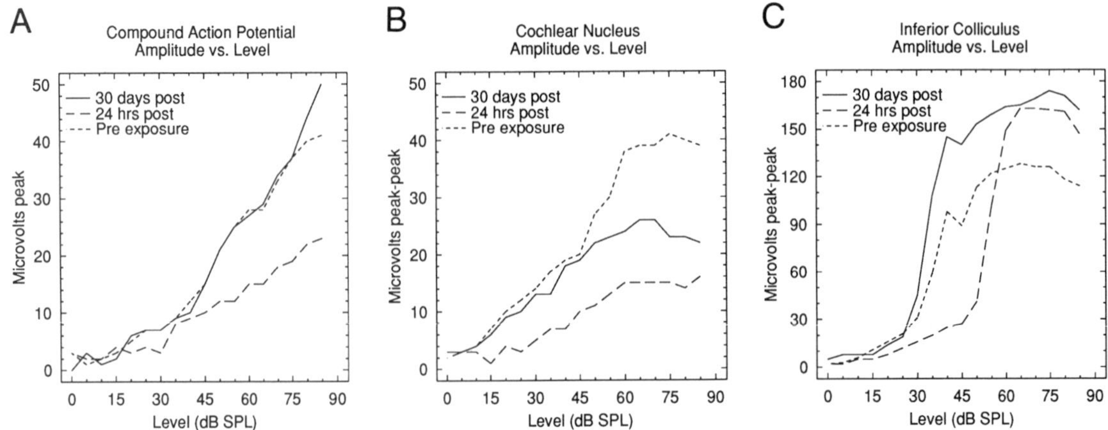


**FIG 4–4.**
Chinchilla 2751. Evoked response amplitude-level functions obtained at 1 kHz from electrodes on the round window **(A),** in the cochlear nucleus **(B),** and in the inferior colliculus **(C).** Amplitude-level functions measured preexposure and 24 hours and 30 days postexposure. (From Salvi RJ et al, in Dancer A et al (eds): *Effects of Noise on the Auditory System*. Toronto, BC Decker, 1991. Used by permission.)

it takes for the enhancement phenomenon to develop. To examine this issue, amplitude-level functions were measured at various times after a 2-hour exposure to a 2.8 kHz tone presented at 105 dB SPL. The exposure resulted in a significant amount of TTS (60 to 75 dB) at the midfrequencies. Amplitude-level functions were then measured at various times following the exposure. Figure 4–5 shows the amplitude-level functions obtained at 1 kHz, 1 hour and 8 hours after the noise exposure. The amplitude-level function measured 1 hour postexposure was shifted to the right owing to a loss in sensitivity of approximately 15 to 20 dB and the maximum amplitude was reduced somewhat. The amplitude-level function measured 8 hours postexposure was also shifted to the right by approximately 15 dB, but its growth (slope of the amplitude-level function) was larger than for the 1 hour postexposure or the preexposure data. Also, the maximum amplitude of the 8-hour postexposure response was consistently larger than the preexposure values at high sound levels. These results indicate that the enhancement phenomenon can develop relatively rapidly.

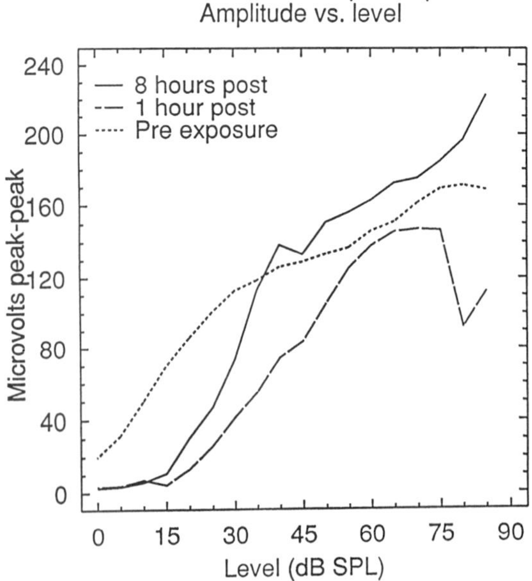


**FIG 4–5.**
Chinchilla 3119. Amplitude-level functions obtained at 1 kHz from an electrode in the inferior colliculus. Amplitude-level functions measured preexposure and 1 and 8 hours postexposure. (From Salvi RJ et al, in Dancer A et al (eds): *Effects of Noise on the Auditory System*. Toronto, BC Decker, 1991. Used by permission.)

## Disinhibition

As mentioned earlier, the evoked response amplitude enhancement was typically seen on the low-frequency edge of the hearing loss. The abrupt change in sensitivity that occurs at the edge of the hearing loss could selectively alter the normal balance between the excitatory and inhibitory inputs that impinge upon individual neurons in the central auditory pathway (see Fig 4–1). For example, if the inhibitory inputs to a subgroup of neurons in the central auditory pathway were selectively eliminated as a result of damage to the auditory periphery, then the excitatory responses from these central auditory neurons might be more effective than normal. The loss of inhibition, or disinhibition, at frequencies bordering the hearing loss could conceivably contribute to the evoked response amplitude enhancement seen in the central auditory pathway.

The ventral cochlear nucleus is the most peripheral level of the auditory pathway where lateral inhibition is observed; thus, it would be interesting to know how the balance of inhibition and excitation is altered with peripheral hearing loss. A selective loss of inhibition could conceivably enhance the excitatory responses in these units. To test this hypothesis, we recorded from single neurons in the CN of anesthetized (ketamine plus xylazine) chinchillas. At the beginning of each experiment, we measured the excitatory and inhibitory response areas (frequency-intensity combinations that caused an increase or decrease in firing rate respectively) of each unit (see Fig 4–1,C and D). Poststimulus time (PST) histograms were also obtained to tone bursts in order to show the neuron's pattern of firing during time when the stimulus was presented. In addition, the

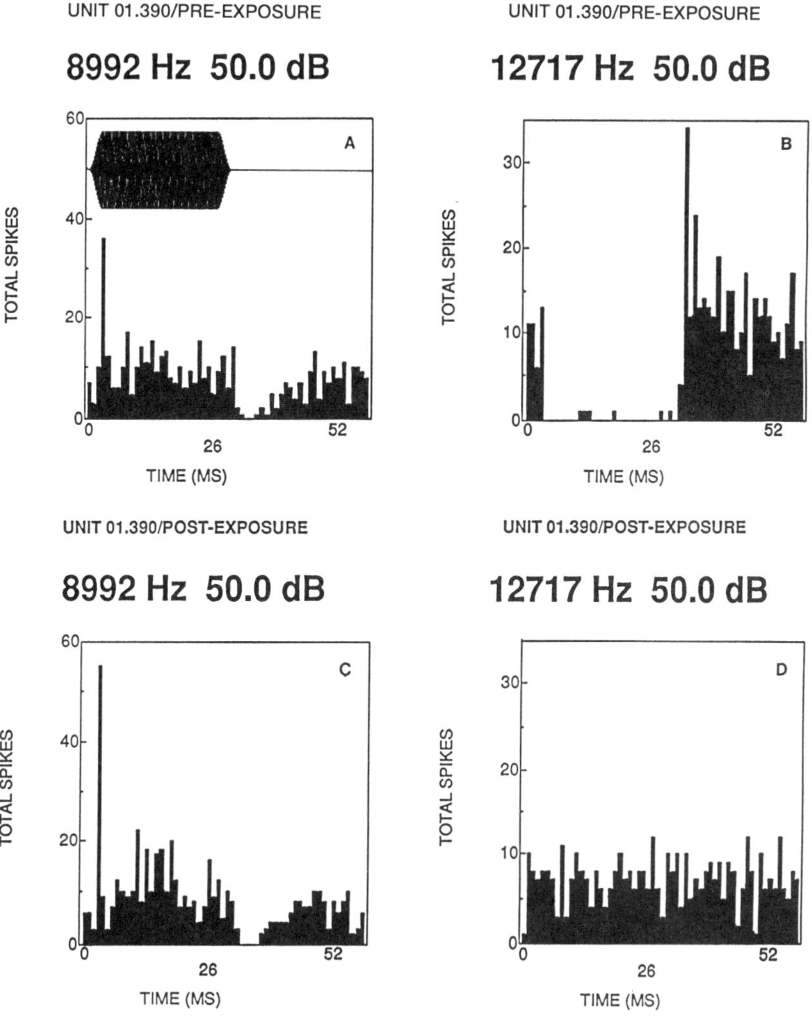


**FIG 4–6.**
PST histograms from a primarylike-notch unit in the CN. Measurements obtained with 30-ms tone bursts (**A**) presented at CF (**A** and **C**) and a half-octave above CF (**B** and **D**). Measurements obtained before (**A** and **B**) and after (**C** and **D**) 5-minute exposure to a 105 dB SPL tone located a half-octave above CF. When a stimulus is excitatory, there is an increase in firing rate during the period of stimulation (**A**); if a stimulus is inhibitory, the firing rate will drop during the period of stimulation (**B**).

neuron's discharge rate as a function of stimulus level was determined. After characterizing the normal discharge patterns, we attempted to selectively damage or eliminate the inhibitory response area by presenting a high-intensity, continuous tone a half-octave above the neuron's CF, i.e., at a frequency located within the inhibitory sideband above CF. Afterwards, all of the single-unit measurements were repeated to determine if there was any change in the maximum firing rate, the excitatory and inhibitory response area, and the shape of the PST histogram. If this method could selectively produce disinhibition, it might be expected that the excitatory response area would become broader and the inhibitory areas to decrease or be eliminated, as illustrated in Figure 4–1,E.

Figure 4–6 shows the results from a neuron with a prominent inhibitory response area located above the excitatory response area. Figure 4–6,A shows the PST histograms collected at CF, i.e., in the excitatory response area. The neuron was classified as a primarylike-notch unit based on the shape of its PST histogram.[41] Figure 4–6,B shows the PST histogram collected with a 50-dB SPL tone presented a half-octave (12,717 Hz) above CF. Note that frequencies above CF inhibited the spontaneous activity of the unit over the duration of the tone burst; however, at the end of the tone burst there was a slight rebound in the neuron's resting rate of activity. After these normal measurements were obtained, a traumatizing tone (105 dB SPL, 12,717 Hz, 5 minutes duration) was presented in the inhibitory sideband located above CF. After the traumatizing exposure, the response to inhibitory tones above CF was greatly reduced. For example, the PST histogram in Figure 4–6,D no longer shows an inhibitory response to 12,717-Hz tone with an SPL of 50 dB SPL. By contrast, the PST histogram to the excitatory tone at CF (see Fig 4–6,C) shows more spike discharges after the exposure.

The effects of the traumatizing exposure on the neuron's discharge rate-level function are more clearly illustrated in Figure 4–7. Before the exposure, the unit's discharge rate was strongly inhibited by the 12,717 Hz tone once the stimulus level exceeded 35 dB SPL (see Fig 4–7, bottom). However, after the exposure, the neuron's firing rate showed little or no decrease when stimulus level was increased. Thus, the traumatizing tone virtually abolished the inhibitory inputs originating above CF. Quite different effects were seen in the excitatory response area. The traumatizing exposure did not affect the unit's spontaneous discharge rate or its threshold at CF; however, the neuron's firing rate showed a significant enhancement at suprathreshold levels after the traumatizing exposure.

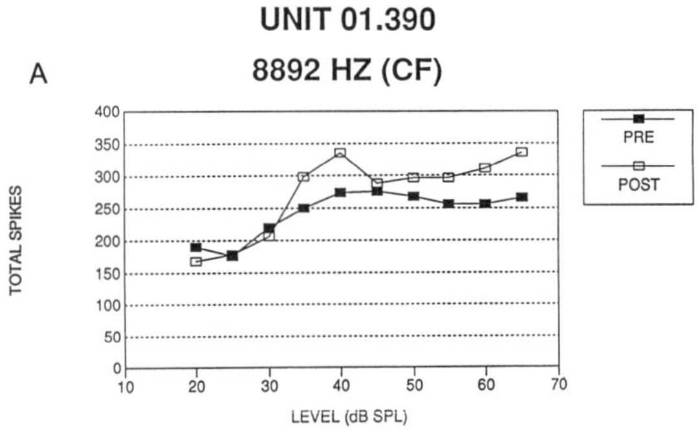


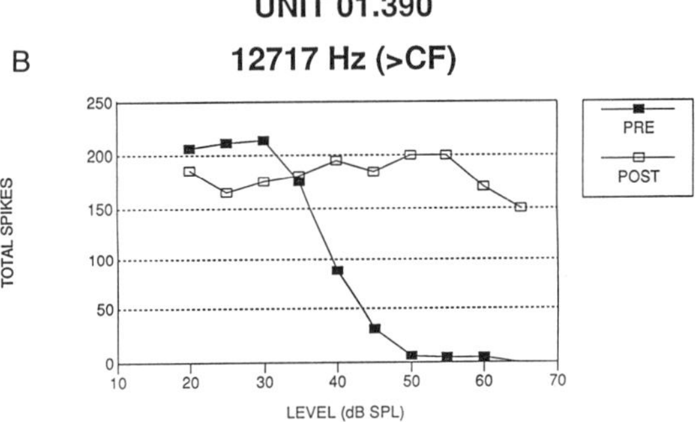


**FIG 4–7.**
Discharge rate-level functions from the primarylike-notch unit shown in Fig 4–6. Measurements obtained before *(filled symbols)* and after *(open symbols)* a 5-minute exposure to a 105-dB SPL tone located a half-octave above CF. **A,** note the increase in the number of spikes to the tone at CF after the exposure. **B,** note the loss of inhibition above CF *(bottom right)* after the traumatizing sound exposure. (From Salvi RJ, et al, in Dancer A et al (eds): *Effects of Noise on the Auditory System.* Toronto, BC Decker, 1991. Used by permission.)

We have so far evaluated data from approximately 90 units in the CN using the paradigm described above and our results can be summarized as follows. If a unit had an inhibitory sideband above CF and if the frequency and intensity of the traumatizing tone were such that it caused a reduction in inhibition, then the neuron almost always showed an increase in its maximum discharge to tones presented at CF. Conversely, if a unit lacked an inhibitory sideband above CF then the traumatizing tone failed to enhance the unit's firing rate at CF.

One question that arises from these experiments is whether the loss of the inhibitory sidebands above CF leads to an expansion of the excitatory response area or a shift in the unit's CF towards the high frequencies. That is, does the loss of the inhibitory sidebands alter the size and shape of the excitatory response area? To explore this issue, we have evaluated the excitatory (Fig 4–8, *black area*) and inhibitory response areas (see Fig 4–8, *stippled area*) of a number of units before and after presenting a traumatizing tone in the inhibitory response area. For the unit shown in Figure 4–8 (CF 2,347 Hz, threshold 18 dB SPL), the traumatizing tone was presented at 3,319 Hz for 5 min at 100 dB SPL, a frequency that clearly inhibited the neuron's spontaneous discharge rate. Even though the traumatizing exposure reduced the amount of inhibition on the high-frequency side of CF, there was no noticeable expansion of the excitatory response area nor was there a shift of CF toward the high frequencies. These results suggest that the tonotopic organization of the CN is not significantly altered by our acute, traumatizing exposures. However, our results should be interpreted cautiously at the present time since we have data from a limited number of CN neurons using a limited range of traumatizing exposures.

## Tonotopic Reorganization in the Auditory Cortex

Studies of the somatosensory system have shown that there is an orderly mapping of the body surface onto the surface of the somatosensory cortex; i.e., there is a well-defined topographic map of the body surface on the somatosensory cortex. When the peripheral afferent inputs from the body surface are removed (e.g., by a local anesthetic or amputation), the region of somatosensory cortex deprived of its inputs does not simply become a "silent region," but instead begins to respond to regions of the skin adjacent to the "lesioned" surface area of the body. These

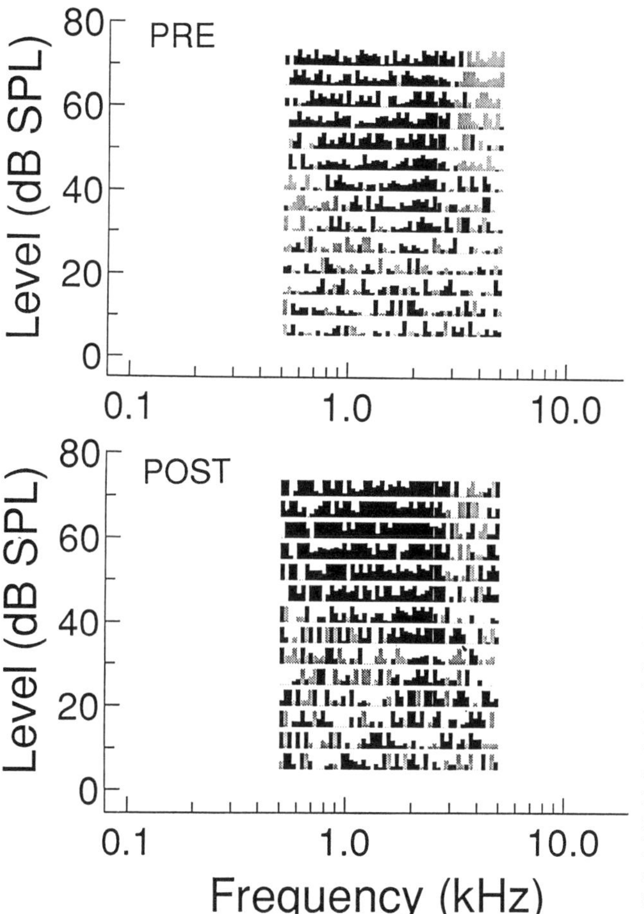


**FIG 4–8.**
Excitatory *(black area)* and inhibitory *(stippled area)* response areas taken before and after the traumatizing exposure. Stimulus intensity varied in 5 dB steps from 5 dB SPL to 80 dB SPL. Frequency swept from approximately 500 Hz to 5,000 Hz in ⅛ octave steps. Height of the bars in each frequency sweep is proportional to the change in discharge rate caused by the stimulus. Note the reduction in the width and amplitude of the inhibitory response area above CF after the traumatizing sound exposure.

results indicate that the adult somatosensory cortex exhibits considerable neural plasticity. Recently, Robertson and Irvine[24] demonstrated that the auditory cortex exhibits a similar type of plasticity following restricted mechanical lesion of the cochlea.

Figure 4–9 shows the frequency organization of the most rostral field of the auditory cortex in a normal guinea pig. The rostral field of the auditory cortex has a frequency organization in which the lowest frequencies are represented in the rostral end and the highest frequencies are represented in the caudal end. Figure 4–9 shows that there is an orderly increase in CF (tonotopic organization) along the rostral-caudal axis of the auditory cortex.

Figure 4–10 shows results obtained from one abnormal guinea pig 71 days after inducing a mechanical lesion in one cochlea. The compound action potential recorded from the round window of the animal revealed a significant threshold shift between 10 and 20 kHz, but normal thresholds at lower and higher frequencies (see Fig 4–10,A). As shown in Figure 4–10,B, the tonotopic organization of the auditory cortex was drastically altered by the cochlear lesion. No responses were obtained from neurons with CFs between 10 and 20 kHz. More importantly, the regions of the auditory cortex that were normally most sensitive to frequencies between 10 and 20 kHz were now tuned to frequencies near the low-frequency edge or high-frequency edge of the hearing loss; i.e., there was an overrepresentation of units with CFs near 10 kHz and an overrepresentation of units with CFs near 20 kHz. Although the CFs appear to have shifted to higher or lower frequencies, the thresholds were nearly identical to those from normal animals. These results indicate that a peripheral hearing loss can significantly alter the frequency organization of the auditory cortex.

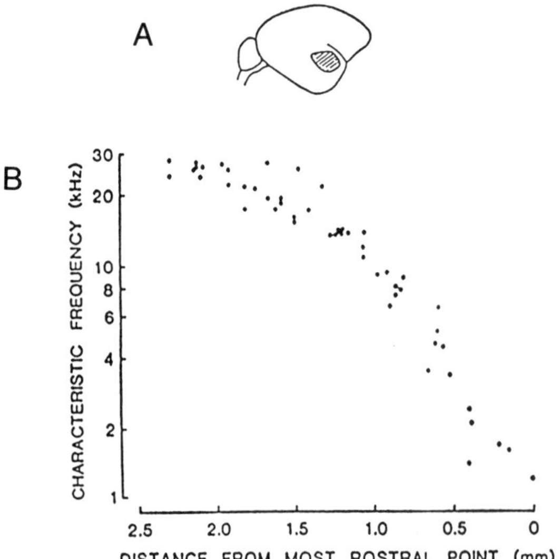


**FIG 4–9.**
**A,** schematic showing a sagittal view of the guinea pig brain. *Stippled area* indicates the location of the auditory cortex. **B,** tonotopic organization of the rostral portion of the auditory cortex of the guinea pig. Note the progressive increase in characteristic frequency along the rostral-caudal surface of the auditory cortex. (From Robertson D, Irvine DRF: *J Comp Neurol* 1989; 282:456–471. Used by permission.)

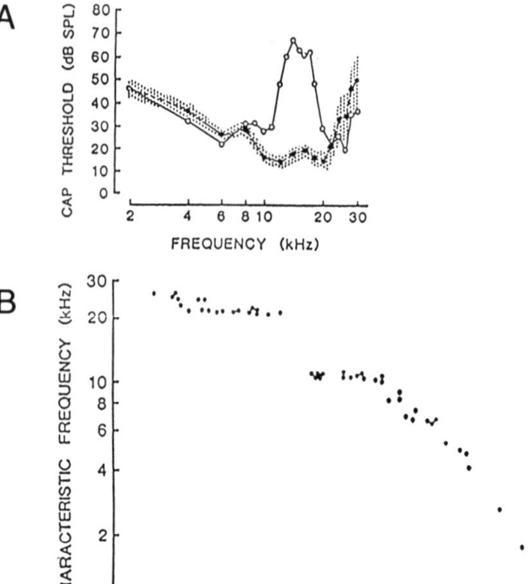


**FIG 4–10.**
**A,** threshold of the auditory nerve compound action potential. *Stippled area* and *filled circles* show the threshold as a function of stimulus frequency in normal guinea pigs. *Open circle* shows the threshold in a guinea pig whose cochlea had been surgically damaged approximately 70 days earlier. Note the large threshold shift between 10 and 20 kHz. **B,** tonotopic organization of the rostral portion of the auditory cortex of the guinea pig. Note the absence of neurons with characteristic frequencies between 10 and 20 kHz. Note the overrepresentation of units with CFs near 10 kHz and 20 kHz. (From Robertson D, Irvine DRF: *J Comp Neurol* 1989; 282:456–471. Used by permission.)

## DISCUSSION

The central auditory system in adult mammals has traditionally been thought of as a "hard-wired" system. However, this view is difficult to reconcile with many studies of the somatosensory system and visual system, which indicate that discrete lesions of the peripheral receptor surface (i.e., cochlea) can drastically alter the functional properties of more centrally located neurons, particularly those neurons that are associated with the receptor surface bordering the peripheral lesion.[2, 3, 16] Removal of the afferent input from a segment of the receptor surface usually causes the deprived areas of the somatosensory or visual cortex to become responsive to stimulation of adjacent regions of the receptor surface.[8, 15, 20, 23] These results suggest that functional changes may also occur in the central auditory system as a result of cochlear damage; however, the full extent of these central changes is only beginning to be understood.

It is now clear that the tonotopic organization of the auditory cortex undergoes significant rearrangement in adult animals as a result of cochlear damage. Neurons in the auditory cortex associated with the damaged regions of the cochlea assume "new" CFs corresponding to frequencies that border the low- or high-frequency edge of the hearing loss. Robertson and Irvine[24] demonstrated that discrete mechanical lesions of the cochlea resulted in an expanded representation on the auditory cortex of sound frequencies adjacent to the damaged region of the cochlear partition. After a recovery period of 35 to 81 days, the thresholds of units at their "new" characteristic frequencies were close to normal, whereas the thresholds were greatly elevated after a recovery period of only a few hours.

The fact that the tonotopic organization of the auditory cortex is altered by cochlear damage does not mean that the primary locus for this plasticity resides in the cortex. Indeed, in other sensory systems, neural reorganization has been observed in the brain stem and spinal cord.[6] Similarly, changes in the tonotopic organization of the central nucleus of the inferior colliculus (ICC) have been observed in C57BL/6 mice, which develop a high-frequency sensorineural hearing loss as a result of aging.[38, 40] The CFs of neurons associated with the high-frequency regions of the ICC shift to lower frequencies and as a result there is an overrepresentation of neurons with CFs bordering the low-frequency edge of the hearing loss.

The overrepresentation of neurons in the ICC with CFs bordering the hearing loss could conceivably give rise to the abnormally large amplitude-evoked responses such as those reported above. Moreover, enhanced evoked response amplitudes begin to develop in the inferior colliculus of deafness-mutant mice as the cochlea begins to degenerate during development.[12] Evoked response amplitude enhancements also have been observed in audiogenic seizure-prone mice that have been primed for audiogenic seizures using intense sounds.[30, 31] After the priming exposure, the mice showed a significant reduction in the amplitude of the cochlear microphonic and the compound action potential from the auditory nerve. By contrast, the amplitude of the evoked response from the CN and inferior colliculus was much larger than normal at high stimulus level.

If the evoked-response amplitude enhancement is in fact a result of tonotopic reorganization, then this would imply that the tonotopic reorganization occurs as far peripherally as the CN. However, we along with others have failed to observe enhanced evoked-potential amplitudes in the CN, but have consistently seen such changes in the inferior colliculus of the chinchilla and cat.[9, 10, 22] There are a number of possible reasons for the discrepancy. One is that locus of the enhancement phenomenon may vary with the age of onset of the hearing loss. A second possibility is that there may be important genetic differences between audiogenic seizure-prone mice and normal animals. Third, the functional characteristics of the subdivisions within the cochlear nucleus are different. Thus, the ability to detect the amplitude enhancement may depend on the location of the recording electrode within the cochlear nucleus. For example, the enhancement phenomenon might be missed if the recording electrode were located near the interstitial nucleus at the point where the auditory nerve enters the cochlear nucleus.

What physiological mechanisms could account for the reorganization of the tonotopic maps and the evoked response amplitude enhancement? One possibility is that these functional changes result from the formation of new synaptic connections within the central auditory pathway. However, such a mechanism seems unlikely to be the principal factor underlying the tonotopic reorganization and the amplitude enhancement since these changes are observed within a matter of hours after cochlear damage has occurred.

An alternative mechanism which could conceivably account for these changes is a loss of central inhibition associated with the damaged regions of the cochlea adjacent to the hearing loss.[38, 39] Willott et al[38, 39] reported a reduction of inhibition among units in the dorsal CN of audiogenic seizure-prone mice and suggested that the loss of inhibition could lead to an increased level of excitability in the inferior colliculus.[40] They suggested that the lack of inhibition might be caused by the loss of inhibitory interneurons, alterations in inhibitory neurotransmitters, or abnormal dendritic morphology. Our preliminary finding from neurons in the ventral cochlear nucleus are consistent with the preceding hypothesis. When the inhibitory drive was reduced or eliminated by presenting a traumatizing tone in the inhibitory sideband above CF, then the maximum excitatory response elicited by a tone at CF increased significantly. One problem with this explanation is that we have not observed evoked potential amplitude enhancement in the CN, although such changes have been seen in the CN of audiogenic seizure-prone mice.[30, 31] In spite of this discrepancy, the proposed mechanism could still provide a satisfactory explanation if the loss of inhibition were to occur proximal to the CN.

Similarly, Robertson and Irvine[24] have suggested that the preexisting anatomical receptive fields within the auditory cortex are actually much wider than those measured physiologically. Accordingly, when the dominant inhibitory inputs to a region are lost because of a peripheral lesion, the preexisting excitatory inputs from adjacent CFs may result in an expansion of the excitatory response area or a shift in CF. We have attempted to evaluate the role of lateral inhibition in shaping the excitatory response area of units in the ventral CN by using intense acoustic stimuli to reduce the inhibitory drive impinging on a neuron. So far, we have not observed an upward shift in CF or an expansion of the excitatory response area in the ventral CN due to the loss of inhibition above CF; however, such changes may occur in other regions of the auditory pathway. Regardless of the specific mechanism(s) that are involved, it is clear that the evoked response amplitude enhancement, the enhancement in single unit discharge rate and the tonotopic reorganization observed in the central auditory system do not simply mirror the pathophysiological changes that emerge from the cochlea.

What clinical or practical significance can one ascribe to tonotopic reorganization and evoked response amplitude enhancement? One possibility is that the abnormally large-amplitude evoked potentials could be related to the problem of loudness recruitment and loudness intolerance that is frequently seen in listeners with sensorineural hearing loss.[5, 10, 13]

Tinnitus is another problem that plagues many listeners with sensorineural hearing loss. Studies of tinnitus performed on listeners with temporary or permanent threshold shift have shown that they match the pitch of their tinnitus to tones located on either the high or low frequency edge of the hearing.[1, 19, 21] The frequency regions associated with the edge of the hearing loss are clearly overrepresented on the tonotopic maps of the auditory cortex[24] and this may make the endogenous activity from such regions of the auditory cortex disproportionately more prominent, thereby providing the neural cue for the perception of tinnitus. This explanation is especially appealing given the fact the auditory-evoked magnetic fields (M100 component of the waveform) from the auditory cortex are abnormally large in tinnitus patients. In fact, it has been suggested that auditory-evoked magnetic fields from the auditory cortex may provide an objective measure of tinnitus.[14]

The functional changes observed in the central auditory system as a result of sensorineural hearing loss may also have important implications for cochlear implants. A common strategy that is used in designing cochlea implants is to build a prosthesis in such a way that it produces essentially the same pattern of neural activity in the auditory nerve as the acoustic stimulus does. This strategy, however, implicitly assumes that the neural circuitry proximal to the cochlea remains intact in individuals who become profoundly deaf after birth. This implicit assumption of a "hard-wired" central auditory system may need to be reevaluated in light of new experimental findings similar to those mentioned above.

**Acknowledgments**

Work supported in part by research grant 2R01DC00368 from the National Institutes of Health. Special thanks to Lin Chen for producing Figure 4–1.

## REFERENCES

1. Atherley GRC, Hempstock TI, Noble WG: Study of tinnitus induced temporarily by noise. *J Acoust Soc Am* 1968; 44:1503–1506.
2. Calford MB, Tweedale R: Immediate and chronic changes in responses of somatosensory cortex in adult flying-fox after digit amputation. *Nature* 1988; 332:446–448.
3. Calford MB, Tweedale R: Interhemispheric transfer of plasticity in the cerebral cortex. *Science* 1990; 249:805–808.
4. Carr CE, Konishi M: Axonal delay lines for time measurement in the owl's brainstem. *Proc Natl Acad Sci USA* 1988; 85:8311–8315.
5. Davis H, Morgan CT, Hawkins JE, et al: Temporary deafness following exposure to loud tones and noise. *Acta Otolaryngol (Suppl)* 1950; 88:1–59.
6. Dostrovsky JO, Millar J, Wall PD: The immediate shift of afferent drive of dorsal column nucleus cells following deafferentation: A comparison of acute and chronic deafferentation in gracile nucleus and spinal chord. *Exp Neurol* 1976; 52:480–495.
7. Evans EF, Nelson PG: The response of single neurones in the cochlear nucleus of the cat as a function of their location and anesthetic state. *Exp Brain Res* 1973; 17:402–427.
8. Frank JI: Functional reorganization of cat somatic sensory-motor cortex (SmI) after selective dorsal root rhizotomies. *Brain Res* 1980; 186:458–462.
9. Gerken GM, Saunders SS, Paul RE: Hypersensitivity to electrical stimulation of auditory nuclei follows hearing loss in cats. *Hear Res* 1984; 13:249–259.
10. Gerken GM, Simhadri-Sumithra R, Bhat KHV: Increase in central auditory responsiveness during continuous tone stimulation or following hearing loss, in Salvi RJ, Hamernik RP, Henderson D, et al (eds): *Basic and Applied Aspects of Noise-Induced Hearing Loss*. New York, Plenum Press, 1986, pp 195–211.
11. Henderson D, Hamernik RP, Woodford C, et al: Evoked response audibility curve of the chinchilla. *J Acoust Soc Am* 1973; 54:1099–1101.
12. Henry KR, Saleh M: Recruitment deafness: Functional effect of priming-induced audiogenic seizures in mice. *J Comp Physiol* 1973; 84:430.
13. Hickling S: Hearing test patterns in noise induced temporary hearing loss. *J Aud Res* 1967; 7:63–76.
14. Hoke M, Feldmann H, Pantev C, et al: Objective evidence of tinnitus in auditory evoked magnetic fields. *Hear Res* 1989; 37:281–286.
15. Jenkins WM, Merzenich MM: Reorganization of neocortical representations after brain injury: A neurophysiological model of the bases of recovery from stroke. *Prog Brain Res* 1987; 71:249–266.
16. Kaas JH, Krubitzer LA, Chino YM, et al: Reorganization of retinotopic maps in adult mammals after lesions of the retina. *Science* 1990; 248:229–231.
17. Liberman MC, Kiang NYS: Acoustic trauma in cats. *Acta Otolaryngol (Suppl)* 1978; 358:1–63.
18. Liberman MC, Dodds LW, Learson DA: Structure-function correlation in noise-damaged ears: A light and electron microscopic study, in Salvi RJ, Hamernik RP, Henderson D, et al (eds): *Basic and Applied Aspects of Noise-Induced Hearing Loss*. New York, Plenum Press, 1986, pp 163–177.
19. Loeb M, Smith R: Relation of induced tinnitus to physical characteristics of the inducing stimuli. *J Acoust Soc Am* 1967; 42:453–455.
20. Merzenich MM, Kaas JH: Organization of mammalian somatosensory cortex following peripheral nerve injury. *Trends Neurosci* 1982; 5:428–436.
21. Penner MJ: Two-tone forward masking patterns and tinnitus. *J Speech Hear Res* 1980; 23:779–786.
22. Powers NL, Salvi RJ: Noise induced enhancement and depression of auditory evoked potentials. *Abstracts of 12th Midwinter Research Meeting, Association for Research in Otolaryngology*, pp 223–224.
23. Rasmusson DD: Reorganization of raccoon somatosensory cortex following removal of the fifth digit. *J Comp Neurol* 1982; 205:313–326.
24. Robertson D, Irvine DRF: Plasticity of frequency organization in auditory cortex of guinea pigs with partial unilateral deafness. *J Comp Neurol* 1989; 282:456–471.
25. Salvi RJ, Hamernik RP, Henderson D: Response patterns of auditory nerve fibers during temporary threshold shift. *Hear Res* 1983; 10:37–67.

26. Salvi RJ, Henderson D, Hamernik RP: Physiological bases of sensorineural hearing loss, in Tobias J, Schubert E (eds): *Hearing Research and Theory,* vol 2. New York, Academic Press, 1983, pp 173–228.
27. Salvi RJ, Perry J, Hamernik RP, et al: Relationships between cochlear pathologies and auditory nerve and behavioral responses, in Hamernik RP, Henderson D, Salvi RJ (eds): *New Perspectives on Noise-Induced Hearing Loss*. New York, Raven Press, 1982, pp 165–188.
28. Salvi RJ, Powers NL, Saunders SS, et al: Enhancement of evoked response amplitude and single unit activity after noise exposure, in Dancer A, Henderson D, Salvi RJ, et al (eds): *Effects of Noise on the Auditory System*. Toronto, 1991, BC Decker, pp 156–174.
29. Salvi RJ, Saunders SS, Gratton MA, et al: Enhanced evoked response amplitudes in the inferior colliculus of the chinchilla following acoustic trauma. *Hear Res* 1990; 50:245–258.
30. Saunders JC, Bock GR, Chen CS, et al: The effects of priming for audiogenic seizures on cochlear and behavioral responses in BALB/c mice. *Exp Neurol* 1972; 36:426–436.
31. Saunders JC, Bock G, James R, et al: Effects of priming for audiogenic seizure on auditory evoked responses in the cochlear nucleus and inferior colliculus of BALB/c mice. *Exp Neurol* 1972; 37:388–394.
32. Schmiedt RA, Zwislocki JJ, Hamernik RP: Effects of hair-cell lesions on responses of cochlear-nerve fibers. I. Lesions, tuning curves, two-tone inhibition and responses to trapezoidal-wave patterns. *J Neurophysiol* 1980; 43:1367–1389.
33. Schreiner CE, Langner G: Periodicity coding in the inferior colliculus of the cat. II. Topographical organization. *J Neurophysiol* 1988; 60:1823–1840.
34. Siegel JH, Kim DO: Cochlear biomechanics: Vulnerability to acoustic trauma and other alterations seen in neural responses and ear-canal sound pressure, in Hamernik RP, Henderson D, Salvi RJ (eds): *New Perspectives on Noise-Induced Hearing Loss*. New York, Raven Press, 1982, pp 137–151.
35. Spoendlin H: Innervation densities of the cochlea. *Acta Otolaryngol* 1972; 73:235–248.
36. Suga N: Auditory neuroethology and speech processing: Complex-sound processing by combination-sensitive neurons, in Edelman GM, Gall WE, Cowan WM (eds): *Auditory Function: Neurobiological Bases of Hearing*. New York, John Wiley and Sons, 1988, pp 679–720.
37. Westrup JJ, Ross LS, Pollak GD: Binaural response organization within a frequency-band representation of the inferior colliculus: Implications for sound localization. *J Neurosci* 1986; 6:962–973.
38. Willott JF: Changes in frequency representation in the auditory system of mice with age-related hearing impairment. *Brain Res* 1984; 309:159–162.
39. Willott JF, Demuth RM, Lu S-M: Excitability of auditory neurons in the dorsal and ventral cochlear nuclei of DBA/2 and C57BL/6 mice. *Exp Neurol* 1984; 83:495–506.
40. Willott JF, Lu SM: Noise-induced hearing loss can alter neural coding and increase excitability in the central nervous system. *Science* 1982; 216:1331–1332.
41. Young ED: Response characteristics of neurons of the cochlear nuclei, in Berlin C (ed): *Hearing Science*. San Diego, College Hill Press, 1984, pp 423–460.
42. Young ED, Brownell WE: Responses to tones and noise of single cells in dorsal cochlear nucleus of unanesthetized cats. *J Neurophysiol* 1976; 39:282–300.

Chapter 5

# Imaging Techniques and Auditory Processing

Judith L. Lauter, Ph.D.

Although most of the nuclei of the classical auditory system are located *between* the periphery and association cortex, our current knowledge of human auditory function is limited almost exclusively to those two extremes. Thus the focus in professional training for audiology is on functional and dysfunctional characteristics of the outer, middle, and inner ear, with some concern with the eighth nerve and still less discussion of cortical bases of auditory perception.

The function of all the portions of the system between the eighth nerve and the region of Brodmann areas 39 and 40, is referred to summarily as "central processing," and when disrupted results in a vague collection of problems called retrocochlear disorders or central auditory disorders (CADs). The diagnostic tests currently in use, are also often described by the acronym CADs, which should properly be read "cortical auditory disorders," since most of these tests are diagnostic only of cortical dysfunction.[18]

There are numerous reasons for our incomplete understanding of the auditory central nervous system (CNS), but foremost among them is the nature of the methods for studying anatomy and physiology. Until recently, most techniques have been highly invasive; for those procedures sufficiently noninvasive to be used with healthy human subjects, the quality of information generated (e.g., via strip-chart electroencephalography) was so crude as to be almost useless for revealing the workings of the auditory CNS.

Rapid progress in computer technology during the last two decades has vastly improved our ability to collect and process the otherwise overwhelming amounts of data required for advanced studies of human behavior and underlying neurophysiology. Recent advances in computer design accompanied by reductions in cost have made it possible not only to study aspects of structure and function previously inaccessible (e.g., the anatomy of deep brain structures in healthy humans), but also to increase the sophistication of experimental questions (e.g., to examine the temporal characteristics of brain processing, and perhaps most importantly, to assess the nature and detail of individual differences).

This brief overview will focus on several methods for noninvasive brain monitoring that were applied beginning in the 1980s to the study of the human auditory CNS. We will begin with a brief comparative overview of the methods, and then proceed in a "bottom-up" direction through the auditory CNS. A checklist of techniques that can be used to study structure and function at each level is provided, with examples from the literature. (For a brief introduction to the methods mentioned here, see Appendix 5–1; for a more complete discussion, including examples of applications to human speech and language, see Lauter,[24] for more examples regarding studies in human hearing, see Lauter.[24a]

The methods to be examined are magnetic resonance imaging (MRI), repeated evoked potentials (REPs), quantitative electroencephalography (qEEG), magnetoencephalography (MEG), and positron emission tomography (PET). Finally, a brief look toward the future will forecast the ways in which improved uses of these methods, together with the addition of new techniques, should rapidly advance our understanding of both normal and disordered central auditory processing.

## OVERVIEW OF THE METHODS

Table 5–1 lists several noninvasive brain-monitoring methods available as of 1990, with comparisons according to a number of features. Because CT and MRI can be used to address questions already formulated for use with older techniques, such as dissection and x-ray, they have enjoyed the widest acceptance. The lack of precedents for the quality of physiological monitoring represented by the other tools has hampered their penetration into research and clinical practice.

The other points of comparison, such as dimensionality and spatial and temporal resolution, highlight the constraints on the type of experimental questions that can be asked with each method. For instance, distinctions based on dimensional representations indicates that for the study of the physiology of subcortical structures, PET and evoked potentials (EPs) are currently more useful than qEEG or MEG. These comparisons are summarized in a checklist form in Table 5–2.

Characterizing these methods according to both temporal and spatial resolution suggests there may be advantages in exploiting their complementarity in order to achieve a more complete version of the brain mechanisms related to auditory processing than could be obtained using any one technique alone. This possibility will be discussed below.

### Methods for Studying the Auditory Brain Stem

In the study of auditory CNS structures from lower pons through midbrain, only MRI and EPs can provide meaningful data, with perhaps the addition of PET for observing activation at the level of the inferior colliculus.

**MRI.**—Examples of MRI imaging of auditory–brain stem structures are provided in a number of reports on MRI applications in

**TABLE 5–1.**

Comparison of Seven Noninvasive Techniques for Monitoring the Brain.

| Technique | Spatial Resolution | Temporal Resolution* | Representation of Brain Provided |
|---|---|---|---|
| STRUCTURAL DATA | | | |
| Computed tomography (CT) | 5 mm | 20 min | 3 dimensions |
| Magnetic resonance imaging (MRI) | 1 mm | 20 min | 3 dimensions |
| FUNCTIONAL DATA | | | |
| Evoked potentials (EPs) | NA | 5 min | Pathways by level |
| Quantitative EEG (qEEG) | 3 cm | 5 min | 2 dimensions |
| Positron emission tomography (PET) | 5 mm | 40 sec† | 3 dimensions |
| Single-photon emission computed tomography (SPECT) | 1 cm | 20 min | 3 dimensions |
| Magnetoencephalography (MEG) | 1 mm | 5 min | 2+ dimensions |

NA = not applicable.
*Time required for single data-collection condition, not time required for entire study.
†Based on use of short–half-life isotope such as $^{15}O$; other isotopes such as $^{18}Fl$ (e.g., $^{18}Fl$ fluorodeoxyglucose) may require as long as 45 minutes for a single scan.

**TABLE 5–2.**
Checklist of Noninvasive Brain-Monitoring Techniques for Application to Four Levels of the Human Auditory CNS

| | MRI | EPs | qEEG | PET | MEG |
|---|---|---|---|---|---|
| Auditory brain stem | + | + | – | (+)* | – |
| Auditory thalamus | + | + | – | + | – |
| Primary auditory cortex | + | + | – | + | + |
| Association auditory cortex | + | + | + | + | + |

*PET is good for only part of brain stem, because of spatial resolution limitations.

otolaryngology.[1a, 3, 6, 36, 49] Features that can be visualized include those on the surface of the brain stem (the eighth nerve as it enters the pons, the quadrigeminal plate protruding toward the overhanging cerebellum), as well as structures within the brain stem (the gray matter of the cochlear nuclei and the two halves of the inferior colliculus).

**EPs.**—An example of a new EP approach to the auditory brain stem is represented by our work with a repeated-measures version of the auditory brain stem response (repeated evoked potentials/auditory brain stem response [REPs/ABR]). These studies reveal that the dramatic individual differences visible in ABR waveform morphology can be represented in simple measures of the stability of waveform parameters such as latency and amplitude.[27–31, 33] For example, although mean values of peak latency (Fig 5–1, *left panels*) show no individual differences or differences associated with ear of stimulation, latency stability profiles (see Fig 5–1, *right panels*) based on calculation of a ratio of mean latency vs. latency standard deviation for each peak, reveal not only between-subject differences, but also within-subject differences according to stimulation condition. Profiles based on amplitude stability have the same types of sensitivity. Such "stability profiles" may also be replicated over time; examples of within-subject replications of both latency and amplitude profiles are presented in Figure 5–2.

When REP stability profiles are calculated at a group level for a number of normal subjects, they can serve as a template against which to compare representatives of clinical populations, such as multiple sclerosis patients[32] or persons with CADs.[22] This comparison can serve as the basis for an objective scoring procedure useful not only for ranking patients within a population, but also to track within-patient changes over time.

**PET.**—Because of resolution limitations, for imaging responses in the auditory brain stem, PET machines available as of 1990 will probably be restricted to the upper-brain stem nuclei, such as the inferior colliculi. An example of a PET image of a response at this level is illustrated in Figure 5–3, representing percent difference comparisons of activation conditions (binaural syllables in the left panel, and right-ear pure tones in the right panel) with resting conditions. Percent-difference images are based on a point-by-point comparison of one image taken during resting conditions (eyes closed, ears plugged, room darkened) vs. one taken during controlled stimulation (e.g., binaural synthetic syllables, monaural right-ear pulsed pure tones). The images in Figure 5–3 are based on the use of $^{15}O$, with data collection completed in only 40 seconds, which allows the subject to be used as her or his own control in a within-subject series of resting and activation conditions tested in the same session. Note that since the separation of the two halves of the inferior colliculus (approximately 2 cm center-to-center) is greater than the 1.5-cm spatial resolution of the imaging system, the response to the monaural as well as to the binaural condition appears simply as a midline area of activation.

## Methods for Studying the Auditory Thalamus

Reference to Tables 5–1 and 5–2 suggests that using current techniques, only MRI, EPs, and PET are useful for studying thalamic responses to auditory stimulation, which may be divided between the classical auditory nuclei (medial geniculate nuclei or MGN) and the pulvinar nucleus of the thalamus, which receives direct collaterals from the MGN.

**MRI.**—In the articles and atlases cited above regarding MRI applications in neurology, examples are provided of images visualizing structures on the surface of and within the thalamus. For example, the medial geniculate nuclei and auditory radiations to the cortex can be identified, as well as the interior extent of the gray matter of the pulvinar, important for auditory processing in that

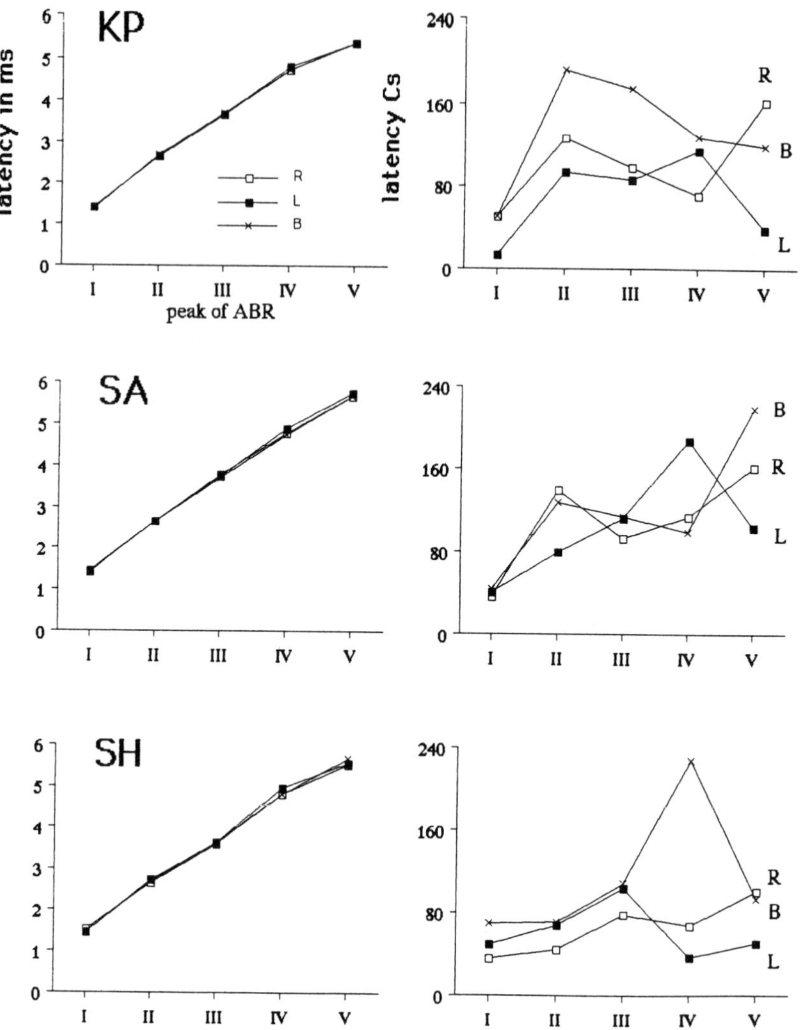


**FIG 5–1.**
Comparison of two measures of the latency characteristics of peaks of the auditory brain-stem response (ABR) based on a within-subjects, repeated-measures design (repeated evoked potentials or REPs): mean latency *(left panels)* vs. latency stability values *(right panels),* for each of three individual subjects.[30] Each set of data is based on eight separate waveforms per ear condition. Testing parameters are standard, with the single exception the collection of repeated waveforms. Stability is plotted in terms of the coefficient of stability (CS), calculated as the ratio of mean divided by standard deviation (over eight waveforms per ear per subject). Note that while the mean latency values on the left reveal neither individual differences nor distinctions according to ear, both types of detail are clearly visible in the latency stability values, suggesting that this simple index of stability provides a much more sensitive measure of evoked-potential characteristics than do mean values of peak parameters such as latency and amplitude.

it receives direct collaterals from the MGN. There are obvious applications to identifying the location of lesions within these structures for diagnosis in persons presenting with central auditory dysfunction owing to thalamic insult, and for tracking the signs of recovery within such patients over time.

**EPs.**—Building on the large body of literature regarding auditory middle latency responses (MLRs), we have begun exploring the usefulness of an REPs protocol for this time window of auditory averaged responses, and comparing it with REPs/ABR characteristics. For example, contrasts of within-subject vs. between-subject consistency

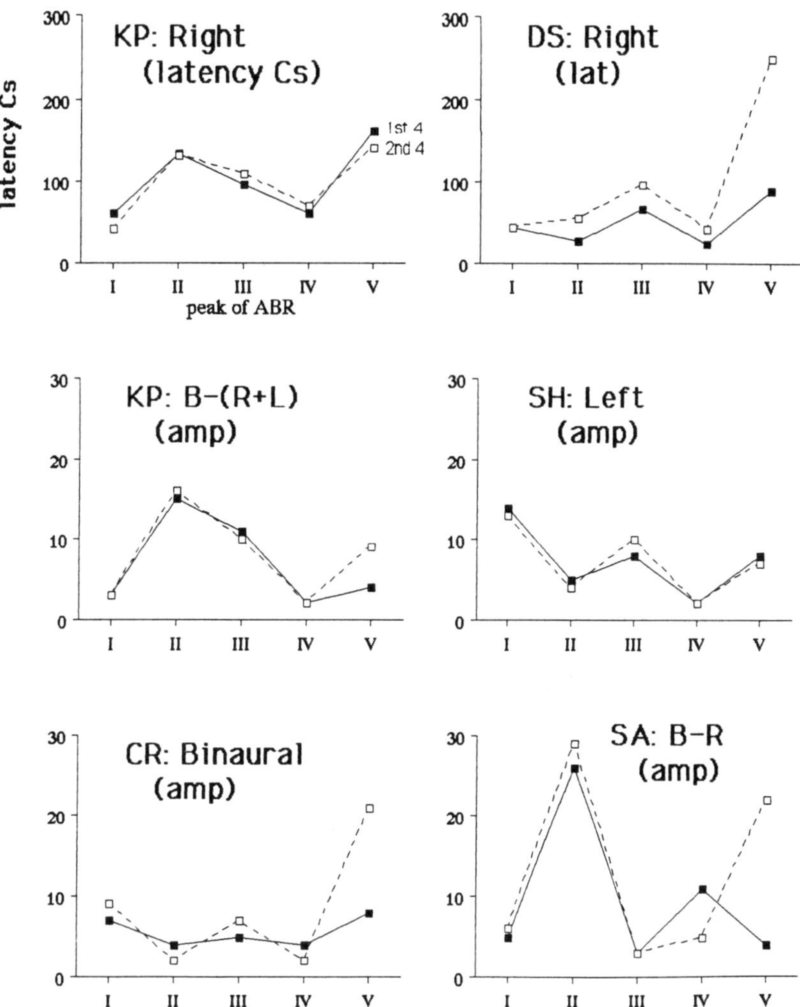


**FIG 5-2.**
Examples illustrating within-subject replicability of "stability profiles" such as those illustrated in Figure 5-1, representing a variety of ear conditions in different subjects. Each graph compares stability profiles calculated for a first 4 test weeks, at a rate of 1 waveform per ear per week *(filled symbols with solid lines),* with profiles for a second four-week series *(open symbols with broken lines).* Note that stability-profile replicability can be demonstrated for measures of peak latency, amplitude, and derived amplitude comparisons (e.g., binaural amplitude minus the sum of both monaural peaks).

of ABR vs. MLR peak latencies indicates that the within-subject latency stability values for MLR peak $N_0$ are *intermediate* between those for ABR peak V and those for later MLR peaks. Such a relation might be interpreted as corroborating other types of evidence which indicate that MLR peak $N_0$ depends primarily on brain-stem generators.[28, 29]

**PET.**—Due to the large size of MGN combined with pulvinar, responses in auditory thalamus are easily visualized on PET. At this level of the auditory system, the wide separation between left-side vs. right-side nuclei enables clear distinctions between responses to monaural vs. binaural stimulation, as well as identification of a clear contralateral dominance for monaural input. Figure 5-4 presents the auditory-thalamic data for the subjects whose images were shown in Figure 5-3: contralateral (left-sided) response to the right-ear pure tones shown in the right panel, and bilateral response to the binaural syllables in the

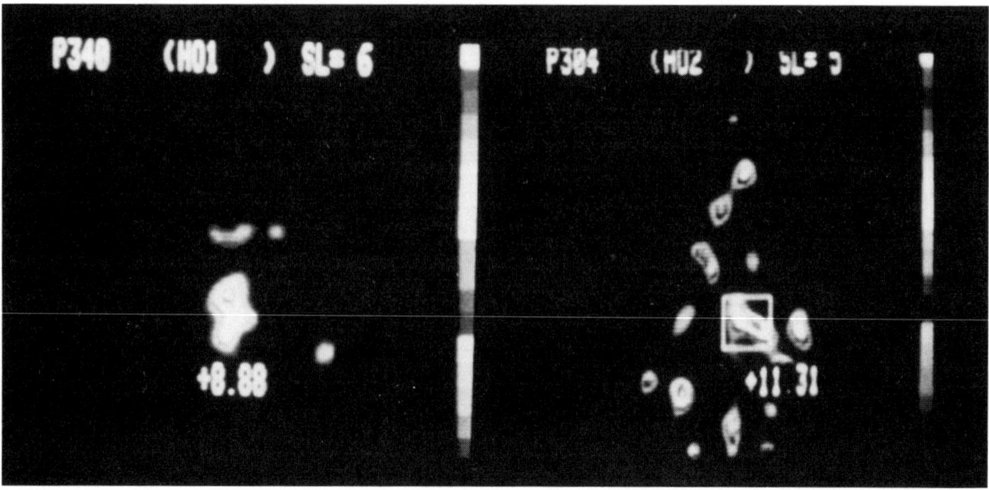


**FIG 5–3.**
Percent-difference PET images at the level of the midbrain from two subjects tested under two auditory conditions, illustrating the topography of changes in regional cerebral blood flow (rCBF) comparing a resting condition with an activation condition. Images were created with an eight-ring PETT VI system with injected $^{15}$O-labeled water and 40-second scan time.[25, 26] *Left panel*, response in subject No. 340 to binaural synthetic syllables; *right panel*, response from subject No. 304 to right-ear monaural pulsed pure tones (see citations for stimulus details). Since the 1.5-cm resolution of this system is approximately equal to the separation of the two halves of the inferior colliculus, the hypothetical contralateral response to monaural stimulation cannot be distinguished from bilateral response to binaural stimulation; both responses are visualized simply as an activation at approximately midline.

lcft pancl. Thc magnitude and extent of the changes illustrated here suggest that they represent responses not only in MGN, but in the pulvinar as well.

## Methods for Studying Primary Auditory Cortex

At this level, all methods reviewed except qEEG are available for studying auditory CNS structure and function. We have omitted qEEG from the available methods here owing to the physical characteristics of EEG (referential recording, volume conduction artifact) that limit its spatial resolution. Under conventional recording and analysis procedures, an electrode placed over "auditory cortex" (locations T3 and T4) should be considered as monitoring a wide region of cortex, presumably including association as well as primary areas. Thus qEEG responses to auditory stimulation recorded at T3/4 will be described under association cortex, below.

**MRI.**—Our example of MRI applications to the study of primary auditory cortex is related to the measurement of anatomical asymmetries in perisylvian regions, such as the area of the planum temporale.[5, 44, 50] Figure 5–5 presents a schematic illustration of two measures used by Plante and colleagues[43–45] to study children with specific language impairment (SLI): whole-hemisphere volume and the volume of perisylvian areas.

As the reports by Plante and colleagues[43–45] demonstrate, abnormal patterns of such asymmetries, including relations between whole-hemisphere vs. perisylvian volumes, may be used to characterize the target children, siblings, and parents in these families. Current work in the Coordinated Noninvasive Studies (CNS) Project (discussed below) makes use of similar measures to quantify individual characteristics of auditory processing asymmetries in normal young adults[17, 19, 21, 35] and to describe anatomical and physiological characteristics of individuals diagnosed as having CADs.[20, 22]

**EPs.**—The literature on cortical evoked auditory potentials attributed to primary cortex (EP peaks N1–P2) is large and merits a separate survey.[38] Preliminary experiments exploring the sensitivity to individual characteristics provided by

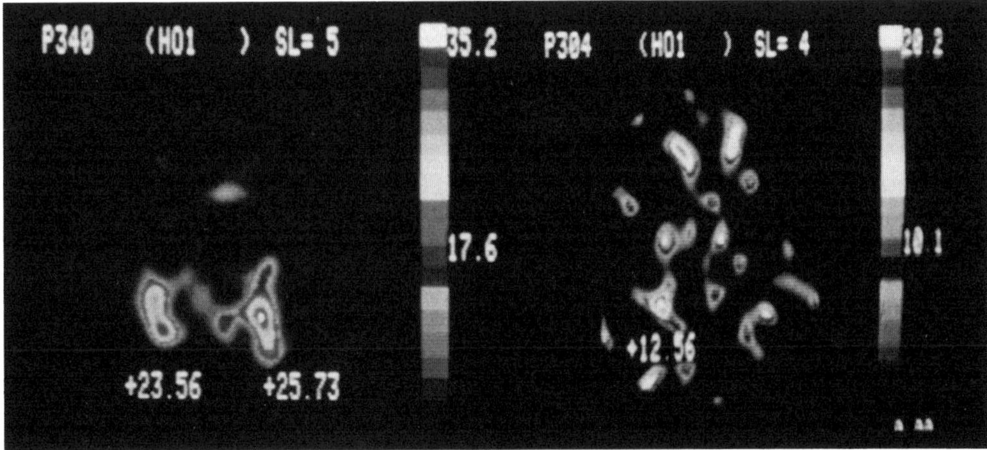


**FIG 5–4.**
Percent-difference PET images at the level of the auditory thalamus (MGN and pulvinar) taken from the image series of the same two subjects tested under the same conditions as described for Figure 5–1. *Left panel,* binaural synthetic syllables evoke a bilateral change response that is large in both magnitude and extent and quite symmetrical; *right panel,* right-ear pure tones evoke a primarily contralateral response.

the REPs procedure[28, 29] group cortical peaks N1 and P2 with later MLR peaks, corroborating earlier suggestions that generators of all these peaks are related. Also, comparisons of between-subject vs. within-subject latency stability measured for early, middle, and late responses indicate that for all three levels of the auditory system, individuals are more like themselves than they are like each other. This is true even in cortex, where early attempts to use the N1–P2 waveform clinically were abandoned owing to the lability (i.e., within-subject variability) of the response.[46]

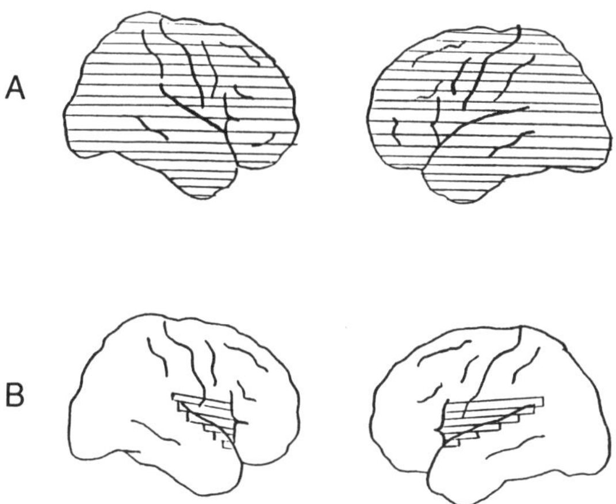


**FIG 5–5.**
Schematic illustrating two MRI measures of brain anatomical asymmetries used in studies of children with specific language impairment (SLI) by Plante and colleagues[43–45] and for characterizing patterns of auditory asymmetries in normal young adults tested in the CNS Project.[17, 19, 21, 35] **A,** whole-hemisphere volume. **B,** volume of perisylvian regions.

**MEG.**—As Naatanen and Picton[38] point out, experimental as well as technical procedures for much of MEG research have been borrowed from research on cortical EPs. Thus MEG data are collected on an averaged basis, to generate evoked fields (EFs), and results are interpreted in terms of peak polarity latency and amplitude. The primary difference is that the greater spatial resolution of MEG, enabling source identification to within 1 mm, makes it possible to map responses over an area of cortex and to identify accurately the sources of responses to families of stimuli, such as pure tones of different frequencies.

Workers at two laboratories have been interested in combining the high spatial resolution of MRI (for anatomy) and MEG (for physiology) to obtain functional-anatomical localization of responses in primary auditory cortex. Papanicolaou and colleagues[41] compared responses to contralateral vs. ipsilateral stimulation; Pantev and coworkers[40] mapped EFs for a number of pure-tone frequencies. Figure 5–6 presents a schematic of the grid of data-collection points used by Pantev et al[40] in their mapping procedure. These authors have also developed a method for anatomical localization of the EFs collected from one subject displayed on the same subject's MRI scan, which

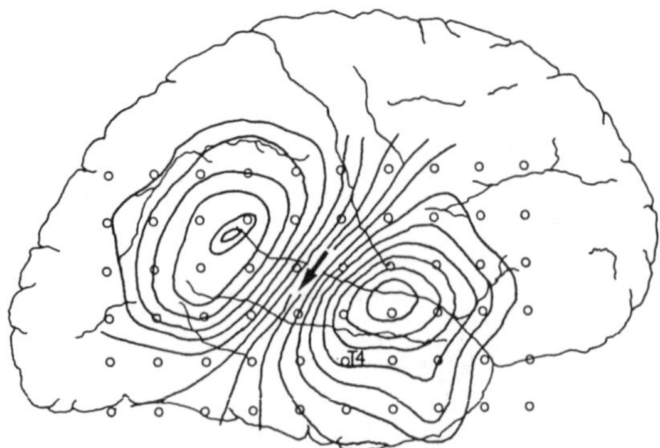


**FIG 5–6.**
Schematic of data-collection locations (indicated by *open circles*) reported by Pantev and co-workers,[40] to map cortical MEG responses to pure tones of different frequencies, combined with isofield contours used to identify the source of response to the series of pure tones. (From Pantev C, et al: *Electroencephalogr Clin Neurophysiol* 75:173–184. Used by permission.)

has allowed them to show, for example, that all analyzed sources lie on the superior temporal plane.[40]

**PET.**—The area of Heschl's gyrus (a single gyrus potentially as large as 4 × 1 cm), combined with PET 5-mm spatial resolution suggests that tonotopic organization might also be demonstrable with PET. Using a PETT-VI generation scanner and $^{15}O^{12}$, combined with a method for individualized anatomical localization based on skull bony landmarks,[4] we found discrete local changes in regional cerebral blood flow (rCBF) that were correlated with the side of stimulation as well as the frequency of a pure tone[25] with distribution of responses similar to those seen with more invasive procedures in nonhuman animals as well as those described above using MEG. It was also observed[26] that while both monaural pure tones and binaural synthetic syllables (Fig 5–7) evoked responses in primary auditory cortex, the response to the syllables was focused in the region responsive to lower rather than high-frequency tones. This was interpreted as indicating a type of "frequency analysis" reflected in the rCBF patterns, since the acoustical energy in the syllables was in fact concentrated in the lower frequencies.

## Methods for Studying Association Auditory Cortex

For the regions of cortex which extend outward in concentric rings from primary auditory areas, eventually meeting similar extensions from other types of cortex, both sensory and motor, all

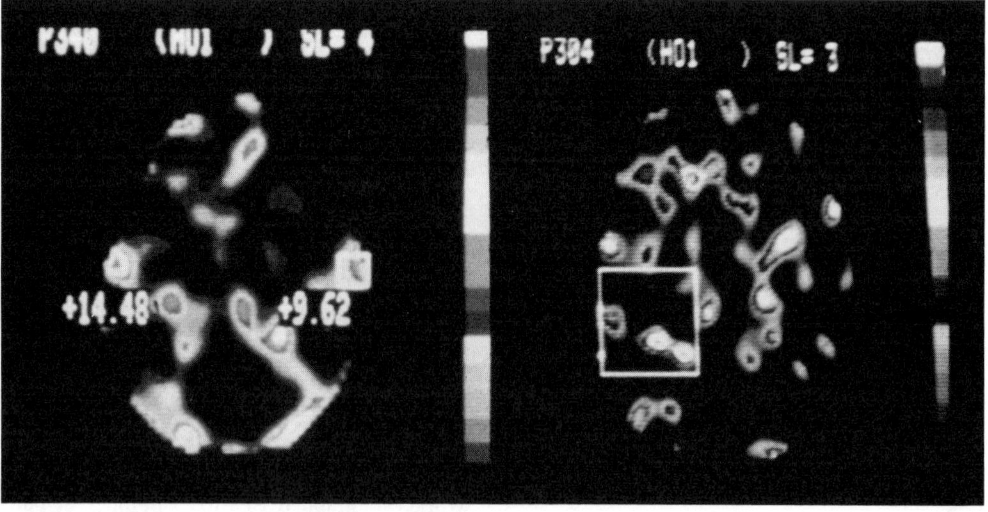


**FIG 5–7.**
Percent-difference PET images from the series illustrated in Figures 5–1 and 5–2, at the level of primary auditory cortex. *Left panel,* binaural synthetic syllables evoke responses on both sides; *right panel,* right-ear 500-Hz pure tones evoke discrete response only on the left side, which in this case consists of a strip of activation extending at approximately a 45-degree angle from anterior-lateral toward posterior-medial.[25] Activation by the low-frequency-predominating syllables is focused in a region which would respond best to low-frequency rather than to high-frequency tones, indicating a "frequency analysis" represented in this physiological response.

methods reviewed provide potentially powerful tools for studying the details of brain structure and function.

**MRI.**—Beyond measures of hemispheric asymmetry, little has been reported using MRI to examine association auditory cortical structure in either healthy persons or to correlate changes in these regions with disorders in people with brain damage. One study[39] reported observations combining CT with qEEG in a case of aphasia acquired during balloon angioplasty. The details of the time course of the appearance of the lesion under anatomical vs. physiological monitoring suggests that, as in the MRI/MEG studies described above, using these noninvasive methods to match structure to function may provide insights into the physiology of brain damage not obtainable in any other way.

**EPs.**—While it is possible that some of the literature on event-related potentials (ERPs)[1] is relevant to function in association auditory cortex, the contribution of sensory factors to these and other late potentials is poorly understood and it is difficult to interpret the results of the cognitive designs of many of these experiments in a way that is relevant to auditory processing. Techniques for assessing late potentials, such as the Contingent Negative Variation (CNV), based on many more electrodes and dynamic analysis of changes in electrical activation recorded across the surface of the scalp over time, may eventually prove more illuminating.[8, 9]

It is particularly important that experimental design for EP studies of association as well as primary auditory cortex take account of the methodological considerations outlined by Gevins and co-authors.[7, 10] In these articles, the authors attribute our ignorance of electrophysiological correlates of human brain function to poor experimental control of stimulus, task, and subject variables. Certainly the study of late cortical potentials, such as those which might be attributable to association areas, must be able to account for the contributions of such basic variables if we are ever to acquire a sophisticated understanding of the function of these complex areas of the brain. This is especially crucial for studies of the effects of brain damage on auditory function, where a basic need is to understand the extent to which such variables differentially affect responses from primary vs. association areas.

**qEEG.**—The great advantage of "running" qEEG for studying behavioral neurophysiology at the cortical level is that there are no time constraints on either stimulus or response, as with EPs. Thus subjects can be monitored during relatively "natural" dynamic behavior, such as performing motor gestures, watching pictures, or listening through earphones.

Many questions related to processing in the auditory CNS may be addressed with qEEG. For example, following methodological guidelines,[7, 10] subjects may be monitored successfully for electrophysiological "activation asymmetries" observed over auditory cortex during dichotic-listening tasks, and the resulting electrophysiological "hemisphere advantages" compared with the same subjects' behaviorally-measured "ear advantages."[23]

qEEG also may be used to measure "resting asymmetries" in auditory cortex. For evaluating auditory function these measures may prove even more crucial than activation asymmetries. First, the relation between this physiological "resting bias" of auditory cortex and underlying anatomical asymmetries not only can aid in objective classification of subjects according to "sidedness" characteristics[35] but also may have diagnostic import.[20]

In addition, it is possible that meaningful interpretation of behavioral tests of central auditory function can be made only in the context of a "resting CNS profile" for each subject. At minimum, this profile would consist of cortical anatomical asymmetries (MRI) combined with subcortical (REPs/ABR) and cortical (qEEG) physiological asymmetries. Eventually such a "central audiogram" may be considered as important a component of the audiological workup, particularly for evaluating central function, as an audiogram of peripheral hearing acuity.

**MEG.**—The state of ERP-type research with MEG may be described in much the same terms as for electrophysiological studies; much basic work remains to be done in order to understand the contribution of a number of independent variables to the response in healthy brains, before the promise of MEG's fine spatial resolution, recorded under both time-locked and "running" conditions, can be realized for study of persons with damage to association auditory cortex.

**PET.**—Perhaps the most striking finding reported in PET studies of auditory responses to date is the clear distinction between responses in association areas to pure tones vs. syllables[25, 26] (Fig 5–8). At this level, approximately 1.5 cm above the sylvian fissure, no response to the monaural pulsed pure tones *(right panel)* is observed, but a clear bilateral response to the binaural syllables does occur—which appears to be accompanied by an added predominance of response on the left side. Thus Figures 5–7 and 5–8 illustrate a contrast in activation at two pathway levels to two types of sounds; while responses in primary cortex are comparable for both pure tones and syllables (see Fig 5–7), the presence or absence of a response at an association level clearly distinguishes between the sound types, perhaps dependent on characteristics of temporal and spectral complexity (see Fig 5–8).

The striking asymmetry apparent in Figure 5–8 in the response to the binaural syllables cannot be accounted for in this case by any physical difference in the sounds presented to the two ears, or by a simple variable such as asymmetrical hearing loss. However, in order to interpret this result as a reflection of a hemispheric processing asymmetry, more information is required. For example, the individual's pattern of "resting asymmetries" must be taken into account (described for both qEEG[23] and PET[34, 42]). Also, other individual characteristics such as those provided by more in-depth "asymmetry profiles" (see descriptions of the CNS Project, discussed below), and responses observed during other types of activation conditions may affect the interpretation of PET data on asymmetries. The preliminary results illustrated here do suggest, however, that there are many possibilities for detailed, sophisticated studies employing the excellent spatial and temporal resolution of $^{15}O$ PET to study responses in auditory association cortex in both normal persons and those with CADs.

## COMBINATIONS OF METHODS

It is possible that the most powerful use of the new noninvasive methods is not in isolation, as they are most often used, but in combinations that take advantage of their multifaceted complementarity. As suggested in Tables 5–1 and 5–2, many features of the methods compare and contrast in ways suggesting that by combining methods, more information might be forthcoming about functional correlates of brain anatomy, and

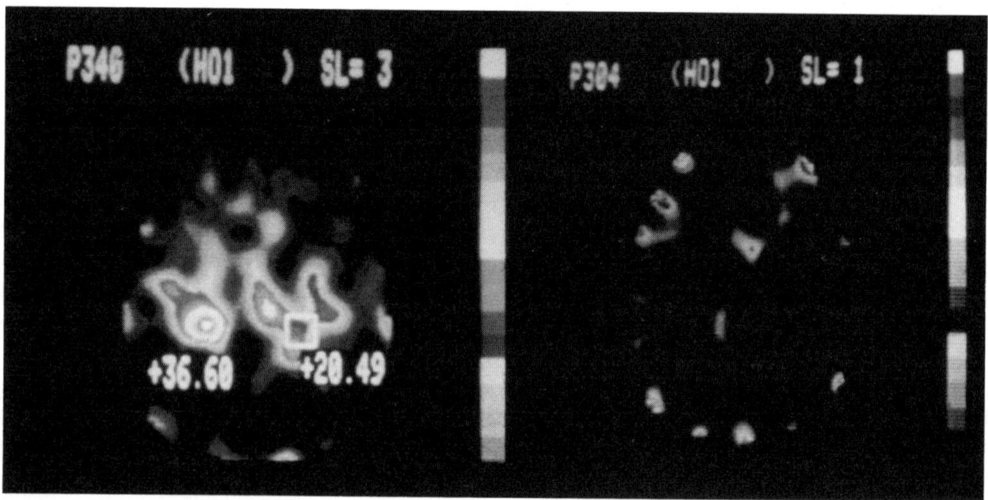


**FIG 5–8.**
Percent-difference PET images from the series described above, at a level 1.5 cm above primary auditory cortex. *Left panel,* binaural synthetic syllables evoke bilateral responses, with an apparent predominance on the left side; *right panel,* right-ear pure tones seem to evoke no response at this level.

connections between structure, function, and behavior, than could be obtained from using any one method alone.

As we have seen, there are already precedents for a "coordinated" use of the noninvasive methods which suggest the power of this approach; for example, the combination of MRI and MEG.[40, 41] In addition, preliminary results in the CNS Project further support the viability and potential of combining methods for within-subject studies of brain mechanisms underlying certain types of behavior.

In the initial stages of this project, the focus is on brain asymmetries.[16, 17, 19, 21] First, individuals are tested using behavioral techniques for dichotic listening[13–15] to determine ear advantages for two sets of complex sounds. This series of behavioral test sessions not only serves to provide a behavioral "hypothesis" for each subject to be tested by means of the various anatomical and physiological measures, but also trains the individual in the target tasks, so that subsequent brain monitoring will be conducted during learned, asymptotic performance.

Next, each subject is tested using MRI to measure anatomical asymmetries in auditory cortex, and in a REPs/ABRs session to establish brain stem ear dominance. Then, in separate sessions on qEEG, PET, and MEG, the individual is monitored during resting as well as several activation conditions while performing tasks very similar to those tested behaviorally, such as listening to monaural presentations of each of the sound sets and attending to different ears during dichotic conditions.

To compare asymmetry measures across techniques, results on all tests are expressed in terms of percent differences comparing measures from the two hemispheres, plotted in an asymmetry space which provides for easy visual comparison not only within, but also across subjects. Findings for a subset of such tests conducted with a total of 15 normal subjects tested to date[21] indicate: (1) dramatic individual differences, (2) good "internal consistency" for each subject comparing anatomical and all physiological measures, and (3) suggestions for transformation rules relating structural and functional asymmetries to the behavioral measures of performance. For example, qEEG "hemisphere advantages" observed during dichotic testing show good agreement with behavioral "ear advantages" measured in the same subjects[23] and there are clear relations comparing the magnitude and direction of anatomical asymmetries in auditory cortex measured with MRI with physiological asymmetries in resting qEEG.[35]

Figure 5–9 presents a sample of data collected for two normal persons with data from a person diagnosed as having central auditory disorder. Results displayed include: (1) behavioral ear advantages (EAs) for two sets of sounds, synthetic syllables *(black bar)* and tone patterns *(white bar);* these data are plotted in the asymmetry space as though indicating processing focused in the contralateral hemisphere; (2) "resting qEEG asymmetry" comparing power in the qEEG beta bandwidth (12 to 20 Hz) measured over left-side vs. right-side auditory cortex during a resting condition *(dotted box at qEEG);* (3) "activation qEEG asymmetries" in qEEG beta over T3/4 observed during dichotic test conditions, e.g., right-ear attention during dichotic syllables *(black bar at qEEG)* vs. left-ear attention during dichotic tone patterns *(white bar);* (4) whole-hemisphere volume asymmetry measured with MRI *(dotted box at MRI);* and (5) perisylvian volume asymmetry *(striped bar at MRI).*

Note the clear individual differences that distinguish the data for the two normal subjects, who also have contrasting sidedness characteristics (the subject in panel A is "personal right-sided, familial right-sided, pRFR," wheras the subject in panel B is "personal left, familial left, pLfL"). Note also that their results are internally consistent. For example, in each, the size and direction of the perisylvian anatomical asymmetry *(the MRI striped bar)* is reflected in the size and direction of the physiological asymmetry indicated by the resting qEEG measure *(dotted box).* This degree of internal consistency is typical of the normal subjects tested to date.[35]

The crucial details in the central patient's data are related to the departures from this normal pattern: (1) the EA scores are "backward" for his sidedness characteristics; and (2) there is no physiological concomitant (in resting qEEG) of his large anatomical perisylvian asymmetry. The "physiological failure" indicated by this last characteristic is further supported by the fact that his REPs/ABR data reveal a clear abnormality in the response to right-ear clicks suggestive of physiological dysfunction in left auditory cortex.[20]

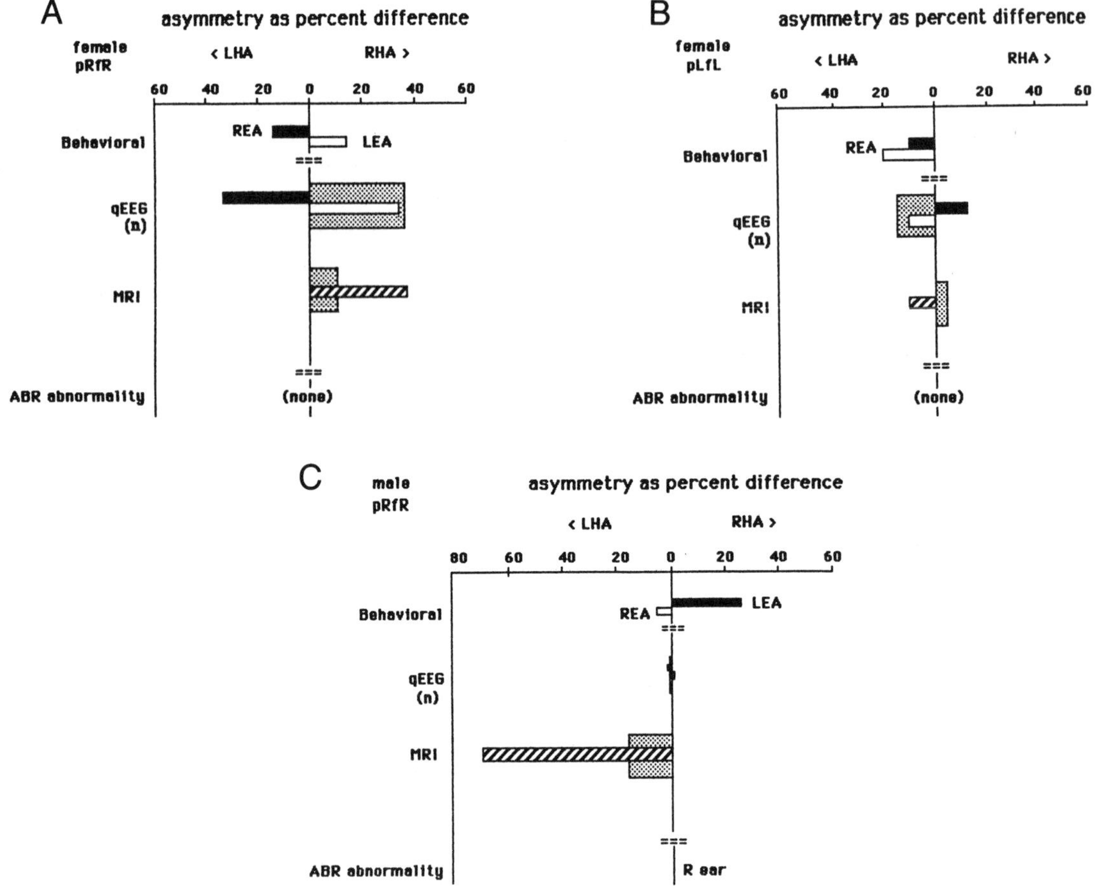


**FIG 5–9.**
"Asymmetry profiles" for two normal subjects (**A** and **B**) and one with central auditory disorder (**C**) tested in the CNS Project.[17, 19, 21] Percent-difference values for a variety of measures range from ear advantages *(Behavioral)* through auditory brain stem asymmetries *(ABR)*. Behavioral results represent "hypotheses" about underlying structure and function, tested via examination with the various noninvasive techniques. Note that while the two normal profiles differ dramatically from each other, the differences are entirely in keeping with their distinctions expressed in terms of "sidedness" characteristics, and also that the degree of "internal consistency" observed in the two normal subjects is not matched in the results for the "central" profile in panel **C**. (See text for more discussion.)

## LOOKING TO THE FUTURE

During the 1990s ("decade of the brain") and beyond, in the first years of the 21st century, we can expect to see more sophisticated use of the techniques already available, such as coordinated combinations of methods, as well as the introduction of new methods, particularly for physiological monitoring.

### Modifications of Current Methods

New versions of existing technologies are already available. Among these are a combination of contrast agents used with MRI; these will provide much more flexibility in terms of selective highlighting of a variety of physical characteristics in both normal and pathological tissue. Also, flash MRI techniques will streamline data collection, enabling the collection of higher-resolution image series in the same amount of time or providing a greater variety of angles of view. The use of dynamic data analysis applied in a range of techniques will result in better temporal resolution as well as allow for tracking the vectors of brain activation over space through time.[8, 48] Finally, we can expect further developments in the extension of MRI proton spectroscopy into chemical shift imaging documenting the distribution of substances other than hydrogen, in applications referred to as magnetic resonance spectroscopy (MRS), which promise to open new windows on hitherto unavailable details relating to neurochemistry and neurophysiology in the living human brain.[37, 47]

### New Methods

One example of a new technique is transcranial magnetic stimulation, a reverse MEG, in which a magnetic field is applied to the brain via coils on the surface of the scalp and electrical activity induced in the underlying tissue. As described in a collection of papers published in 1990,[2] this innocuous type of stimulation can evoke activity in individual muscles, interrupt speech, and suppress visual perception. While there are only preliminary reports regarding the evocation of sensory percepts with this technique, the relevant physics and physiology do not preclude such possibilities. Accurate control of the direction and strength of the applied field should make such experiments viable, even involving targeting of subcortical structures.

### Improvements in Experimental Design

From a more general standpoint, future developments in noninvasive brain monitoring can be also expected to include methodological improvements directed toward maximizing the information obtained. Some of these will be along the lines defined much earlier in critical reviews of EEG research on higher cortical functions[7, 10]; which concluded that after decades of such work, "little fundamental knowledge has been uncovered," owing in part to "inadequate experimental designs."

Of particular interest will be application of principles of signal detection theory,[11] focus on individual characteristics, and use of repeated-measures, within-subjects experimental designs.

**Signal Detection Theory.**—Clearly, in a testing situation where the nature of the dependent variable is an unknown (such as brain responses to sound observed with PET), great care should be taken to rigorously quantify and control all independent variables. It is to be expected that any interpretation of the results of such experiments that does not take into account the contribution of variables such as temporal resolution, perceptual components of complex tasks, and amount of subject training will only result in a continuing lack of fundamental knowledge regarding human brain function—in spite of the fact that such powerful tools are now available to fill this void. More specifically with regard to the auditory system, new tests exploiting the richness of nonspeech sound design[18] should provide new insights into functional and dysfunctional characteristics of auditory nuclei between lower brain stem and association cortex.

**Individual Characteristics.**—The new brain machines provide consistent evidence of the dramatic nature of individual differences. It is to be expected that the promise of the noninvasive techniques will only be realized by taking advantage of the detail which they reveal, rather than by ignoring it—detail which certainly must be accounted for in any sophisticated set of theories regarding the relations between brain and behavior. Only by remaining open to new insights into the "repertoire" of ways in which brain anatomy and physiology are related to behavior will we realize the promise of these new "windows on the brain."

**Repeated-Measure Designs.**—Finally, the strategy that holds the most promise for investigations into auditory processing as well as other types of human behavior is the use of repeated-measures experimental designs. Aspects of such an approach include (1) within-subject testing under identical conditions, to exploit the sensitivity of variability measures as expressions of individual characteristics[30]; (2) within-subject testing under different conditions on the same device, in order to interpret brain responses under a particular condition in the context of responses under related conditions; and (3) within-subject testing on a variety of methods, to establish individual profiles articulated in terms of anatomical, physiological, and behavioral characteristics.

## CONCLUSION

The brain-monitoring devices that are already available, their extensions, and new devices that should emerge in the near future provide an unparalleled opportunity to observe directly how details of brain structure and function are related to performance. It is to be expected that as we learn to use these methods to explore the repertoire of ways in which the anatomical and physiological design of the human auditory system is expressed in behavior, our currently vague notions of central auditory processing will undergo basic changes, becoming at once more detailed and more comprehensive.

Such a revolution in concepts regarding the rules of normal central auditory function should in turn provide the basis for a "new audiology," characterized by diagnosis based on a combination of sophisticated experimental design, high-resolution brain monitoring, and in-depth study of individuals. Assessment focus can be expected to shift from general categorization of problems arising from damage affecting the auditory periphery, to more complete, customized descriptions of dysfunction considered within an overall profile of savings, formulated for each individual in terms of a combination of anatomical, physiological, and behavioral details.

Finally, it is possible that such advances in diagnostic detail could provide the basis for new intervention strategies. Improved behavioral testing and brain-monitoring techniques could be used to explore the dynamic characteristics of auditory disorders, documenting the ways in which anatomical, physiological, and behavioral aspects of auditory disorders change over time. Evaluation of spontaneous changes as well as assessment of the effects of therapy should eventually lead not only to new formulations of how damage to any and all parts of the auditory system contribute to auditory disorders, but more generally, to a new appreciation of the complexity and elegance of the auditory central nervous system and the ways in which it accomplishes the everyday miracles of comprehending the patterns of speech and music.

## ACKNOWLEDGMENT

Work supported by a grant from the U.S. Air Force Office of Scientific Research.

## REFERENCES

1. Brunia CHM, Mulder G, Verbaten MN (eds): Event-Related Brain Research. *Electroencephalogr Clin Neurophysiol* 1991; suppl 42.
1a. Bydder GM, Steiner RE, Thomas DJ, et al: Nuclear magnetic resonance imaging of the posterior fossa: 50 cases. *Clin Radiol* 1983; 34:173–188.
2. Chokroverty S (ed): *Magnetic Stimulation in Clinical Neurophysiology*. Boston, Butterworths, 1990.
3. Cure JK, Cromwell LD, Case JL, et al: Auditory dysfunction caused by multiple sclerosis: Detection with MR imaging. *Am J Neuroradiol* 1990; 11:817–820.
4. Fox PT, Perlmutter JS, Raichle ME: A stereotactic method of anatomical localization for positron emission tomography. *J Comput Assist Tomogr* 1985; 9:141–153.
5. Galaburda, AM, Geschwind N: Anatomical asymmetries in the adult and developing brain and their implications for function. *Adv Pediatr* 1981; 21:271–292.
6. Gentry LR, Jacoby CG, Turski PA et al: Cerebellopontine angle-petromastoid mass lesions: Comparative study of diagnosis with MR imaging and CT. *Radiology* 1987; 162:513–520.
7. Gevins AS: Analysis of the electromagnetic signals of the human brain: Milestones, obstacles, and goals. *IEEE Trans Biomed Eng* 1984; 31:833–850.
8. Gevins AS, Bressler SL, Morgan NH, et al: Event-related covariances during a bimanual visuomotor task. I. Methods and analysis of stimulus- and response-locked data. *Electroencephalogr Clin Neurophysiol* 1989; 74:58–75.
9. Gevins AS, Morgan NH, Bressler SL et al: Human neuroelectric patterns predict performance accuracy. *Science* 1987; 235:580–585.
10. Gevins AS, Schaffer RE: A critical review of electroencephalographic (EEG) correlates of higher cortical functions. *CRC Crit Rev Bioeng* 1980; 4:113–164.
11. Green DM, Swets JA: *Signal Detection Theory and Psychophysics*. Huntington, NY, Krieger, 1974.
12. Herscovitch P, Markham J, Raichle ME: Brain blood flow measured with intravenous H2-015. I. Theory and error analysis. *J Nucl Med* 1983; 24:782–789.
13. Lauter JL: Dichotic identification of complex sounds: Absolute and relative ear advantages. *J Acoust Soc Am* 1982; 71:701–707.

14. Lauter JL: Stimulus characteristics and relative ear advantages: A new look at old data. *J Acoust Soc Am* 1983; 74:1–17.
15. Lauter JL: Contralateral interference and ear advantages for identification of three-element patterns. *Brain Cogn* 1984; 3:259–280.
16. Lauter JL: Asymmetries in Complex-Sounds Processing. Conference on Auditory Pattern Recognition, Evanston, Ill, 1987.
17. Lauter JL: Functional organization of normal human auditory central nervous system observed with noninvasive techniques: Year one of the CNS Project. *J Acoust Soc Am* 1989; 86:S46.
18. Lauter JL: Auditory system, in Pearlman AL, Collins RC (eds): *Neurobiology of Disease*. New York, Oxford University Press, 1990; pp 101–123.
19. Lauter JL: The Coordinated Noninvasive Studies (CNS) Project. St Louis, Society for Neuroscience, 1990.
20. Lauter JL: Central auditory dysfunction: qEEG and MRI correlates of individual differences in ear advantages and REP/ABR results. *J Acoust Soc Am* 1991; 90:2292.
21. Lauter JL: The Coordinated Noninvasive Studies (CNS) Project. Washington, DC, American Association for the Advancement of Science, 1991.
22. Lauter JL: MacCAD and REP/ABRs: A new test battery for central auditory dysfunction. *J Acoust Soc Am* 1991; 89:S47.
23. Lauter JL: Processing asymmetries for complex sounds: Comparisons between behavioral ear advantages and electrophysiological asymmetries based on quantitative electroencephalography (qEEG). *Brain Cogn,* in press.
24. Lauter JL: Visions of the brain: New noninvasive imaging techniques and their applications to the study of human speech and language, in Winitz H (ed): *Human Communication and its Disorders*. Norwood, NJ, Ablex Publishing Co, in press.

24a. Lauter JL: Windows on hearing: Noninvasive methods for studying the human auditory system, in preparation.

25. Lauter JL, Herscovitch P, Formby C, et al: Tonotopic organization in human auditory cortex revealed by positron emission tomography. *Hear Res* 1985; 20:199–205.
26. Lauter JL, Herscovitch P, Raichle ME: Human auditory physiology studied with positron emission tomography, in Syka J, Masterton RB (eds): *Auditory Pathway*. New York, Plenum, 1988, pp 313–317.
27. Lauter JL, Karzon RG: Individual differences in auditory electric responses: Comparisons of between-subject and within-subject variability. III. A replication, and observations of individual vs. group characteristics. *Scand Audiol* 1990; 19:67–72.
28. Lauter JL, Karzon RG: Individual differences in auditory electric responses: Comparisons of between-subject and within-subject variability. IV. Latency-variability comparisons of early, middle, and late responses. *Scand Audiol* 1990; 19:175–182.
29. Lauter JL, Karzon RG: Individual differences in auditory electric responses: Comparisons of between-subject and within-subject variability. V. Amplitude-variability comparisons in early, middle, and late responses. *Scand Audiol* 1990; 19:201–206.
30. Lauter JL, Loomis RL: Individual differences in auditory electric responses: Comparisons of between-subject and within-subject variability. I. Absolute latencies of brainstem vertex-positive peaks. *Scand Audiol* 1986; 15:167–172.
31. Lauter JL, Loomis RL: Individual differences in auditory electric responses: Comparisons of between-subject and within-subject variability. II. Amplitudes of brainstem vertex-positive peaks. *Scand Audiol* 1988; 17:87–92.
32. Lauter JL, Lord-Maes JM: Repeated-measures ABRs in multiple sclerosis: Demonstration of a new tool for individual neurological assessment. *J Acoust Soc Am* 1990; 88:S18.
33. Lauter JL, Oyler RF: Individual differences in ABR latency variability in children 10–12 years of age. *Br J Audiol,* in press.
34. Lauter JL, Plante E: Global brain asymmetries in regional cerebral blood flow (rCBF) during resting conditions observed with positron emission tomography (PET): Establishing a baseline for experiments in brain asymmetries and complex sounds in the CNS Project. *J Acoust Soc Am* 1989; 85:S69.
35. Lauter JL, Plante E: Quantitative electroencephalographic (qEEG) correlates of anatomical asymmetries in human auditory cortex; in preparation.
36. Mawhinney RR, Buckley JH, Worthington BS: Magnetic resonance imaging of the cerebellopontine angle. *Br J Radiol* 1986; 59:961–969.
37. Mettler FA Jr, Muroff LR, Kulkarni MV (eds): *Magnetic Resonance Imaging and Spectroscopy*. New York, Churchill Livingstone, 1986.
38. Naatanen R, Picton T: The N1 wave of the human electric and magnetic response to sound: A review and an analysis of the component structure. *Psychophysiology* 1987; 24:375–425.
39. Nuwer MR: Quantitative EEG: II. Frequency

analysis and topographic mapping in clinical settings. *J Clin Neurophysiol* 1988; 5:45–85.

40. Pantev C, Hoke M, Lehnertz K, et al: Identification of sources of brain neuronal activity with high spatiotemporal resolution through combination of neuromagnetic source localization (NMSL) and magnetic resonance imaging (MRI). *Electroencephalogr Clin Neurophysiol* 1990; 75:173–184.
41. Papanicolaou AC, Baumann S, Rogers RL, et al: Localization of auditory response sources using magnetoencephalography and magnetic resonance imaging. *Arch Neurol* 1990; 47:33–37.
42. Perlmutter JS, Powers WJ, Herscovitch P, et al: Regional asymmetries of cerebral blood flow, blood volume, and oxygen utilization and extraction in normal subjects. *J Cereb Blood Flow Metab* 1987; 7:64–67.
43. Plante E: MRI findings in the parents and siblings of specifically language-impaired boys. *Brain Lang* 1991; 41:67–80.
44. Plante E, Swisher L, Vance R: Anatomical correlates of normal and impaired language in a set of dizygotic twins. *Brain Lang* 1989; 37:643–655.
45. Plante E, Swisher L, Vance R, et al: MRI findings in boys with specific language impairment. *Brain Lang* 1991; 41:52–66.
46. Reneau JP, Hnatiow GZ: Evoked response audiometry: A topical and historical review. Baltimore, University Park Press, 1976.
47. Smith ICP: Magnetic resonance spectroscopy in biology and medicine. *Clin Biochem* 1989; 22:69–76.
48. Ter-Pogossian MM, Ficke DC, Mintun MA et al: Dynamic cerebral positron emission tomographic studies. *Ann Neurol* 1984; 15:S46–S47.
49. Van der Poel JC, Jones SJ, Miller DH: Sound lateralization, brainstem auditory evoked potentials and magnetic resonance imaging in multiple sclerosis. *Brain* 1988; 111:1453–1474.
50. Witelson SF: Bumps on the brain: Right-left anatomic asymmetry as a key to functional lateralization, in Segalowitz SJ, Whitaker HA (eds): *Language Functions and Brain Organization*. New York, Academic Press, 1982, pp 117–144.

## APPENDIX 5-1

### Selected Noninvasive Methods for Human Neuroscience

*Magnetic resonance imaging (MRI)* refers to a particular form of magnetic resonance spectroscopy (MRS) focusing on the distribution of hydrogen atoms in a part of the body, such as the brain. The technique depends on certain physical properties of atoms when placed in a strong magnetic field. Its major attractions for human neuroscience are (1) flexibility in data collection parameters such that different tissues can selectively receive different highlighting, e.g., cerebrospinal fluid may be shown as very dark, compared with white-toned white matter, or vice versa; (2) multiple angles of view for visualizing structures at different orientations; and (3) spatial resolution of approximately 1 mm. Magnetic resonance imaging is quite noninvasive, requiring neither radiation nor injected materials, although contrast materials are used in some applications. Risks to the subject are limited to claustrophobia from lying inside the test cylinder, and exposure to the relatively loud pulsing low-frequency noise associated with data collection.

New methods for monitoring brain electrical activity with surface electrodes such as *quantitative electroencephalography (qEEG)* and *repeated evoked potentials (REPs)* combine old and new methodologies. Commercially available systems for qEEG, known as "brain mappers," combine old-style EEG recording with updated computer systems fitted with high-capacity storage, such as optical disks, and software for offline spectral analysis of the collected waveforms. Results of the analysis provide measures such as absolute power and power asymmetry as observed at different electrode locations over the surface of the brain over time, expressed either quantitatively in tables, or qualitatively as color-coded "brain maps." Attractions for human neuroscience include (1) "real-time" versions of brain activity (as opposed to the time-locked variants required in evoked potentials); and (2) ease of contrasting the electrical topography of the brain during resting vs. a variety of activation conditions.

*Repeated evoked potentials (REPs)* refers to a family of protocols based on standard methods for collecting evoked potentials, developed by Lauter and colleagues.[27–31, 33] The crucial departure from conventional EP practice is use of a within-subject, repeated-measures design, such that several waveforms are collected under each condition and the results are analyzed not only in terms of absolute values of peak characteristics such as latency and amplitude, but also in terms of the stability of these values. The attractions of this method derive from the dramatic increase in sensitivity compared with conventional methods, including documentation of clear individual differences even in normal subjects, and ear differences. Greater sensitivity renders the test useful for studying details of auditory CNS function in normal subjects, as well as for evaluating brain stem integrity in a range of patient groups, from individuals presenting with auditory CNS pathology to a variety of neurological populations.[20, 22, 32]

Since the subject interface for both qEEG and REPs is limited to application of electrodes, both techniques are considered to be quite noninvasive and show excellent subject acceptance.

*Magnetoencephalography* is a method by which tiny magnetic fields generated as a side-effect of brain electrical activity may be monitored at the surface of the scalp. The data-collection device is referred to as a superconducting quantum interference device (SQUID), and works via superconducting transducers housed in a cylindrical "dewar" which is placed against the scalp overlying the part of the brain of interest. Testing procedures are borrowed from scalp-recorded electrophysiology and include both collection of resting magnetic field topography, as well as "evoked fields," for which changes in field strength and polarity are time-locked to a stimulus and averaged over time. Attractions for human neuroscience include (1) high degree of noninvasivity, since not even electrodes are required; and (2) fine spatial resolution, of approximately 1 mm, since none of the conduction artifacts associated with EEG are involved. The few channels on the systems available through the 1980's necessitated laborious data-collection, requiring great patience on the part of subject and experimenter; new many-channel machines should redress this single disadvantage of the technique.

*Positron emission tomography (PET)* refers to a form of autoradiography in which positron-emitting isotopes of different substances (such as Fluorine, Carbon, and Oxygen) are administered to a subject either via inhalation or injection, and their process of decay is monitored from outside the body. On current devices, spatial resolution is approximately 5 mm, while temporal resolution is largely dependent on the half-life of the isotope used; for example, with $^{15}O$, a complete three-dimensional scan of the entire cranial central nervous system can be completed in as little as 40 seconds. The short exposure time reduces dosage to the subject, and enables experimental designs in which each subject is used as her/his own control, and a typical session contrasts responses during resting and a variety of contrasting activation conditions. The advantages of PET for human neuroscience include (1) three-dimensional simultaneous physiological detail; (2) excellent spatial and temporal resolution; (3) ease of comparing physiological topography at various levels of the brain during both resting and activation conditions. For students of the auditory system, the combination of the "vertical" organization of the auditory CNS with PET's three-dimensional capability makes it possible to visualize simultaneous reactions in several auditory nuclei during the same stimulation condition. Risk of PET procedures to the subject includes a small amount of radioactivity, no more than 640 mCi during an eight-condition session. Arterial blood sampling, considered a greater risk than the minimal radioactivity, is typically no longer done for studies of normal function.

# PART III

# BASIC CONSIDERATIONS

Chapter 6

# Classification of Auditory Processing Disorders

Jack Katz, Ph.D.

Auditory processing disorders have been difficult to conceptualize, both for those who appreciate their importance and even more so for those who are convinced that speech requires little processing to be understood. A need to have a better understanding of what constitutes our major auditory processing faculties led to the work reported here. Clinicians often express frustration in relating central auditory test findings to the myriad of academic, communicative, and behavioral problems of the client. While they find the work to be useful in aiding children and adults with their problems, they do not understand why their tests are sensitive to those with disorders of reading, spelling, speech, and language. Furthermore, professionals may not know how to group the test findings and disorders to make useful applications of their results. Importantly, without a reasonable theoretical base, we do not know how to improve our tests or how to design better management strategies.

In 1985 I tried out a categorization scheme for central auditory processing disorders (CAPDs). The framework for understanding central auditory processing (CAP) was established based on Staggered Spondaic Word (SSW) test signs and 30 years of work with those who have CAPD. The SSW test is a well known, standard procedure for studying central auditory nervous system (CANS) disorders and CAPD.[2]

A student was asked to randomly go through the files to find examples of children who were referred for CAPD and who had certain signs on the SSW. If they *did not* have the presumed problems in academic and communicative activities and if the CAP test results *did not* cluster as predicted, this would have ended this line of reasoning; however, because the results were on target for the most part, the attempt to categorize CAPD went forward. Two studies were carried out to try to validate the three category system. Each of the studies provided us with new associations and concepts and suggested a fourth category and a subcategory. These will be discussed later in this paper.

## STAGGERED SPONDAIC WORD TEST FINDINGS—THE BASIS OF THE CATEGORY SYSTEM

The SSW test, a 10-minute procedure, has been in use by audiologists for many years.[10] It was originally employed to study site-of-lesion in adults with tumors and strokes. Later on, when interest turned to CAPD in learning-disabled children, the test was pressed into service to identify auditory processing disorders.[16, 26] Some of the signs that were noted on the SSW test in brain-damaged adults were also found in the results of learning-disabled children. This provided a potential opportunity to relate the auditory processing disabilities of learning-disabled children to an anatomical-physiological model based on the work with patients with brain lesions. In this way the aberrant behaviors noted in a client or in a group of subjects could be analyzed to see if they corresponded to limitations associated with a specific cerebral region. While this model in no way suggests that the CAPD was caused by brain damage, abnormal test results could represent slower development or different patterns of neural operation in the associated region (or in other regions that might be responsible for these behaviors). An effective model would then permit us to predict related problems and to understand better how to deal with the deficits.

In the SSW test, different words are presented to the two ears in a partially overlapped fashion through earphones. Each item is introduced by the question, "Are you ready?" Figure 6–1 shows the first two items of the test. The first item starts in the right ear and ends in the left (a right-ear–first or REF presentation), the second is routed the opposite way (a left-ear–first or LEF presentation). In each case the first word is noncompeting (i.e., there is no competing word in the other ear), the second and third words compete with one another in opposite ears, and then the final noncompeting word is presented to the second ear. The basic analysis is based on performance on the four SSW conditions: (1) right noncompeting (RNC), (2) right competing (RC), (3) left competing (LC), and (4) left noncompeting (LNC). More complete descriptions of the SSW test are available in the literature.[2,11,21]

The number of errors for the four REF words and the four LEF words can be scored and analyzed separately to provide somewhat different information about the person's site-of-lesion and/or auditory processing deficits. Figure 6–2 shows eight columns representing REF and LEF words. These eight "cardinal numbers" can be combined to provide the percentage of error for the RNC, RC, LC, and LNC conditions; e.g., combining columns A and H will give the RNC errors. In addition, we can combine them in other ways. For example, we can combine the first two REF conditions (columns A + B) with the first two LEF conditions (E + F) to see how the person performs at the beginnings of items compared to the performance at the ends of items (columns C + D + G + H). This comparison is referred to as order effect. If there are significantly more errors at the end of the items than the beginning, then this is called an order effect low/high. On the other hand if there are significantly more errors at the beginning, this is called an order effect high/low.

Order effects, ear effects, and type A patterns are referred to as response biases. These are specific error patterns that are calculated from the eight cardinal numbers. Reversals are also a form of response bias, but they are not based on the eight cardinal numbers.

| | | TIME SEQUENCE | | |
|---|---|---|---|---|
| | | 1 | 2 | 3 |
| A | RIGHT EAR | up | stairs | |
| | LEFT EAR | | down | town |

| | | TIME SEQUENCE | | |
|---|---|---|---|---|
| | | 1 | 2 | 3 |
| B | LEFT EAR | out | side | |
| | RIGHT EAR | | in | law |

**FIG 6–1.**
The first two items of the SSW test. **A,** first item, which begins in the right ear (REF) and ends in the left. The words in time sequence No. 2 compete with one another in opposite ears. **B,** second item, which follows the same general format as the first item except that the words begin in the left ear (LEF).

## Order Effect

If the number of errors on the second halves of test items exceeds the number of errors on the first halves by five (in adults) then this constitutes a significant order effect low/high. This finding in patients with brain lesions is associated with involvement of the posterior temporal region[12] (i.e., Heschl's gyrus and the auditory cortex). Functionally, this region appears to provide for phonemic decoding[22] and is involved in receptive language functions.[24] In the initial studies, when there was an order effect low/high (or other SSW signs that are associated with this region, e.g., ear effect H/L), we made an assumption that this represented poor or slow phonemic decoding. For

| Right First | R-NC | R-C | L-C | L-NC |
|---|---|---|---|---|
| 1. | up | stairs | down | town |
| 3. | day | light | lunch | time |
| 39. | race | horse | street | car |
| TOTAL | 1 | 6 | 4 | 2 |
| | | (CARDINAL NUMBERS) | | |
| Right First | (A) R-NC | (B) R-C | (C) L-C | (D) L-NC |

| | L-NC | L-C | R-C | R-NC |
|---|---|---|---|---|
| 2. | out | side | in | low |
| 4. | wash | tub | black | board |
| 40. | green | house | string | bean |
| TOTAL | 1 | 5 | 8 | 2 |
| | | (CARDINAL NUMBERS) | | |
| | (E) L-NC | (F) L-C | (G) R-C | (H) R-NC |

**FIG 6–2.**
Portions of the scoring form, including some of the earlier and later items. Odd-numbered items are REF and even-numbered items LEF. **Columns A–D** represent REF items starting with the right noncompeting (RNC) condition. Total errors are shown at the bottom for half of the RNC words in column A. **Columns E–H** show the LEF results, starting with the left noncompeting (LNC) condition. The errors in columns A–H constitute the eight cardinal numbers from which most of the SSW calculations are made.

purposes of simplicity we will discuss order effect only, instead of both order and ear effects.

The opposite error pattern, the order effect high/low is associated with the anterior half of the brain.[12] Damage to the frontal and anterior temporal lobes is generally accompanied by expressive language, memory, or behavior problems.[9, 25] One way to think about the order effect high/low is that the person has more difficulty in remembering the first spondee than remembering the second spondee (i.e., a fading memory effect). Efron and his colleagues[5] point out that the anterior temporal region is associated with auditory figure-ground function (referred to here as speech-in-noise). Thus, my assumption was that the order effect high/low and other SSW signs (e.g., ear effect low/high), implicating this region would be considered as probable evidence of speech-in-noise and/or fading memory disabilities.

### Type A Pattern

The type A pattern on the SSW is based on the eight cardinal numbers. When column F (or B) is much poorer than the others (the specific criteria are age related[14]), this may be considered a type A pattern (Fig 6–3). This pattern of errors has been found quite frequently in patients with classic dyslexia, that is, those with severe reading and spelling dysfunction. In these cases diagnostic tests have often implicated the temporal-parietal-occipital (angular gyrus) region or possibly the posterior portion of the corpus callosum. Both of these regions are known to be important for reading and spelling.[3, 27] Furthermore, we have found the type A pattern in one third of the cases with verified corpus callosum tumors. Because of the close association of the type A region with severe reading and spelling disorders we initially considered this pattern as a sign of severe auditory-visual integration deficit.

### Reversals

The fourth SSW sign, reversals, was not part of the original sampling because it was not clear whether this peculiarity represented a category that could stand by itself or whether reversals were a general finding in CAPD cases (not anatomically specific). A reversal on the SSW is a response in which the word order of an item is changed (and there is no more than one error on the item). For example, if the person says "downtown, upstairs" for "upstairs, downtown" this would be a reversal. Both Luria[23] and Efron[4] have discussed sequencing problems in brain damaged populations. They have associated this characteristic with midportions of the cerebrum (the frontal-temporal-parietal and premotor regions). On the SSW, in brain lesion cases with significant reversals, the suspected region encompasses both of the above regions as well as the rolandic region in the frontoparietal area.[17]

## TEST BATTERY

In an ongoing study[18] the two order effects, the type A pattern, and significant reversals on the SSW test served as the criteria for the cate-

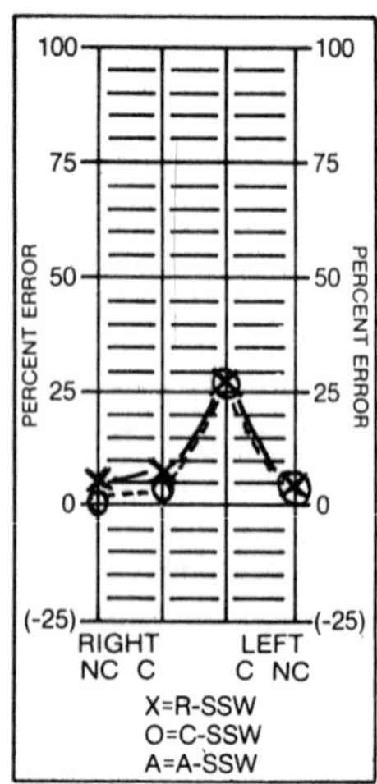


| TOTAL | 1 | 2 | 1 | 0 | | TOTAL | 2 | 10 | 1 | 1 |
|---|---|---|---|---|---|---|---|---|---|---|
| | | (CARDINAL NUMBERS) | | | | | | (CARDINAL NUMBERS) | | |
| Right First | Ⓐ R-NC | Ⓑ R-C | Ⓒ L-C | Ⓓ L-NC | | | Ⓔ L-NC | Ⓕ L-C | Ⓖ R-C | Ⓗ R-NC |

**FIG 6–3.**
SSW-gram of a case with a type A SSW pattern. It is usually seen as a rather sharp peak of errors in the left competing (LC) condition. The eight cardinal numbers that are combined to produce these values are shown in the form below. The totals for the four conditions are multiplied by 2.5 to obtain the R-SSW scores (percent error). When these values are corrected for the percentage of error on the standard discrimination test, the C-SSW scores result. Sometimes when a sharp peak of errors is noted, the values may not quite meet the criteria for type A. Especially in young children, we would be inclined to consider the prominent LC as evidence of a potential type A.

gory system. From this point of departure we were able to further elaborate on the central test findings, academic difficulties, speech and language problems as well as the common behaviors that were closely associated with each category. It should be emphasized that the categories are not mutually exclusive. In at least half of patients with auditory processing problems we find evidence of two or three categories of dysfunction operating when using just three tests of central function.

Three tests that we have used (in various forms) over the past 25 years provide the information needed to categorize CAP problems. In addition to the SSW test, we use the Phonemic Synthesis (PS) test and a speech-in-noise task.

The PS (DLM, Allen, Texas) is a recorded test in which words are presented sound by sound at a comfortably loud level, usually at about 50 dB above threshold. Familiar monosyllabic words make up the test items. For example, /n-o-z/, which is presented with lengthened sounds and long pauses, requires (1) discrimination of the speech sounds, (2) retention of these images, and (3) synthesis of the sounds into words while maintaining the proper sequence.[13] As in the case of the SSW test we can gather further information by noting reversals and delayed or quick responses.

The speech-in-noise task, as applied at the University at Buffalo Speech and Hearing Clinic, is a monaural procedure using the Hirsh W-22 recording (Technisonic Studios, St. Louis) at 40 dB SL with ipsilateral competing speech spectrum noise at 30 dB SL. Each ear is tested separately.

The four categories, which were derived from the four SSW signs, will be discussed below. For each category we will consider the fundamental processing difficulty, the related academic, communicative, and behavior problems, as well as the diagnostic signs that are generally found (in some combination) in these cases.

## DECODING CATEGORY

The decoding category attempts to isolate auditory processing that breaks down at the phonemic level. One might speculate that the problem is one of vague engrams (mental concepts) of some of the phonemes. Often adults with this problem tell us how surprised they are to find out that "this is what the T-sound (or L-sound) sounds like." Because of this vague notion, we presume that it takes these persons longer to process speech because they are not always clear about what they have heard. Without extra time to resolve their uncertainty they would appear confused and frustrated or demonstrate errors in discrimination. In addition, they would be deficient in remembering phonemes and manipulating them (e.g., on tasks such as reading, spelling, and phonics as well as phonemic synthesis or analysis).

We have found those who show audiometric signs of poor decoding generally have difficulty in reading and spelling skills that depend on phonics. It is especially noticeable when the person reads aloud. Spelling is often very challenging for them because they hear a word and must figure out from the sounds how to spell it. Poor decoders are aided if they have good visual memory.

Children who are poor phonemic decoders are often found to have articulatory errors involving the /r/ and /l/ sounds. The /l/, which can be learned from a placement approach, generally clears up quickly in speech therapy, but the /r/, which is highly dependent on good auditory skills, often remains misarticulated. It is not surprising that those with poor decoding skills perform poorly on receptive language tests. When an individual is working hard simply to keep up with the flow of sounds in normal communication, it is likely that an unfamiliar word or atypical phrasing will throw him or her off. Rapid speech or other challenges may result in confusion of otherwise simple verbal concepts.

One can consider decoding problems from an anatomical-physiological standpoint as well. Figure 6–4 shows that the posterior temporal region is associated with decoding dysfunction.[23] This region also constitutes a major portion of Wernicke's area, which serves receptive language functions.

Some of the SSW decoding signs, which are associated with involvement of the area shown in Figure 6–4, are significant errors on the RC and LNC conditions and order effect low/high. The depressed performance on the RC condition is interesting. In the brain-damaged population we would take poor RC performance to be evidence of left posterior temporal impairment. If the left hemisphere is executive for interpreting speech phonemes, then we might infer that a significant RC error peak in those with CAPD represents a deficit involving the phonemic area of the left posterior temporal lobe (or Wernicke's area).

Not surprising, poor decoders often have significant delays on the SSW and other tests that require rapid processing. When presented with individual speech sounds on the PS test, they are often unable to respond with the blended word. Sometimes only the individual sounds are repeated back. This "nonfused" response is a useful (but not exclusive) clue for classifying decoding cases.

**DECODING CATEGORY**

Limitation: Utilizing Phonemic Information

**SSW Test Signs of Decoding Category in Brain Damaged Subjects is Associated with Region of Brain Shown Below:**

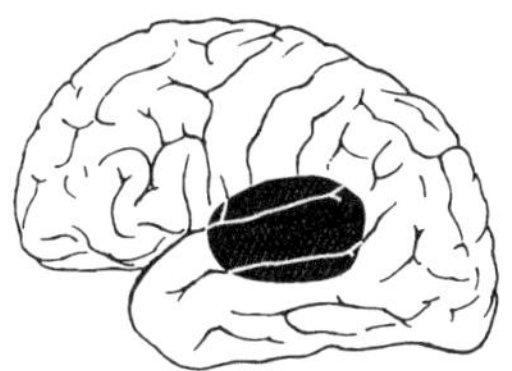

**Associated Problems**

Reading (phonics and difficulty sounding out word), spelling, receptive language and articulation

**Remedial Approaches to AP Problem**

Improve knowledge of phonemes of the language. Can use commercial programs such as Phonemic Synthesis (DLM) and Auditory Discrimination in Depth (ADD) (DLM) or sound blending

**FIG 6–4.**
Summary of the decoding category.

## TOLERANCE-FADING MEMORY (TFM) CATEGORY

The TFM category focuses on two symptoms that are often found together. We know of no functional bond between poor auditory memory and poor figure-ground skills. However, in about 75% of the TFM cases, both deficits are present. Perhaps an anatomical-physiological model (Fig 6–5) may suggest why difficulty understanding speech in a background of noise and a rapidly fading memory are characteristics that are often found together.

One explanation is that the anterior temporal region contains both the hippocampus and amygdala, important organs associated with memory.[6, 8] A damaged anterior temporal region is also associated with auditory figure-ground dysfunction.[5]

Other limitations are also associated with damage to the frontal lobes. In a recent study, animals that had lesions of the frontal lobes were unable to perform different responses when either

**TOLERANCE- FADING MEMORY (TFM) CATEGORY**

Limitation: Listening in noise and generally short term memory

**SSW Test Signs of TFM Category in Brain Damaged Subjects is Associated with Region Shown Below:**

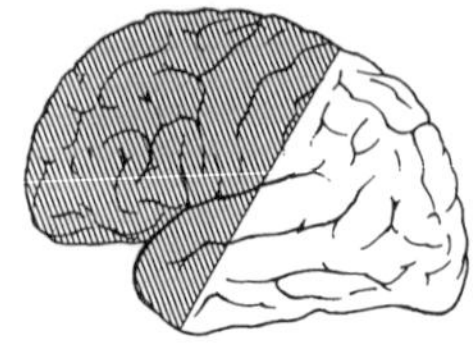

**Associated Problems**

Reading comprehension, expressive language, handwriting, easily distracted, fearful

**Remedial Approaches to AP Problem**

Speech-in-noise desensitization (gradually increasing tolerance), also commercially available programs such as Listening to the World (AGC) and Auditory Perception Training-Auditory Figure-Ground (DLM), use of assistive listening device

**FIG 6–5.**
Summary of the tolerance-fading memory (TFM) category.

of two stimuli were presented to them. Nevertheless, they were able to perform normally if a single stimulus was employed requiring a single response.[25] The inability to act differentially to different stimuli may not seem to be related to the speech-in-noise task, however; when listening in noise, one must deal with one auditory signal and ignore the others. Children with speech-in-noise problems seem to be as attentive to background noise as they are to the foreground speech; that is, they seem to respond the same way to both the foreground and background instead of differentially.

Not surprisingly, the subjects who have TFM problems have reading comprehension difficulties. While they can generally sound out words and know what the words mean, when they have finished reading a paragraph or a short story they are unable to tell what they have read. Perhaps their poor memories or their high levels of distractability can account for their limitation in reading comprehension. Figure 6–5 summarizes the TFM category.

Many children with TFM have expressive problems: they have trouble making themselves understood orally and in written form and they often have poor handwriting that tends to be sloppy and poorly planned. The anatomical-physiological model may help to explain these results. Expressive language is associated with the inferior frontal region (e.g., Broca's area). In addition, the posterior frontal region is important for motor programming (e.g., for writing and articulatory movements); thus, dysfunction associated with this portion of the TFM region might further limit the effectiveness of expression.

We have often observed people in this group respond quickly to SSW and PS items. This is not surprising given their rapidly fading memories. When we consider that damage to the frontal region of the brain may produce difficulty in responding to one part of a message without responding to all other parts, this could help explain why there is a tendency for patients with TFM to respond to the "Are you ready?" which precedes the item, even though they know that it should not be repeated or answered. "Tongue-twisters" are responses that we also see in this group (e.g., "chee chain" for "key chain"). These may be associated with poor motor programming.

## INTEGRATION CATEGORY

At the present time we do not have as much information about this category and about the following one as we do about the two previous categories. The marker that we used initially to identify this group was the type A SSW pattern. This pattern generally identified a group of severely learning-disabled individuals. However, from the early category studies it became clear that, unlike the other groups, the integration cases were not as homogeneous. Some cases varied markedly in their central test results from those who had severe scholastic problems. For example, type A patients had among the poorest and among the best PS scores, and some in the group had quite normal speech-in-noise performance while others had very poor performance. Because of the variations within the integration group, it was necessary to divide it into two types.

Later we expanded our criteria for the integration group. We accepted sharp peaks of errors in the LC condition as indicative of potential type A cases who had not matured sufficiently to show the type A pattern. This decision was based on the finding that the type A pattern is not seen in 6-year-old children who have overall poor SSW performance. When the children get older the type A pattern can show up as other limitations (even those that are quite normal for their age) are resolved.

Behaviorally, patients with integration disabilities seem to display difficulty in bringing information together. For example, auditory-visual integration was one of the first deficits that we noted. Other problems were then observed that suggested additional types of impaired integration. Some individuals appeared to show a lack of connection between their emotional affect and their speech and some required very long periods of time to answer questions. Interestingly, despite the inordinately long delays, they showed no apparent struggle in getting the correct answers and generally spoke them matter-of-factly.

While patients with both types 1 and 2 of integration disabilities demonstrate type A patterns, or at least show sharp peaks of errors in the LC condition on the SSW graph, other characteristics differ. For the most part the type 1 cases resemble the decoding group in their test scores and in their classroom difficulties, while the type 2 cases are much like the TFM group in these respects.

## Integration Type 1

Patients with the type 1 integration disabilities have the classic pattern of severe reading and spelling problems. They are so impaired in these skills that they are often considered dyslexics. These patients display evidence of poor phonemic knowledge (e.g., extreme difficulty in phonics). Furthermore, the type 1 group appears to have severe problems both in auditory and visual perception. Their drawings of geometric shapes generally show poor form and the angle may be rotated. Left-right orientation problems (e.g., writing "b" for "d") are often seen. We have noted that some of these people have better skills in cursive than in printed writing. Figure 6–6 summarizes the integration type 1 category.

**INTEGRATION CATEGORY TYPE 1**

Limitation: Combining auditory and visual information

**SSW Test Signs of Integration (Type 1) Category in Brain Damaged Subjects is Associated with the region shown Below:**

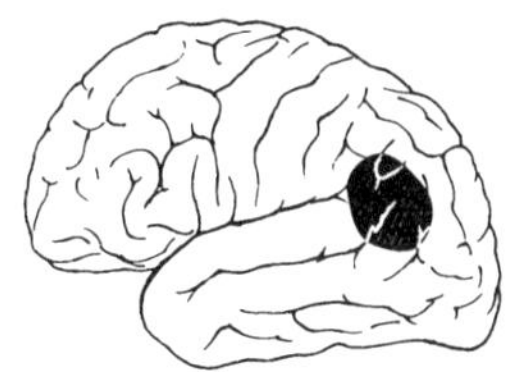

**Associated Problems for Type 1**

Severe reading and spelling disability, extremely poor handwriting (person sometimes labeled dyslexic)

**Remedial Approaches for Type 1**

Strengthen phonemic knowledge. Can use commercial programs Phonemic Synthesis (DLM) or Auditory Discrimination in Depth (ADD) (DLM) or sound-symbol training

**FIG 6–6.**
Summary of the integration type 1 category. Insufficient information is available at this time to include a chart on integration type 2.

Type A patterns are not well localized in any one part of the brain. Perhaps this explains why we see so much diversity in the behaviors of CAP patients who have type A patterns. For example, this finding was common among patients with corpus callosum lesions.[15] One third of our patients with confirmed corpus callosum tumors had type A patterns. Other type A cases were brain-damaged persons who were diagnosed as dyslexics and had abnormalities suggesting involvement of the parieto-occipital region. These facts are important for our model because the posterior corpus callosum and the angular gyrus of the parieto-occipital region, with which it is associated, are closely linked to dyslexia.[1,3,27] Because of the linkage of these regions with dyslexia in brain lesion cases, for purposes of this model we considered one or both of these areas to be impaired in the type 1 cases.

Other than the type A patterns or the sharp LC peaks, the type 1 patients perform much like the poor decoders on central tests. For example, they have depressed scores in PS and often demonstrate nonfused responses. Their speech-in-noise scores vary from individual to individual; however, they are not severely depressed and on occasion, unlike poor decoders, they may be quite good in blocking out background noise.

Perhaps it is worth mentioning that there may be a subgroup of integration type 1 patients who have spelling problems, but are satisfactory in their reading ability.[19] This may be akin to cases of agraphia without alexia, or vice versa.[1] Children with this condition may not be seen by professionals because many school districts do not consider an academic problem limited to spelling to be a learning disability.

### Integration Type 2

Persons who are classified as integration type 2 differ importantly from the type 1 cases in that they often have less difficulty in school subjects and they may not display auditory-visual integration problems. These patients often have sloppy handwriting unless great care is taken. As in the case of the TFM group, such problems may be associated with poor motor planning skills. It is not the severe writing impairment that is seen in type 1 cases. Type 2 cases sometimes are mistakenly thought to have nonorganic problems because they may respond more poorly to faint (and sometimes not so faint) tones than to faint speech. These children may appear willful or possibly "nonorganic."

Behavior in type 2 cases may be associated with dysfunction of the anterior region of the brain. In addition, because the type A pattern is closely associated with commissural pathways, we could suggest that the anterior portion of the corpus callosum and/or the anterior commissure are the probable sites of this problem.

Some extreme delays on central tests are not uncommon in this subgroup. In this respect they resemble the type 1 cases. However, their speech-in-noise scores are generally quite poor with good performance on the PS test. Because we have found relatively few type 2 cases, much remains to be learned about them and how they might differ from TFM and integration type 1 cases.

## ORGANIZATION CATEGORY

We have by far the least amount of information about the organization CAP category because we have identified relatively few pure cases, and have only recently begun studying this group. The two identifying test characteristics are significant word reversals on the SSW and speech sound reversals on the PS test. Lucker[20] made an excellent observation when he reported that those who have reversals on the SSW tend to be disorganized. Logically, a person who has difficulty maintaining a proper sequence (without compensating by using great effort or attention) is likely to follow confused or inefficient paths (much like certain professors do). At the present time we are trying to find out what communicative, behavioral, and academic characteristics may be associated with the organization group. Our current information on the organization category is tentatively suggested in Figure 6–7.

**ORGANIZATION CATEGORY**

Limitation: Maintaining sequence and organizing information

**SSW Test Signs of Organization Category in Brain Damaged Subjects is Associated with Region Shown Below:**

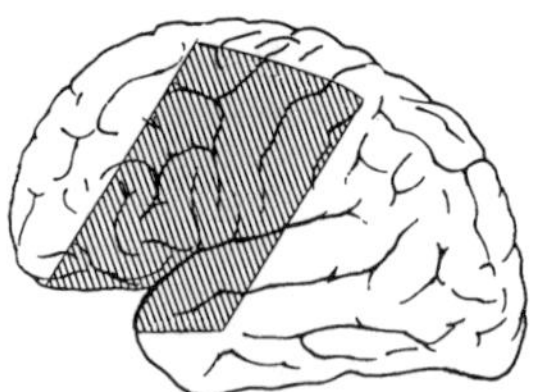

**Associated Problems**

Disorganized at school and at home, reversals in spelling and in reading, poor handwriting

**Remedial Approaches**

Sequencing activities, written outlines and lists

**FIG 6–7.**
This chart summarizes the information about the organization category.

For purposes of our model, the work on sequencing problems by Efron[4] and Luria[23] provides a suitable anatomical region as the suspected area of disability. This is the same general region that has been associated with SSW reversals (see Fig 6–7). The region of the "reversal strip" may be seen to overlap part of the TFM region and is immediately adjacent to the decoding area. Therefore, we should not be surprised to find considerable overlap of the organization group with these other two categories.

## DISTRIBUTION OF CENTRAL AUDITORY PROCESSING DISORDER CATEGORIES IN LEARNING-DISABLED CHILDREN

Katz and co-workers[18] tested a group of 94 children, 6 to 12 years of age (mean = 8.8 years). The children were referred because of concern about a CAP disorder, usually associated with learning problems. They had to demonstrate both normal hearing in the speech frequencies (500, 1,000, and 2,000 Hz) and normal tympanograms (or patent ventilation tubes) at the time of test. The study included a central test battery (SSW, PS, and speech-in-noise tests) as well as two questionnaires (i.e., one for the parent and one for the classroom teacher). We have begun to evaluate the results and can report on some of the basic information.

First a brief description of the sample. The subjects were evaluated primarily at three centers by audiologists experienced in central auditory testing. The three settings and locations were (1) a community speech and hearing center in the greater Buffalo area; (2) a rehabilitation center in St. Catherine's, Ontario; and (3) a large medical center in Princeton, N.J.

The sample was made up of 35% females and 65% males, which represents about two-thirds males. This is a typical sex ratio in learning disabled populations. All of the subjects had thresholds of <20 dB HL (ANSI-1969) with speech frequency averages of 7 dB in the right ear and 6 dB in the left. Discrimination scores ranged from 68% to 100% with averages for the right and left ears of 94% and 93%, respectively. Ninety subjects had normal tympanograms bilaterally, while the remaining four had patent ventilation tubes.

The subjects were first classified as either normal-CAP or not normal, based on the central auditory test results. If the results were not normal, their primary (most dominant) category of dysfunction was assessed. Complete agreement among three investigators was generally obtained. When there was not complete agreement then the majority decided the category. Following the assessment of the primary category, the secondary category was considered in the same way and finally the tertiary category.

Figure 6–8 shows the percentage of subjects assigned to each of the primary categories (decoding, TFM, integration type 1, integration type 2, or organization). If the results were not clearly supportive of any category, then the subject was classified as "other."

The data gave us some surprises. We were impressed that only one child (1%) out of the 94 subjects passed each of the tests both quantitatively and qualitatively. The major surprise was

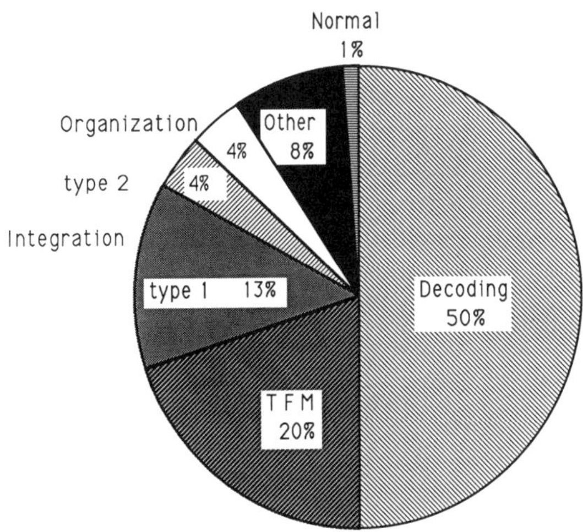


**FIG 6–8.**
This chart shows the percentage of 94 learning-disabled children who were classified into the four categories. The integration group was divided into the type 1 and type 2 cases. Children who had significant findings on CAP tests but could not be classified into one of the four categories were placed in the "other" group. One child performed normally on all of the CAP tests and was therefore placed in the "normal" group.

that 50% of the group showed evidence of a primary decoding disorder. We had anticipated that TFM would be the most common area of dysfunction judging from our informal impressions. It will be interesting to see if the decoding category remains the major one when we undertake our second sample of cases.

The second most frequent category of dysfunction was TFM. Twenty percent of the subjects were so classified as having this primary CAP problem. A total of 17% of the sample was classified as having an integration problem as the primary area. As expected, type 1 was the more common subcategory of the integration group (13% of the total sample) with only 4% in the type 2 subgroup. A scant 4% of the sample had organization as their primary category. The remaining 8% of the sample could not be classified as having any one of the four categories of dysfunction and therefore were placed in the Other group. Generally speaking these were subjects who had relatively few abnormal CAP test results and the signs did not support any problem in particular.

In 52% of the cases there was sufficient difficulty in two or more CAP areas that a secondary category was agreed upon. TFM was the most common of these with 26% of the total sample. Poor decoding was judged to be present in 16% and organizational difficulty specified in 10%. Only 5% of the 94 subjects were judged to have a third area of deficit. For the tertiary category, 4% of the total group was classified as having an organization problem and 1% had TFM.

Table 6-1 summarizes the results of the categorization phase of our research. It is clear that decoding and TFM represented the most frequent categories. When we studied the data further we found that if a child had difficulties in more than one significant category (in 52% of these cases) it involved both decoding and TFM. Decoding and organization problem combinations came in second with 19%. In each of the five cases in which there were three significant categories, the catego ries were decoding, TFM and organization (not necessarily in that order).

In our study we found 91% of the subjects could be classified as having one of the four categories as their primary problem. Eight percent with some CAP deficit could not be classified specifically and one subject was considered to have normal CAP functions. Half of the subjects had a second significant area of deficit and a small percentage had three problem areas. With regard to management, we found that once the underlying problems were identified, it was not difficult to develop remedial strategies. Of the four categories, we have found the decoding problem to be the easiest auditory deficit to remediate.

## SUMMARY

The purpose of this chapter is to propose a categorical system to classify and account for behaviors that are seen in people who have CAP problems. SSW indicators, based on the results of site-of-lesion studies, permitted us to divide up learning disabled cases into a number of CAP categories. The behaviors that we found in children

**TABLE 6-1.**
Evidence of CAP Categories in 94 Children Referred for CAP Evaluation*

| Category | Primary | Secondary | Tertiary | Total |
|---|---|---|---|---|
| Decoding | 50 | 16 | 0 | 66 |
| TFM | 20 | 26 | 1 | 47 |
| Organization | 4 | 10 | 4 | 18 |
| Integration | | | | 17 |
| Type 1 | 13 | 0 | 0 | (13) |
| Type 2 | 4 | 0 | 0 | (4) |
| Other | 8 | 0 | 0 | 8 |
| Normal | | | | 1 |
| | 99 | 52 | 5 | 157 |

*Percentage of children classified as having one of the CAP dysfunction categories as their primary, secondary, or tertiary problem. One child was entirely normal.

with CAPD generally corresponded with the expected findings in speech, language, and academic subjects, based on the anatomical model.

Four major categories—decoding, tolerance-fading memory, integration, and organization—were identified in a total of 91% of the children in the sample. The most frequently noted deficit was that of phonemic decoding, followed by tolerance-fading memory dysfunction.

The proposed system appears to be useful in classifying the vast majority of learning-disabled subjects when three CAP tests (SSW, PS, and speech-in-noise) were used. The categorization has been helpful in understanding the underlying problems presented by our clients. In addition, knowledge of the categories has aided us in planning remedial approaches.

The category system has been used successfully for the past five years by a number of audiologists. However, more needs to be learned about them and their subcategories. In addition, wider clinical validation must be undertaken to be sure that the method holds up in a variety of clinical settings.

## REFERENCES

1. Ajax E, Schenkenberg T, Kosteljanetz M: Alexia without agraphia and the inferior splenium. *Neurology* 1977; 27:685–688.
2. Arnst D, Katz J: The SSW test: Development and clinical use. San Diego, College-Hill Press, 1982.
3. Damasio A, Damasio H: The anatomic basis of pure alexia. *Neurology* 1983; 33:1573–1583.
4. Efron R: Temporal perception, aphasia, deja vu, in Mishelevich DJ, Chase RA (eds): *Interdisciplinary Seminar Program, Temporal Lobe Function in Man. II. Language and Speech, Part 2*. Baltimore, Neurocommunications Laboratory, Department of Psychiatry, Johns Hopkins University School of Medicine, 1965.
5. Efron RP, Crandell P, Koss B, et al: Central auditory processing. III. The "cocktail party" effect and temporal lobectomy. *Brain Lang* 1983; 19:254–263.
6. Ellis M: Amygdala norepinephrine involved in two separate long-term retrieval processes. *Brain Res* 1985; 2:126–136.
7. Fuster J: *The Prefrontal Cortex*. New York, Raven Press, 1980.
8. Isaacson R, Pribram K: *The Hippocampus,* vol 4. New York, Plenum Press, 1986.
9. Ivnik R, Scharbough F, Laws E: Effects of anterior temporal lobectomy on cognitive functions. *J Clin Psychol* 1987; 43:128–137.
10. Katz J: The use of staggered spondaic words for assessing the integrity of the central auditory nervous system. *J Aud Res* 1962; 2:327–337.
11. Katz J: The SSW test: An interim report. *J Speech Hear Disord* 1968; 33:132–146.
12. Katz J: *SSW Workshop Manual*. Buffalo, NY, Allentown Industries, 1978.
13. Katz J: Phonemic synthesis, in Lasky EZ, Katz J (eds): *Central Auditory Processing Disorders: Problems of Speech, Language and Learning*. Austin, Tex, Pro-Ed, 1983, pp 269–295.
14. Katz J: *The SSW Test Manual,* ed 3. Vancouver, Wash, Precision Acoustics, 1986.
15. Katz J, Avellanosa AA, Aguilar-Markulis NV: Evaluation of corpus callosum tumors using SSW, CES and PICA. Paper presented at American Speech-Language Hearing Association convention, Detroit, 1980.
16. Katz J, Illmer R: Auditory perception in children with learning disabilities, in Katz J (ed): *Handbook of Clinical Audiology*. Baltimore, Williams & Wilkins, 1972, pp 540–563.
17. Katz J, Pack G: New developments in differential diagnosis using the SSW test, in Sullivan M (ed): *Central Auditory Processing Disorders*. Omaha, University of Nebraska Press, 1975, pp 84–107.
18. Katz J, Smith PS, Kurpita B, et al: Categorizing test findings in children referred for auditory processing deficits. *SSW Rep* 1992; 14:1–6.
19. Lucker JR: Diagnostic significance of the type A pattern of the staggered spondaic word (SSW) test. *Audiol Hear Educ* 1980; 6:21–23.
20. Lucker JR: Interpreting SSW results of learning disabled children. *SSW News* 1981; 3:1–3.
21. Lukas RA, Lukas JG: Spondaic word procedures, in Katz J (ed): *Handbook of Clinical Audiology,* ed 3. Baltimore, Williams & Wilkins, 1985, pp 383–396.
22. Luria AR: *Higher Cortical Functions in Man*. New York, Basic Books, 1966, pp 103–113.
23. Luria AR: *Traumatic Aphasia*. The Hague, Mouton, 1977, pp 176–178.
24. Penfield W, Roberts L: *Speech and Brain Mechanisms*. Princeton, NJ, Princeton University Press, 1959, pp 119–137.
25. Struss D, Benson F: Neuropsychological studies of the frontal lobes. *Psychol Bull* 1984; 95:3–25.
26. Stubblefield JH, Young CE: Central auditory dysfunction in learning disabled children. *J Learn Disabil* 1975; 8:32–37.
27. Weisberg L, Wall M: Alexia without agraphia: Clinical-computed tomography correlation. *Neuroradiology* 1987; 29:283–286.

# CHAPTER 7

# Auditory Processing of Speech

**Ray D. Kent, Ph.D.**

The poetic phrase "words written on water" evokes an ephemeral and transitory image. Speech is no less ephemeral, no less transitory. The spoken message is a rapidly decaying acoustic disturbance in an ocean of air. The listener who would try to capture this signal must follow its temporal course in environments that are often noisy, reverberent, and otherwise disruptive. Speech survives this adversity through a robust resistance to interference. This resistance to disruption is based partly on the redundancy of spoken language and partly on the acoustic envelope of the speech signal, giving speech its coherence in a world of acoustic competition. A substantial amount of evidence points to the conclusion that speech is perceived both on the basis of the acoustic signal and predictions based on its context and familiarity. The relative contributions of these information sources is of course circumstantial.

The spoken message is always history. After the acoustic event has passed, a neural image is retained to support its linguistic interpretation, and if necessary, its reinterpretation. The trick is to maintain an adequately detailed history for a sufficient interval while keeping up with the ongoing flow of speech. Henry Ford was supposed to have defined history as "just one damn thing after another." The prevailing view among those who study speech perception seems to be that it is "just one segment after another." However, there is considerable disagreement on exactly what the segment is. Suggestions range from some small acoustic segment to phonemes to a sound sequence of about 200 msec duration to syllables to words. For that matter, there are those who have proposed the phrase or clause as a decision unit. The unit question is taken up in the following section, which summarizes some contemporary theories of speech perception.

## MODELS OF SPEECH PERCEPTION AND WORD RECOGNITION

Disagreement over the size of the decision unit is not the only area of uncertainty in attempts to understand speech perception. Table 7–1 gives a summary of some major features of contemporary models of speech perception and word recognition. The dimensions that are compared and contrasted are the (1) processing unit, (2) sources of knowledge available to the model, and (3) primary recognition process.

The first column lists the various candidates for processing unit. As already noted, the units vary considerably, from short-term spectra, to phones and allophones, to syllables, to whole words. Some models allow different sizes of units to interact. For example, the interactive activation model recognizes distinctive features, phonemes

**TABLE 7–1.**
Models of Speech Perception and Word Recognition*

| Model | Processing Units | Knowledge Sources | Recognition Process |
|---|---|---|---|
| Logogen (Morton[54–56]) | Whole words | Interactive | Passive-threshold devices to recognize words |
| LAFS (Klatt[26]†) | Context-sensitive spectra | Direct bottom-up hypothesization of word candidates | Passive matching to templates based on short-term spectra |
| Cohort (Marslen-Wilson[33, 34, 36]) | Acoustic-phonetic "sound sequences" | Interactive | Activation of "word-initial cohort" (words that share an initial sound sequence) |
| Autonomous Search (Forster[12]) | Phonetic segments (phonemes) | Noninteractive | Mediated bottom-up processing |
| Interactive activation (McClelland and Elman[40]‡) | Distinctive features phonemes, words | Interactive | Active threshold device using networks |
| Phonetic refinement (Pisoni[54]) | Phones & allophones | Interactive | Activation of phonetic sequences in networks to form a transcription |
| LAME (Warren[62, 63]) | "Multiple engrams" (several units) | Interactive (parallel) | Adaptive simultaneous pattern perception |
| Auditory-perceptual (Miller[45, 46]) | Sensory responses based on acoustic spectra | Interactive | Perceptual "space" for phonemic representation |
| Motor (revised) (Liberman and Mattingly[31]§) | Syllable | Noninteractive | Modular detection of motor "gestures" |
| FLMP (Massaro[38]) | Features and segments | Interactive | Feature evaluation, feature integration, and pattern classification |
| Vector analysis (Fowler and Smith[14]) | Phones | Interactive | Use natural lines of coarticulation to form vectors |

*Modified from Pisoni DB: Acoustic-phonetic representations in word recognition. *Research on Speech Perception,* Progress Report No. 10, Speech Research Laboratory, Dept of Psychology, Indiana University, Bloomington, 1984, pp 129–152.
†A companion module, SCRIBER, also is described.
‡See also Watrous[64] for a report on phoneme discrimination using connectionist networks.
§A collection of papers on modularity and motor theory is available in Mattingly and Studdert-Kennedy.[39]

and words. The LAME model also proposes that several different units operate, with the relative contribution of any given unit depending on the cognitive skills of the listener, stimulus properties and environment.

The column headed Sources of Knowledge basically distinguishes models that allow interactivity of knowledge sources from those that do not. For those models that possess interactivity, a further question is how this interactivity comes about. The interactivity-noninteractivity question has important implications for the auditory processing of speech. Interactive models assume that phonetic or word recognition draws on various sources of information available to the listener. In "top-down" strategies, these information sources enable prediction, hypothecation and (dis)confirmation. A listener's linguistic knowledge is particularly important, but sources of knowledge also include context, communicative goals and attributes of the speaker. The interactivity-noninteractivity question is closely related to the proposal that speech is modular. One criterion for a modular process is that it is characterized by "informational encapsulation," i.e., the process cannot be influenced by other sources of information.

The final column gives a capsule description of the primary process by which the units of the message are recognized. The models vary greatly in this respect, some relying on passive-threshold (Logogen model) or passive-matching decisions (LAFS), while others call upon active strategies (e.g., autonomous search). This column is particularly telling: it shows that among these theories there is preciously little consensus on the nature of auditory processing for speech.

The "unit" question is central to this conference and to inquiries into the temporal processing of speech. If we knew with certainty what the unit is, much (but not necessarily all) of the dissonance in Table 7–1 would disappear. Experimental evidence of various kinds has been presented for all of the units listed in the table. It is not surprising, therefore, that some investigators have suggested that more than one unit is involved in processing. Warren[63] takes the extreme view in this regard. He proposed that we turn the usual vertical scheme of processing (verticality being implicit in our "bottom-up" and "top-down" strategies) on its side to permit parallel processing with several units acting simultaneously. An appealing feature of this proposal is that a unit would be identified depending on the sufficiency of cues for that unit. Conceivably, two listeners attending to the same speech signal might process it with different units. One listener might use primarily word-sized units, whereas the other might rely on phoneme-sized units. For example, the young child might use different units than the adult listener.

## PARTICLE, FIELD, AND WAVE IN AUDITORY PERCEPTION

It is doubtful if any one unit satisfactorily accounts for all of the data on speech processing. If this assessment is true, then there are two primary directions to take toward resolution of the problem. First, two or more units can be considered as potentially involved. Then the different units either can interact, or one of them can be selected depending on their relative suitability in a given listening situation. Second, a very different view can be taken: We might propose that auditory processing is not strictly and solely a matter of sequential unit recognition. That is, auditory processing is not simply or essentially a strategy of "just one segment after another." Rather, auditory processing convolves the unit, or discrete element, with the continuous, or the flowing event. The idea, which can be traced back to Pike,[53] is to consider the processing of language as involving particle, field and wave.

Physics has come to view reality in essentially this way—as both particle and wave, as both discrete element and continuous field. The physicist can demonstrate the particle-wave dualism of light with an interferometer. This device shows that light has wavelike properties such as refraction and reflection, but it also has particle-like properties such as quantum effects in energy absorption. The particle of light is the photon but light is also a wave phenomenon.

What does this have to with auditory processing of speech? Simply this: the segment, analogous to the particle in physics, is a condensate and consolidate of the energy-event complex of speech. That is, the segment emerges as a consolidation of properties that appear in the physical signal of speech—a signal that is inherently continuous. The properties that define a segment may even have different time courses, so that they overlap one another but do not necessarily share exactly the same temporal intervals. The segment and the flowing pattern cohere in a common understanding of auditory processing. As the flowing pattern of sound is processed, the extracted information gives rise to segmental decisions. The size of segment can vary with the signal properties, the listener's cognitive resources, the listening task, and the availability of contextual information. Mere discrimination of an acoustic cue is not prima facie evidence of segmental perception. Discrimination of acoustic cues for speech has been demonstrated for nonhuman species.[28] It would seem that linguistic experience is required to organize the discriminable cues into units that correspond with the phonetic structure of a language.[38, 58]

To add flesh to the admittedly stark bones of this argument, let us consider the phenomena of speech perception against a backdrop of particle, field, and wave. To show how these concepts apply to speech perception, various phenomena of speech perception are collected in Appendix 7–1. These phenomena can be explained largely as particle effects (App 7–1,A), field effects (App 7–1,B), and wave effects (App 7–1,C) and represent much of what is known (or needs to be explained) about speech perception. These are the facts or observations of the field of study.

The *particle* denotes segments or units in speech perception. These effects represent phenomena of condensation, in which segments are derived from an appropriate combination of cues extracted from the acoustic signal. The optimal cues for segment recognition are brought into relief by experiments on prototypicality.[20] These experiments basically reveal that not all of the stimuli that give rise to a common phonetic interpretation are created acoustically equal. To paraphrase George Orwell from *Animal Farm,* all segments within an equivalence classification are equal (i.e., interpreted as the same sound), but some are more equal than others (in the sense of being better members of the category). The best exemplars of a phonetic classification represent segmental excellence. These notions become sensible with a relativistic interpretation that involves fields or decision spaces.

A given stimulus can be judged differently depending largely on contextual factors that serve to define a decision space. If a segment were defined on the basis of invariant cues, then a given set of stimulus properties would always give rise to the same segmental decision and no other decision. But such is not the case, and the phenomena listed under *field effects* in Appendix 7–1,B are a summary of the counterevidence. The notion of *field* accounts for these relational and contextual effects in perception. Writers on speech perception frequently refer to perceptual decisions occurring in a space or volume in which auditory events are represented. A common and simple example is the F1-F2 chart, or the acoustic space defined by a speaker's first- and second-formant frequencies. In a recent application of this idea, Miller proposed a spatial representation based largely on ratios of formant frequencies.

Units are identified within their context (fields of occurrence) and the fields are in turn identified within a larger temporal context (the continuing flow of speech). The wave indicates streams and a listener's continuously unfolding inductions. The phenomena listed in Appendix 7–1,C as *wave effects* pertain to processes that extend over time and give both coherence and interpretative bases for the components of the speech signal. In important respects, the acoustic waveform of speech is in fact a stream. When we view speech as waveforms or spectrograms (or as the underlying articulatory movements, as in the case of an x-ray motion picture), we are continually struck by the difficulty of delineating units of almost any size. Many investigators have stressed that the acoustic structure of speech is aptly characterized as having a shingled effect, in which adjacent segments frequently overlap in their acoustic properties. Listeners seem to hear out these overlaps and can use this kind of information to anticipate upcoming segments in a phonetic string. Whalen[65] noted that coarticulatory effects in speech have a magnitude and range that exceed the physiological requirements of adjacent segments. That is, articulation is overlapped more than what is minimally necessary to articulate abutting phones. Whalen surmises the reason: "It seems, then, that coarticulation is geared toward making speaking easier and/or *enhancing the effectiveness of the speech stream for the listener* (emphasis added)."[65]

A variety of phenomena on speech perception are listed in Appendix 7–1. The phenomena are most appropriately explained by the concept in question. This is not to say that explanations cannot span two or more concepts, for they often do. The appendix demonstrates that the particle-field-wave nature of perception embraces phenomena that are not easily captured by any one of the models summarized in Table 7–1. It should be emphasized that the particle or unit achieves its definition in both a field and a wave. The latter two are also in mutual dependency. For example, the field or decision space may change in character during the flow of speech. Some of these changes reflect production characteristics, as when a speaker produces an utterance with pitch declination (a generally falling fundamental frequency over the course of the utterance), with articulatory movements that gradually assume smaller ranges over the utterance (a kind of articulatory declination), and with a general attenuation of the intensity envelope. The listener can adapt to these changes because of the mutual dependencies among unit, field and wave. The mutual dependency of the triune is not restricted to speech. Stream formation for acoustic events is based largely on pitch-duration ratios.[4, 25] When the elements of a tonal series are close in frequency, they tend to be heard as a single stream. But as the tones are separated in frequency so as to form a high-pitched and low-pitched series, two streams will be heard in relation to the pitch divergence.

This conception also accommodates recent recommendations that speech perception theories account for stimulus variability related to differences in talkers.[51, 52, 55] Although much of the work on speech perception has been directed at finding decision unit criteria that are unaffected by speaker differences (e.g., normalization strategies), it is becoming clear that these differences can be important and that the listener does not immediately discard information from the speech signal. It has been argued that canonical phonetic representations are less than optimal for human speech perception and machine speech recognition because these representations are not consistent with the principle of "delayed commitment," that is, retaining the acoustic information in the speech signal until it no longer holds potential value in the decision process.[26, 27, 55] But because many theories of speech perception have been developed primarily to identify canonical decision units such as phonemes, they often neglect important questions about the residual information in the speech wave. If, on the other hand, segmental decisions are regarded as condensate phenomena, the acoustic context of these decisions remains available for perceptual processing in the field and wave characteristics of the signal.

To see how units can be recognized within this conception, it is useful to review selected phenomena associated with the recognition of units. The word will be emphasized because of space limitations in this paper and because the word has special prominence in contemporary accounts of speech perception (Table 7–1) and clinical audiology.

## THE WORD AS UNIT

A substantial portion of recent research has emphasized the word as the unit of decision or recognition. Related to these research efforts has been the development of models of word recognition, some of which are included in Table 7–1. The word also has been a highly favored unit in clinical tests of speech recognition, speech discrimination and central auditory testing. Speech audiometry is closely identified with word lists such as the NU-CHIPS, NU-6, PB-50, SSW, W-2, W-22, and so on. The chapters by Katz and Stecker in this volume describe word lists that have been used to assess central auditory processing. To a significant degree, speech audiometry is known by its word lists.

Given this historical focus on the word, it is appropriate to summarize what we know about word recognition. Some general conclusions drawn from the recent literature are as follows.

1. Words apparently are recognized one at a time, serially, and word-onsets seem to be particularly important in directing the word-recognition process.[6, 36]
2. Word recognition can be strongly influenced by frequency of word usage and contextual predictability.[21, 43]
3. Word recognition takes into account the rate of speech, and it appears that the listener knows "fast rate" rules.[47]
4. Words excised from their spoken contexts and presented in isolation are sometimes poorly identified.[29, 60]
5. Words often can be recognized from only a time-gated portion of the full acoustic signal. Recognition generally is better for forward time gating (beginning with word onsets) than for backward time gating (beginning at word offsets).[9, 21, 36]
6. Recognition of time-gated words varies with subject age. Teenaged listeners recognize words with shorter gates than do younger children and older adults.[11] It also has been reported that young adults achieve word recognition at shorter gates than older adults.[8]
7. Time-gated word-recognition scores are lower than conventional word-recognition scores even when the entire word is included in the time-gated presentation.[9]
8. Short monosyllabic words, particularly those that occur with low frequency in the language, may remain unrecognized when preceded by low-predictability contexts.[1, 21, 57]
9. Words in context may be identified even when a portion of the word has been replaced by nonspeech energy; listeners may be unaware of the replacement.[61]
10. Listeners' ability to monitor for target words in a string is affected by syntactic factors.[2, 35] Baum[2] reported that reaction times were significantly longer

when even a single syntactic rule was broken.

11. Copy synthesis, based on the assembly of word strings from stored words often yields an unsatisfactory result.[22] In some cases, the successive words seem to come from several different sources rather than a single source. In other words, they lack coherence even if they have semantic and syntactic appropriateness.

In summary, at various times, listeners (1) recognize a word when only part of its acoustic pattern is present, (2) fail to recognize a word even when its entire acoustic pattern would appear to be available, (3) recognize a word differently depending on its acoustic-phonetic context, (4) recognize a word when part of its acoustic pattern has been replaced by nonspeech energy, and (5) monitor words with attention to the syntactic frame in which they appear. These phenomena are difficult to reconcile with a view that the word as recognition unit is wholly and sufficiently evident as a discrete portion of the acoustic signal. They are compatible with the view espoused here that the word emerges as a kind of condensate from the flowing wavelike pattern of speech. In this view, the acoustic cues for unit recognition are contained in the signal but their selection and interpretation depend on properties that can extend over considerable portions of the utterance preceding and following the word itself.

## THE SEGMENT AS UNIT

Similar phenomena have been reported in respect to the phonetic segment or phoneme as recognition unit. This topic cannot be reviewed in detail in this paper, but a few brief observations are in order, beginning with the classic Haskins Laboratory research on synthetic CV syllables.[7, 10] When synthetic formant transitions were presented in isolation, listeners heard them as nonspeech chirps. But when the same transitions were connected to steady-state vowel formants, listeners heard consonant-vowel syllables. The formant transitions apparently were integrated with the formant steady-states to yield a phonetic recognition of the overall pattern. Similar experiments with stimuli consisting of a noise burst followed by steady-state formants also indicated a vowel dependency in the interpretation of the consonantal cue.[7] The phonetic identity of consonants also has been shown to be influenced by speaking rate[47] and by lexical factors.[18]

In short, the segment, like the word, does not appear to have an invariant appearance within a prescribed temporal interval of the acoustic signal. This issue underlies the long-standing problem of *segmentation,* or the assumption that segments can be identified in the speech wave as successive, discrete elements. Segmentation can be conceptualized as a spectrogram in which lines drawn perpendicular to the time axis mark the boundaries of segments. But visualizing the concept is much easier than actually implementing it. Fowler and Smith[14] (also see Fowler[13]) recognized this conclusion in their proposal of vector analysis theory, which identifies segments using "natural lines of coarticulation" rather than assuming the usual notion of well-defined sequences of segments. They recognized that the component features of phonetic elements often overlap in their temporal pattern, or, as Fujimura[15] observed, "events do not occur synchronously among different articulatory dimensions." This overlap confounds attempts to segment the stream of speech. Fowler and Smith propose the hypothesis that "information for segmentation and its complement, coherence, is not solely temporal succession and simultaneity."[14] Therefore, acoustic events that are temporally concurrent will not necessarily form a unitary percept (e.g., two sounds that occur together are not necessarily fused into one auditory percept). Further, some successive events will be heard as coherent, e.g., in the sense of primary streams.[4]

The present conception differs from that of Fowler and Smith[14] in several ways, but especially in that it is not based solely on the idea that underlying articulatory processes define the natural lines of coarticulation from which segments can be induced. The present claim is more general, extending to acoustic patterns in which coarticulatory evidence is minimal and perhaps not present at all in the usual sense. For example, sinusoidal synthesis generates acoustic patterns that consist of co-occurring sinusoids adjusted to the approximate center frequencies of formants.

Given the proper instructions, listeners can perceive these sinusoidal streams as one stream interpretable as speech.[56] Similarly, most of us have had the experience of confusing nonspeech sounds (a babbling brook, a vocalizing animal, clattering factory noises) as speech. It wasn't coarticulation that fooled us. Rather, it was a sound pattern that triggered our perception of a coherent acoustic stream containing enough acoustic variety to trigger a search for segmental cues.

Nor is it coarticulation that causes listeners to "hear" the missing sound in Warren's phonemic restoration experiments.[61] Expectations based on natural coarticulatory patterns should immediately alert us to the unnatural presence of a nonspeech noise in the acoustic stream. But in phonemic restoration, listeners are unaware of the violence done to the acoustic signal. However, it is notable that listeners typically are aware of another kind of acoustic manipulation—excised portions of the acoustic signal. Such gaps of silence are readily detected. This tells us that listeners follow the continuous pattern of speech in the expectation of deriving segmental information, which, when coupled with other information sources, allows an understanding of the message. Minor acoustic disruptions are neglected so long as the listener is reasonably confident that the message was understood.

Some portions of the acoustic signal probably have a higher informational value than others. Furui[16] showed that a brief "transition" portion of syllables carried substantial information for the recognition of both initial consonant and vowel. This result further reinforces skepticism about segments as necessarily serial events and encourages us to examine the speech signal as a coherent source of information for simultaneous decisions.

## IMPLICATIONS FOR ASSESSMENT OF AUDITORY PROCESSING

The core idea of the present perspective is that the auditory processing of speech involves the selection of acoustic cues from a flowing pattern. The structure of the pattern probably directs the listener's selection of acoustic cues for an efficient auditory processing. The relevant structural information is largely temporal and is related in part to coarticulation[13, 14, 65] and in part to patterns of stress and rhythm distributed across the syllables of an utterance. The temporal coherence of speech seems to be related to stress patterns and rhythmic patterns expressed over syllable sequences. The ear seems well suited to hear syllable crests. Lauter and Hirsh[30] pointed out that auditory discrimination for amplitude modulation, which is optimal at about 4 Hz, is closely matched to the typical syllable rate in speech, which is about four per second. Syllable peaks and margins are a major influence in shaping the wave or stream of speech. The effect is largely precessional, giving an impression of connectedness or coherence to the pattern. Martin[37] demonstrated that the rhythmic structure of speech permits the listener to make predictions about temporal patterns over sentences. Predictivity implies coherence. Contained within these patterns is a variety of acoustic cues from which units may be identified. The cues for a given unitary decision are often complementary and redundant. For example, a stop consonant might be recognized from the stop burst spectrum, from the formant transitions into a following vowel, and perhaps even from its voice-onset time.

A listener's understanding of speech can be strongly affected by its predictability, which is based to some degree on the coherence of the signals. Temporal structure alone carries information, as can be demonstrated with speech-modulated noise. This noise signal carries a residual intelligibility, apparently based on the richness of the preserved temporal information. The temporal structure also may help to direct auditory processing to the efficient use of spectral cues for unit recognition.

Predictability of the message varies with situation, speaker, semantic-syntactic cues, and the cognitive resources of the listener. Interest in the factor of predictability has led to two primary procedures in intelligibility testing. First, in the SPIN test, predictability has been manipulated so that the test sentences take either a high-predictability form or a low-predictability form. The difference in identification between the two sentence types is taken as an index of a listener's use of context. The other approach is to measure predictability from comparisons of word and sentence recognition. Benoit[46] proposed that linguistic complexity could be quantified as the ratio

$$r = \log(p_s) / \log(p_r)$$

where $p_s$ is the probability of sentence recognition and $p_r$ is the probability of recognition for the individual words comprising the sentence. Low values of *r* are expected for high-contextual information and high values of *r*, for low-contextual information. It would also be expected that a listener who fails to use contextual information would tend to have constant values of *r* for different levels of contextual information. An appealing feature of Benoit's proposal is that it permits a comparison of single-word recognition (the odds-on favorite in clinical audiology) and sentence recognition (a frequently suggested alternative to word tests).

## A RESEARCH AGENDA

Even a cursory review of the literature on auditory processing is sufficient to identify a chorus of calls for attention to time. Hirsh[23] emphasized the importance of auditory pattern recognition, defining an auditory pattern as a "sequence of events whose properties are those of the sequence rather than the traditional acoustic properties of the individual sounds." This remark emphasizes the point that the temporal sequence needs to be understood as more than a simple concatenation of sound elements. Watrous[64] observed that "Speech communication is an inherently *temporal* process; time is the independent variable that orders the process of speech production and perception."

To account for speech, as both a productive and perceptual behavior, we must understand its temporal course. Specifically, speech perception is in large part temporal information. Michon and Jackson[44] presented evidence that temporal information (1) is equivalent to topical information, (2) draws on a subject's limited processing resources, and (3) is processed deliberately rather than automatically. Tompkins et al[59] underscored the complexity of the information-processing when they wrote, "Lower-level psychophysical and auditory information processing functions are inextricably linked with higher cognitive operations." Finally, Remez et al[56] concluded from their experiments on sinusoidal synthesis of speech (in which speech is represented as elemental sinusoidal patterns) that the "time-varying coherence of the spectrum bears phonetic information, apparently independent of the elements that compose the dynamic patterns."

If the arguments in this paper come close to the truth, then the understanding of the auditory processing of speech has a threefold objective—segment, field, and wave. This is by no means a formal theory of auditory processing for speech but rather an outline for such a theory. The outline presents a perspective on the way in which the human listener extracts essential acoustic information from the speech signal to enable linguistic and other cognitive faculties to interpret the speaker's intended message. The auditory processing involves complementary operations described as particle (or unit), field, and wave.

Disorders of auditory processing would be approached with the same conception. It would enable the interpretation of phoneme recognition, word identification and sentence understanding in a common framework. This conception points to a number of directions for future study. The immediate task that a listener faces is to establish an auditory stream for acoustic events. This ability seems to be taken mostly for granted, but research on persons with aphasia indicates that stream segregation (the ability to separate co-occurring auditory streams) itself might be impaired. Gaddie[17] showed that aphasic people were less effective than language-normal controls in the recognition of interleaved melodies, i.e., two melodies played so that their respective notes alternate with one another. Specifically, the aphasic subjects required a greater frequency separation of the tonal components to achieve the same degree of melody recognition as the control subjects. This result prompts the question of whether the disturbance in aphasia is not only in the language domain but rather a more comprehensive domain of information processing.[41, 42]

Michon and Jackson[44] went beyond the concept of auditory streaming to propose the concept of *cognitive streaming*. This concept is particularly important for the linguistic interpretation of the spoken speech signal. Auditory streaming gives perceptual order to complex acoustic environments, which we hear in the rigid one-dimensionality of time—everything in an ongoing successional pattern. But we can separate the various sources, even if they emerge from a single loudspeaker, into imputed or inferred origins. In so doing, we make auditory sense of acoustic chaos. The auditory stream of speech, once established, enables the listener to establish a cognitive stream. This involves categorization, prediction and other cognitive resources to extract from the auditory stream the immediately relevant and necessary information. Once the cognitive purpose is served and the listener is reasonably confident of the intended message, the particular auditory stream behind that message is indeed history. Of course, the continuing cognitive stream persists in preparation for resumption of the auditory stream of speech.

## CONCLUSION

It is proposed that the auditory processing of speech involves complementary operations involving the particle (unit), field (space), and wave (stream). Within the ongoing stream of speech, the listener detects the various acoustic cues which define the phoneme, the word, and other units. These cues can vary from situation to situation, depending on speaker, signal quality, and predictability of the message. The available cues in the stream are consolidated into unitary decisions and it is from their patterns of simultaneity and succession that segments emerge as a condensate. Relativistic or contextual effects in perception are largely accounted for as field and wave phenomena.

### Acknowledgments

Work supported in part by U.S. Public Health Service research grant DC00319 from the National Institute on Deafness and Other Communication Disorders. I thank Malcolm McNeil of the University of Wisconsin–Madison for his comments on a draft of this paper. Professor Jack Katz, co-editor of this volume, helped to make the words fit the ideas.

## REFERENCES

1. Bard EG, Schillcock RC, Altman GTM: The recognition of words after their acoustic offsets in spontaneous speech: Effects of subsequent context. *Percept Psychophys* 1988; 44: 395–408.
2. Baum S: On-line sensitivity to local and long-distance syntactic dependencies in Broca's aphasia. *Brain Lang* 1989; 37:327–338.
3. Benoit C: An intelligibility test using semantically unpredictable sentences: Towards the quantification of linguistic complexity. *Speech Commun* 1990; 9:293–304.
4. Bregman AS: Auditory streaming: Competition among alternative organizations. *Percept Psychophys* 1978; 23:391–398.
5. Cole RA (ed): *Perception and Production of Fluent Speech*. Hillsdale, NJ, Erlbaum, 1980.
6. Cole R, Jakimik L: A model of speech perception, in Cole R (ed): *Perception and Production of Fluent Speech*. Hillsdale, NJ, Erlbaum, 1980, pp 133–203.
7. Cooper FS, Delattre PC, Liberman AM, et al: Some experiments on the perception of synthetic speech sounds. *J Acoust Soc Am* 1952; 24:597–606.
8. Craig CH: Real-time speech understanding among elderly listeners. Paper presented at the Annual Convention of the American Speech-Language-Hearing Association, Seattle, November, 1990.
9. Craig CH, Kim BW: Effects of time gating and word length on isolated word recognition performance. *J Speech Hear Res* 1990; 33:808–815.
10. Delattre PC, Liberman AM, Cooper FS: Acoustic loci and transitional cues for consonants. *J Acoust Soc Am* 1955; 27:769–773.
11. Elliott LL, Hammer M, Evan K: Perception of gated highly familiar spoken monosyllabic nouns by children, teenagers and older adults. *Percept Psychophys* 1987; 42:150–157.
12. Forster KI: Accessing the mental lexicon, in Wales RJ, Walker E (eds): *New Approaches to Language Mechanisms*. Amsterdam, North-Holland, 1976.
13. Fowler CA: Segmentation of coarticulated speech in perception. *Percept Psychophys* 1984; 36:359–368.
14. Fowler CA, Smith RA: Speech perception as vector analysis: An approach to the problem of invariance and segmentation, in Perkell JS, Klatt DH (eds): *Invariance and Variability in Speech Processes*. Hillsdale, NJ, Erlbaum, 1986, pp 123–139.

15. Fujimura O: Methods and goals of speech production research. *Lang Speech* 1990; 33:195–258.
16. Furui S: On the role of spectral transition for speech perception. *J Acoust Soc Am* 1986; 80:1016–1025.
17. Gaddies A: The perception of interleaved melodies by aphasic adults. Master's thesis, University of Wisconsin-Madison, Madison, Wis, 1985.
18. Ganong WF III: Phonetic categorization in auditory word perception. *J Exp Psychol Hum Percept Perform* 1980; 6:110–125.
19. Garman M: *Psycholinguistics*. Cambridge, England, Cambridge University Press, 1990.
20. Greiser D, Kuhl P: The categorization of speech by infants: Support for speech-sound prototypes. *Dev Psychol* 1991; 25:577–588.
21. Grosjean F: Spoken word-recognition processes and the gating paradigm. *Percept Psychophys* 1980; 28:267–283.
22. Harris CM: A study of the building blocks in speech. *J Acoust Soc Am* 1953; 25:962–969.
23. Hirsh IJ: Temporal aspects of hearing, in Tower DB (ed): *The Nervous System: Human Communication and Its Disorders,* vol 3. New York, Raven Press, 1975.
24. Jackson A, Morton J: Facilitation of auditory word recognition. *Mem Cognit* 1984; 12:568–574.
25. Jones R: Time, our lost dimension: Toward a new theory of perception, attention and memory. *Psychol Rev* 1976; 83:325–355.
26. Klatt DH: Speech perception: A model of acoustic-phonetic analysis and lexical access. *J Phonet* 1979; 7:279–312.
27. Klatt DH: Review of selected models of speech perception, in Marslen-Wilson WD (ed): *Lexical Representation and Process*. Cambridge, Mass, MIT Press, 1989, pp 169–226.
28. Kuhl PK: Auditory perception and the evolution of speech. *Hum Evolut* 1988; 3:19–43.
29. Ladefoged P, Broadbent DE: Information conveyed by vowels. *J Acoust Soc Am* 1957; 29:98–104.
30. Lauter JL, Hirsh IJ: Speech as temporal pattern: A psychoacoustic profile. *Speech Commun* 1985; 4:41–54.
31. Liberman AM, Mattingly IG: The motor theory of speech perception revised. *Cognition* 1985; 21:1–36.
32. Luce PA, Pisoni DB: Speech perception: New directions in research, theory and application, in Winitz H (ed): *Human Communication and Its Disorders: A Review,* vol 1. Norwood, NJ, Ablex, 1987.
33. Marslen-Wilson WD: The temporal structure of language understanding. *Cognition* 1980; 8:1–71.
34. Marslen-Wilson WD (ed): *Lexical Representation and Process*. Cambridge, Mass, MIT press, 1989.
35. Marslen-Wilson W, Tyler L: The temporal structure of spoken language. *Cognition* 1980; 13:361–392.
36. Marslen-Wilson WD: Functional parallelism in spoken word recognition, in Frauenfelder UH, Tyler LK (eds): *Spoken Word Recognition*. Cambridge, Mass, MIT Press, 1987, pp 71–102.
37. Martin JG: Rhythmic (hierarchical) versus serial structure in speech and other behavior. *Psychol Rev* 1972; 79:487–509.
38. Massaro DW: Multiple book review of *Speech Perception by Ear and Eye: A Paradigm for Psychological Inquiry*. *Behav Brain Sci* 1989; 12:741–794.
39. Mattingly IG, Studdert-Kennedy M (eds): *Modularity and the Motor Theory of Speech Perception*. Hillsdale, NJ, Lawrence Erlbaum, 1990.
40. McClelland J, Elman J: The TRACE model of speech perception. *Cognit Psychol* 1986; 18:1–86.
41. McNeil MR: Aphasia: Neurological considerations. *Top Lang Disor* 1983; 3:1–19.
42. McNeil MR, Kimelman MDZ: Toward an integrative information processing structure of auditory comprehension and processing in adult aphasia, in LaPointe LL (ed): *Seminars in Speech and Language. Aphasia: Nature and Assessment*. New York, Thieme-Stratton, 1986, pp 123–147.
43. Mehler J, Segui J, Carey P: Tails of words: Monitoring ambiguity. *J Verb Learn Verb Behav* 1978; 17:29–35.
44. Michon JA, Jackson JL: Attentional effort and cognitive strategies in the processing of temporal information, in Gibson J, Allan L (eds): *Timing and Time Perception*. *Ann NY Acad Sci* 1984; 423:298–321.
45. Miller JD: Auditory processing of the acoustic patterns of speech. *Arch Otolaryngol* 1984; 110:154–159.
46. Miller JD: Auditory-perceptual interpretation of the vowel. *J Acoust Soc Am* 1989; 85:2114–2134.
47. Miller JL: Effects of speaking rate on segmental distinctions, in Eimas PD, Miller JL (eds): *Perspectives on the Study of Speech*. Hillsdale, NJ, Erlbaum, 1981, pp 39–74.
48. Miller JL, Kent RD, Atal BS (eds): *Reprint Collection in Speech Communication. Vol 2: Speech Perception*. Woodbury, NY, Acoustical Society of America, American Institute of Physics, 1991.
49. Morton J: A preliminary functional model for language behavior. *Int Audiol* 1964; 3:216–225.
50. Morton J, Broadbent DE: Passive versus active recognition models, or is your homunculus really

necessary? in Wathen-Dunn W (ed): *Models for the Perception of Speech and Visual Form*. Cambridge, Mass, MIT Press, 1967, pp 103–110.
51. Mullennix JW, Pisoni DB: Stimulus variability and processing dependencies in speech perception. *Percept Psychophys* 1990; 47:379–390.
52. Mullennix JW, Pisoni DB, Martin CS: Some effects of talker variability on spoken word recognition. *J Acoust Soc Am* 1989; 85:365–378.
53. Pike KL: Language as particle, wave and field. *Texas Q* 1959; 2:37–54.
54. Pisoni DB: Acoustic-phonetic representations in word recognition. *Research on Speech Perception,* Progress Report No. 10, Speech Research Laboratory, Dept of Psychology, Indiana University, Bloomington, 1984, pp 129–152.
55. Pisoni DB: Effects of talker variability on speech perception: Implications for current research and theory, in Fujisaki H (ed): *Proceedings of the 1990 International Conference on Spoken Language Processing*. Kobe, Japan, Nov 18–22, 1990, in press.
56. Remez RT, Rubin PE, Pisoni DB: Coding of the speech spectrum in three time-varying sinusoids. *Ann NY Acad Sci* 1983; 405:485–489.
57. Rubenstein H, Pollock I: Word predictability and intelligibility. *J Verb Learn Verb Behav* 1963; 2:147–158.
58. Studdert-Kennedy M: Language development from an evolutionary perspective, in Krasnegor N, Rumbaugh D, Schiefelbusch D, et al (eds): *Language Acquisition: Biological and Behavioral Determinants*. Hillsdale, NJ, Erlbaum, in press.
59. Tompkins CA, Jackson ST, Schulz R: On prognostic research in adult neurogenic disorders. *J Speech Hear Res* 1990; 33:398–401.
60. Verbrugge RR, Strange W, Shankweiler DP, et al: What information enables a listener to map a talker's vowel space? *J Acoust Soc Am* 1976; 60:198–212.
61. Warren RM: Auditory illusions and perceptual processes, in Lass NJ (ed): *Contemporary Issues in Experimental Phonetics*. New York, Academic Press, 1976, pp 389–417.
62. Warren RM: Mode of representation in production and perception. Chairman's comments, in Myers T, Laver J, Anderson J (eds): *The Cognitive Representation of Speech*. Amsterdam, North Holland, 1981, pp 34–37.
63. Warren RM: Multiple meanings of "phoneme" (articulatory, acoustic, perceptual, graphemic) and their confusions, in Lass NJ (ed): *Speech and Language: Advances in Basic Research and Practice,* vol 9. New York, Academic Press, 1983, pp 285–311.
64. Watrous RL: Phoneme discrimination using connectionist networks. *J Acoust Soc Am* 1990; 87:1753–1772.
65. Whalen DH: Coarticulation is largely planned. *J Phonet* 1990; 18:3–35.

## APPENDIX 7–1

### Speech Perception Phenomena*

***A. Particle (Unit) Phenomena: Condensation or Consolidation Effects***

*Segmentation*—Ability of listeners to assign serially ordered segments to the speech signal (phonetic transcription is a good example).

*Categorization*—A listener's tendencies to rely on equivalence classes for speech sounds. The members of a class may differ acoustically; e.g. a stop consonant may have different formant-frequency transitions in different vowel contexts. (It is sometimes said that identification categories predict discrimination performance.)

*Protypicality*—"Best" cases, or exemplars, can be determined for an equivalence class of sounds. That is, some sounds are better examples of a sound class than others, although they all might be classified in the same phonetic category. For example, five sounds might all be heard as [s], but one of them is a better [s] than the others.

*Cue integration or trading*—Integration of cues for a single segment, or the trading of such cues within a segment decision, e.g., the cues of silence, burst, and formant transitions all pertain to stop consonants, but these cues may be variably present. The listener can use any available cues.

*Bimodal perception (McGurk effect)*—Visual and auditory cues can be combined in a phonetic decision; the visual cues sometimes can override auditory cues. A stimulus heard unambiguously as [da] when presented auditorily is identified as [ba] when presented with a visual image showing labial closure.

*Coarticulation*—Overlapping of articulatory (and therefore acoustic) properties for sequences of sounds; listeners seem to make phonetic interpretations of acoustic cues distributed across apparent segment boundaries such that information for successive sounds accrues simultaneously.

*Gating effects (some)*—Recognition of sounds, syllables, or words on the basis of partial (temporally gated) information; recognition is better for word-initial segments than for word-final segments and word recognition often can be accomplished on only a gated word-initial segment of about 200 ms or less.

*Duplex perception*—Dual perception of an acoustic cue as speech and nonspeech; e.g., an isolated third-formant transition presented to one ear will be heard as a chirp in that ear but also can be integrated with an incomplete speech stimulus in the other ear to be heard as part of a full syllable.

*Left-hemisphere advantage for brief or rapidly changing stimuli*—Right ear (and inferentially the left hemisphere) outperforms the left ear (and inferentially the right hemisphere) in the recognition of phonetic stimuli that are brief or rapidly changing, e.g., stop consonants.

***B. Field Phenomena: Relational Effects***

*Adaptation effects*—Change in the identification or discrimination of a speech sound occurring with repeated presentation of that sound; wave or streaming effects may also contribute to this phenomenon.

*Stimulus order effects*—Dependency of phonetic identification of one sound on sounds presented earlier, e.g., perception of a synthesized vowel varies with the stimuli that precede or follow it.

*Undershoot*—Phonetic target in context can be identified even if the acoustic pattern undershoots (misses) its target, as often happens with increased rate or reduced stress.

*Language dependency of acoustic correlates of similar phonetic elements*—Languages that share a similar phonetic element (say, a given vowel) may differ in the acoustic correlates for that sound (slightly different vowel formant frequencies).

*Phonetic boundary shift related to linguistic factors*—Boundary for a phonetic feature can be shifted through the influence of linguistic variables, e.g., the VOT boundary for a voiced-voiceless contrast is affected by word-nonword distinction.

*Equivalent spectral patterns*—Effective second formant, F2′, can be used to produce synthetic vowels that are readily identified phonemically. For front vowels, F2′ has a frequency value between natural F2 and F3; for back vowels, F2′ has about the same frequency as the natural F2.

*Language-dependency of acoustic discrimination*—Listener's discrimination of a given

*It is unwieldy to document each phenomenon with an appropriate citation from the experimental literature; however, the interested reader is referred to comprehensive reviews.[5, 19, 32, 34, 48]

acoustic property can vary with language background; e.g., formant-frequency discrimination for vowels is finer for a speaker of a vowel-rich language.

*Resistance of intelligibility to filtering and other spectral distortions*—No single band of frequencies is absolutely necessary for speech intelligibility, and even severely filtered (or spectrally rotated) signals can be understood under certain conditions.

*Long-term spectral correlates of affect*—Certain spectral regions are correlated with affective dimensions, e.g., arousal, control and pleasure.

### *C. Wave Phenomena: Stream or Induction Effects*

*Streaming*—Assignment of sounds to inferred sources; listeners can segregate simultaneous sound sequences according to the time-frequency relations of the components. Under certain conditions of repetition, speech stimuli will "break apart" to form co-occurring streams; e.g., a repeated [sa] will break into a repeated [da] stream and a nonspeech noise stream.

*P-Center*—One of the most reliable aspects of listener perception related to syllable pattern; indicates the perceptual center of a syllable.

*Language rhythms*—Whereas the strict isochronicity hypothesis that speech has regular timing intervals has little support, there is evidence for language-specific tendencies toward isochrony of some unit (e.g., syllable for Spanish, mora for Japanese, and stressed syllable, or stressed-unstressed alternation, for English). These rhythms may be useful in guiding perceptual processing of the speech signal.

*Rate adjustment*—Phonetic interpretation of an acoustic cue can vary with speaking rate (may be a syllable rate phenonemon); the listener knows "fast speech" rules.

*Verbal transformation*—Auditory illusion in which a repeated phonetic sequence is judged to change (even though the physical stimulus is invariant). Upon repeated presentation of a particular word, a listener may suddenly perceive a different word.

*Declination effects*—Range of an articulatory or acoustic variable often declines during the course of an utterance, such that maximal contrastivity is present during the initial portion. Declination is most commonly associated with vocal fundmental frequency, but it appears that declination may also include the intensity envelope and formant movements.

*Phonetic restoration*—Phenomenon in which listeners hear a speech sound that has been physically replaced with an extraneous sound; the effect appears to depend on the adequacy of contextual cues. For example, the underlined sound in "Which speech sound is mi*ss*ing in this sentence?" can be replaced by a nonspeech noise, but listeners will be unaware of the substitution.

*Sinusoidal synthesis*—Synthetic version of speech in which sinusoids are regulated to vary roughly in the manner of the formant frequencies of natural speech. This highly simplified signal frequently can be interpreted as speech.

*Slips of the ear*—Listener's misidentifications of speech are strongly influenced by stress and intonation patterns, phrase and word recognition, and stressed vowels.

*Delayed auditory feedback (DAF)*—Delayed sidetone; at a critical delay interval, it can become difficult to speak under DAF.

*Right hemisphere advantage for prosodic patterns*—Left ear (and inferentially the right hemisphere) outperforms the right ear (and inferentially the left hemisphere) in the recognition of long-term patterns such as melodies and prosodic patterns.

*McGurk effect (discussed under particle phenomena)*—Visual and auditory cues are integrated over the course of an utterance.

Chapter 8

# Auditory Processing Disorder or Attention-Deficit Disorder?

Warren D. Keller, Ph.D.

Symptoms of inattention, distractibility, poor listening skills, and excessive activity are quite common in children. One of my esteemed colleagues, a psychologist who specializes in marital therapy, reminds me often of his sentiments that children are an overrated commodity. He finds them terribly confusing and difficult to understand. While so many of us are intrigued by development, he finds development, especially the very rapid development that occurs throughout childhood, a source of confoundment and confusion. He reminds me that "it's difficult to get a fix on a moving part." My colleague also reminds me that most of his adult clients are much more aware of the source of some of their difficulties. A typical scenario might involve his asking "So, what brings you here to see me today?" and their responding, "Doctor, I'm depressed." If we were to ask one of our children "So, why are you so inattentive, distractible, experiencing such poor listening skills, and so active in school?" I am certain we would all get an "I don't know." Children will behave similarly for a variety of reasons and auditory-processing disorders (APD), attention-deficit disorder (ADD) and a variety of other difficulties can result in symptoms of inattention, distractibility, poor listening skills and hyperactivity. Child psychologists, psychiatrists, and mental health professionals must bear in mind that all that is "hyper" may not be hyperactivity, and speech and language pathologists and audiologists must remember that all that is poor listening may not be APD. The purpose of this chapter will be to sensitize practitioners to the importance of an accurate differential diagnosis between APD and attention-deficit hyperactivity disorder (ADHD).

## ATTENTION-DEFICIT HYPERACTIVITY DISORDER

Attention-deficit hyperactivity disorder, or "hyperactivity," has a long and illustrious history in mental health. As early as the 1900s, the complex of symptoms now referred to as hyperactivity were described as being a "defect in moral control." Later, such terms as postencephalitic disorder, hyperkinesis, minimal brain dysfunction, hyperkinetic reaction of childhood, and ADD with and without hyperactivity were used to describe this disorder. The present terminology as reflected in the *Diagnostic and Statistical Manual of the American Psychiatric Association* is attention-deficit hyperactivity disorder.[1] The terms ADD, ADHD, and hyperactivity will be used synonymously in this chapter.

Hyperactivity is believed to be one of the most common childhood problems referred to child evaluation and treatment centers. Attention-deficit hyperactivity disorder is characterized by inattention, impulsivity, and hyperactivity inappropriate for the chronological age of the child. The child's capacity for sustained attention and concentration is compromised and there is typically an exacerbation of symptoms in situations where physical movement is restrained or where sustained attention and concentration are required. Hyperactive toddlers may scramble out of their car seats when restrained and the hyperactive child in the classroom will become restless and inattentive the longer he or she is required to pay attention. Children with ADHD have difficulty remaining on task and focusing attention. It is believed that they are distractible both auditorially as well as visually; however, their inability to remain attentive might also cause them to seek out distractions. Hyperactive children are impulsive and experience difficulty with delay of gratification. Barkley[3] describes the hyperactive child as having difficulty following rule-governed behavior. Hyperactive children experience difficulty coping with the routine rules to which other children can generally adhere. They experience significant difficulty sustaining appropriate behavior without clear, frequent, and immediate consequences. In addition, they habituate quickly and the effectiveness of rewards and punishments tends to diminish quite rapidly for the hyperactive child. These are children who require significantly greater parental supervision and who provide their parents with frustrating disciplinary dilemmas given their highly oppositional, noncompliant behavior and their seeming inability to profit from experience. It is believed that the prevalence of attention deficit disorder is between 3% and 5% of the school-age population.[3]

Attention-deficit hyperactivity disorder is a chronic, pervasive developmental disorder that is cross-situational and manifests with a variety of secondary features that can be of assistance in making an accurate diagnosis. In addition, the associated features seen in hyperactivity may often become the focus of treatment. The multiple problems associated with ADHD are described in Table 8–1.

Children with ADHD will manifest problems in most situations; while they are at home with their families, while at school with their teachers and peers, while at work, and in many social situations. One of the greatest misperceptions regarding children with ADHD is that they are constantly hyperactive, fidgety, and restless. It is a common belief that if we are able to identify a situation in which the hyperactive child is not "hyperactive" then that child must not be hyperactive. This is not the case. Children with ADHD, when provided frequent reinforcement, strict control, or novelty, will perform much like their nonhyperactive peers. It would not be unusual for a child with ADHD to be able to play video games for an hour or more. Super Mario provides for the child immediate reinforcement and novelty, two behavioral components that will "cure" the hyperactive child. It is believed that an accurate diagnosis of ADHD will be missed approximately 80% of the time if there is an overreliance on observable behavior seen in a brief office visit.

Hyperactive children can be expected to experience difficulties with all aspects of attention. A child who has difficulties with focused attention may be perceived by others as daydreaming. They may seemingly be preoccupied with other thoughts and be perceived by the teacher as lacking in task commitment. A child with impaired selective attention may be easily distracted by extraneous noises in the classroom. The child with impaired divided attention may have difficulty completing two tasks at one time, such as listening during a lecture and taking notes. Children with ADHD may show difficulties with the length of time that they must remain attentive and therefore be unable to sustain their attention. There may also be a deficit with respect to vigilance, or their alertness.

In the school setting, hyperactive children will be described by their teachers as having a short attention span. Since their ability to sustain attention is typically compromised they will often experience difficulty completing academic tasks, especially written independent work. While some children with attentional difficulties will take inordinate amounts of time to complete rather simple assignments, other ADHD children will complete the assignments quickly, impulsively, and therefore very inaccurately. Their impulsivity may also be manifested by shouting out answers in the classroom, excessive interrupting, excessive talking, motor restlessness, and failure to understand directions before beginning assignments.

School achievement is most often compromised in children with ADHD. The incidence of cognitive deficits resulting in specific learning disabilities is believed to be much greater among the

**TABLE 8–1.**
Attention Deficit Disorder

| | |
|---|---|
| General characteristics | Emotional difficulties |
| Inability to sustain attention | Temper tantrums/explosive behavior |
| Impaired focused attention | Low self-esteem |
| Impaired selective attention | Problems interpreting others' emotions |
| Impaired divided attention | Problems modulating behavior based on feedback |
| Impaired vigilance | Low frustration tolerance |
| Impulsivity | Mood swings |
| Distractibility | Hyperactivity/hyperemotionality |
| Symptoms often seen in school settings | Social difficulties |
| Disorganization | Poor peer relations |
| Short attention span | Problems with turn-taking |
| Impulsivity | Impulsiveness |
| Problems completing work | Hyperactivity |
| Work completed impulsively | Aggressiveness |
| Child takes too long to complete work | Noncompliance |
| Chronic academic underachievement | Lying/stealing |
| Variability in academic performance | Poor self-control |
| Messy work, often carelessly done | Poor general social skills |
| Failure to follow instructions | Alcohol/drug abuse |
| Motor restlessness | Physical features |
| Noisy/excessive talking | Poor general health |
| Associated features | Enuresis/encopresis |
| Cognitive deficits | Increased incidence of otitis media |
| Specific learning disabilities | Increased frequency of allergies/food sensitivities |
| Auditory processing disorders | Greater frequency of disturbance in sleep/wake cycles |
| Problems with visual perceptual processing | Poor motor coordination |
| Academic underachievement for intelligence | Suspected underaroused central nervous system |
| | Greater frequency of minor physical anomalies |
| | Familial pattern to the disorder |

population of children with ADHD. The precise relationship, however, between ADHD and learning disability remains somewhat obscured. Safer and Allen[22] found associated problems of hyperactivity in approximately 80% of a population of learning-disabled children. In another study by Halperin and co-workers,[13] only 9% of a sample of ADHD children evidenced a primary reading disability. Generally, it is believed that 25% to 40% of hyperactive children may have specific learning disabilities that will adversely impact their academic achievement. The types of cognitive processing deficits that they experience are diverse and it is not believed that there is any one specific subtype of learning disorder that characterizes all ADHD children. In addition, a substantial portion of children with ADHD do not have learning disabilities; that is, they do not have specific processing deficits that negatively affect their learning. Very often, however, their achievement and performance in the classroom will be compromised owing to the primary attentional problems and behavioral symptoms that are a result of the ADHD. These children when evaluated one-on-one may show strong academic achievement but yet still be failing in the classroom setting.

Children with ADHD also present with a multiplicity of socioemotional disturbances. Hyperactive children will often present as toddlers with difficult temperaments, temper outbursts, and as highly noncompliant, difficult-to-discipline children. Their impulsivity in the classroom setting is also observed in their interactions with other children. ADHD children may have difficulty sharing, following rules in games, and almost invariably need to be "first." Given the behavioral excesses and poor self-control exhibited by children with ADHD, it should come as no surprise that they often meet with rejection from their peers. Pelham and Bender[19] found evidence that hyperactive children are almost uniformly disliked by their peers. The inappropriate social behavior displayed by hyperactive children leads to peer rejection, which may then lead to increased frustration and an increase in the anger experienced by the hyperactive child towards other children. Barkley[3] estimates that the rate of noncompliance to parental commands may be as high as 70% for the ADHD child. Their inattentiveness, noncompliance, and inappropriate behavior have a pronounced impact on the type of child-management procedures that their parents then adopt. Deviant, defiant children elicit parental behavior characterized by a greater number of commands, increased physical discipline, and more controlling and coercive behavior. The child with an ADD is certainly at an increased risk for depression, especially during the adolescent years. Given the multiplicity of problems with which they are confronted across varying situations it is not surprising that many hyperactive children become depressed adolescents. A substantial number of hyperactive children appear to be at great risk for the development of alcoholism and substance-abuse problems.[9] Attention-disordered children who display excessive aggressiveness, antisocial behavior, and poor social development are at greatest risk for a poor outcome with respect to adulthood status. Higher intelligence, higher socioeconomic status, and lower incidence of severe family psychopathology are all correlated with positive outcomes in adulthood.[10]

There are a variety of physical features also seen in children with ADHD. It is believed that one third to one half of hyperactive children may experience difficulties with bladder and/or bowel control beyond the age at which most children have ceased wetting and soiling.[14] Clinically, many of these children appear as if they are too busy to pay attention to the physiological urges that they may experience either to urinate or to defecate. Whether or not these problems might in fact be related to neuromaturational delays is unknown. Overall, hyperactive children seem to experience generally poor health and appear to be at greater risk for upper respiratory infections, allergies, and ear infections. Hagerman and Falkenstein[12] found that in a group of hyperactive children, 94% had a history of three or more ear infections in contrast to only 50% of nonhyperactive children. In the hyperactive group, 69% had a history of more than 10 bouts of otitis media whereas only 20% of the control group experienced more than 10 episodes.

Some research has found that as many as 50% of hyperactive children will experience allergies,[3] although it is not believed that the allergies cause the attentional problems. Although previous research tended to conclude that food colorings and other food additives had little effect on the behavior of hyperactive children[23] more recent research suggests that food sensitivities may be a significant factor affecting many children with ADHD.[7] Many researchers have speculated on the finding that many hyperactive children appear to metabolize glucose differently. In one study approximately 88% of a sample of children with ADHD had abnormal glucose tolerance test results.[7] Conners also finds that sugars may have a variable effect on behavior depending upon which foods are ingested along with the sugar.[7] In one study Conners found that hyperactive children who ate a protein breakfast followed by sugar actually showed better attention than children who were receiving a placebo substitute for the sugar.[7] Chocolate, nuts, citrus fruits, and milk products are believed to be just some of the foods that can exacerbate behavioral difficulties for a select subgroup of attention-disordered children.

Zametkin and colleagues[24] have found additional evidence consistent with previous blood-flow studies[17] indicating reduced glucose metabolism in adults who had been hyperactive since childhood. The largest reductions in metabolism were in the premotor cortex and the superior prefrontal cortex, areas of the brain believed to be involved in the control of attention and motor activity. Zametkin's findings were consistent with speculation of an underaroused nervous system fostering ADD[3] and supported the speculation that the frontal lobes may have a primary role in hyperactivity. The results were also consistent with the results of neuropsychological tests of frontal lobe function in children with ADD.

The relationship between minor physical anomalies and hyperactive behavior has also been investigated. Children with ADHD are more likely to evidence epicanthal folds, hypertelorism or wideset eyes, attached earlobes, or deviations in their hair whorls. Clinodactyly or a markedly curved fifth finger, a single palmar crease, and high-arched palates may also be seen. Whether these minor physical deviations are specific to hyperactivity or increased in samples of learning disabled and/or children with other psychiatric disturbances is still not clear.[20, 21]

## CENTRAL AUDITORY PROCESSING DISORDER

For those reading about the characteristics and associated features of children with ADHD with a background in audiology or speech and language pathology, the parallels between these children and children with auditory processing disorders should be quite apparent. Children with auditory processing disorders will likely evidence difficulties with communication skills or learning problems owing to compromised integrity of their auditory systems. Keith[15] refers to an auditory processing disorder as the "inability or impaired ability to attend to, discriminate, recognize, or comprehend information presented auditorially even though the person has normal intelligence and hearing sensitivity." Auditory perceptual disorders are more pronounced when there are poor listening environments or in the presence of high levels of auditory background noise. It is believed that children with auditory processing disorders are but a subset of the children who experience language and learning disabilities. The child with an auditory perceptual disorder who experiences difficulties with auditory blending, discrimination of phonemes, auditory closure, or auditory memory may well present very similarly to the child with a primary ADD. The behaviors characteristic of children with auditory processing disorders can be strikingly similar to those of the child with an ADHD and a primary learning disability. Table 8–2 describes those characteristics of children who are at risk for APD.[18]

**TABLE 8–2.**
Behaviors of Children At Risk for APD

| |
|---|
| Says "huh" or "what" frequently |
| Gives inconsistent responses to auditory stimuli |
| Often misunderstands what is said |
| Constantly requests that information be repeated |
| Has poor auditory attention |
| Is easily distracted |
| Has difficulty following oral instructions |
| Has difficulty listening in the presence of background noise |
| Has difficulty with phonics and speech sound discrimination |
| Has poor auditory memory (span and sequence) |
| Has poor receptive and expressive language |
| Gives slow or delayed response to verbal stimuli |
| Has reading, spelling, and other academic problems |
| Learns poorly through the auditory channel |
| Exhibits behavior problems |

Not only can the child with ADHD look like the child with APD, the types of classroom management strategies and remediation procedures that are effective for the child with auditory processing disorders can also be quite effective for the child with ADHD.[18] The similarities in the behavioral manifestations of APD and ADD; the distractibility, hyperactivity, short attention span, forgetfulness, restlessness, problems following directions, inappropriate social behavior, excessive talking, and inability to complete assignments have led some to question whether or not APD and ADD may reflect a single developmental disorder.[6, 8] It has been postulated that central auditory processing deficits reflect no more than primary attention deficits. In a relatively small sample of 21 children, it was found that test scores on a standard auditory processing battery significantly improved when the children with presumed APD were provided stimulant treatment. Burd and Fisher[6] have argued that central auditory processing tests do not provide an effective measure of auditory processing abilities since they tend to be very attention-dependent and appear to measure little else other than attention. They questioned whether APD existed independent of ADD.[6]

Audiologists need not feel alone with respect to these attacks. Undoubtedly, critics questioning the existence of ADHD and the most effective treatment approaches recommended by psychologists and psychiatrists have been quite vocal.[4] To my knowledge, no one has yet appeared on the Oprah Winfrey show questioning the existence of auditory processing disorders as they have questioned the existence of ADHD.

## RELATIONSHIP BETWEEN APD AND ADD

The relationship between central auditory processing dysfunction and attention-deficit hyperactivity disorder is not known. Keith[15] certainly acknowledges that ADHD and APD may be related. My impression is that there is a syndrome of symptoms characterized by impulsivity, inattention, and distractibility that we now term ADHD. In addition, some children suffer from inherent auditory perceptual difficulties that we describe as APD. Auditory processing dysfunction, in my opinion, is likely a separate disorder that may occur in conjunction with ADHD or may occur independently.

Baker and Cantwell[2] have found that a significant percentage of children who as toddlers presented with speech and language problems developed symptoms of inattention and hyperactivity. The increased incidence of behavioral difficulties in children with speech and language delays is well known.[16] Clearly, the relationship between auditory and language dysfunction and behavioral disorders appears to be an intimate one.

In making a differential diagnosis of ADHD in a youngster one must be cautious that a primary depressive disorder, anxiety disorder, or oppositional disorder is not mimicking ADHD. Children with specific developmental disorders, or learning disabilities, can also present as being inattentive and distractible and share many symptoms characteristic of ADHD children. In addition, chaotic disorganized family situations or the situational stresses that might co-occur with traumas such as divorce might also result in symptoms similar to ADHD. There is no mention in *Diagnostic and Statistical Manual of Mental Disorders, Third Edition Revised* of the fact that auditory perceptual difficulties can present as ADHD as well. Similarly, in one of the most comprehensive and practical texts available on the assessment and treatment of ADHD[5] there is little mention of auditory processing disorders and their possible comorbidity with ADHD.

## SOME THOUGHTS ON DIFFERENTIAL DIAGNOSIS OF APD AND ADD

I believe that all too often the differential diagnosis of APD or ADD may be determined largely by whether or not the family first consults with an audiologist or psychologist.

When initially asked to write this chapter, the question was raised how, as a practicing child psychologist, I was able to accurately refer children with auditory processing disorders to audiologists based on my evaluations. The fact that a good deal of my practice is focused on the diagnosis and treatment of hyperactive children is likely testimony to the fact that there exists a close relationship between APD and ADD. In addition, I believe, like Gordon,[11] that comprehensive evaluation leads to the most effective treatment. Nearly all children whom I evaluate are administered the *Goldman Fristoe Woodcock Test of Auditory Discrimination,* the *Selective Attention Test,* or more recently the *SCAN,* and during the past 10 years I have been impressed by the numbers of children whom I have evaluated because of school and behavior problems who experience so much difficulty on these types of tasks. The child whom I would typically refer for further auditory perceptual testing is the child with a history of recurrent otitis media, with perhaps some speech articulation difficulties, with poor performance on a measure of auditory discrimination in quiet or noise who did *not* present with the complex of symptoms and associated features also characteristic of ADHD. Children who perform poorly on the Speech Sounds Perception Test or the Rhythm Test from the *Halstead Reitan Neuropsychological Battery* would also be candidates for further central auditory testing. Those children who on neuropsychological examination showed evidence of left-hemisphere dysfunction and poor reading and language skills would also be referred for further central auditory testing. The possibility of auditory processing deficits is increased when these children do not present on standardized measures of personality and behavioral functioning as characteristic of ADHD children.

Despite warnings to the contrary, suppressed performance on the Distractibility Factor of the Wechsler Intelligence Scale for Children Revised will often be interpreted by psychologists as suggestive of "hyperactivity." The Distractibility Factor comprises the Arithmetic, Digit Span, and Coding subtests of the Wechsler Intelligence Scale for Children Revised. While poor concentration and "distractibility" can certainly result in poor performance on these measures, these subtests of the Wechsler Scales also provide sensitive measures of auditory memory and the child's ability to retain and interpret lengthy auditory input. It is quite likely that suppressed performance on these subtests, especially the Arithmetic and Digit Span subtests, can be sensitive markers for central auditory processing disturbance. Poor performance on the "Distractibility Factor" can be indicative of a primary learning disorder or APD as well as an ADHD.

A diagnosis of ADHD should not be made without first ruling out the possibility that APD might be mimicking ADHD. I have had the opportunity to evaluate children who I believe were erroneously provided stimulant treatment, who did not benefit from the medication, and who had auditory perceptual disorders without ADHD. When stimulant treatment was stopped, there was no change in their behavioral functioning or school performance. Very often, these have been children who have undergone minimal evaluation prior to beginning methylphenidate therapy with little medication follow-up. On the other hand, like Burd and Fisher,[6] I often see children whose poor performance on a measure such as the Noise subtest of the *Test of Auditory Discrimination* appears to be the result of inattention and distractibility secondary to ADHD and whose performance significantly improves when they are provided stimulant treatment. Performance on measures of auditory distractibility and, I suspect, on other measures of central auditory processing capabilities can provide useful supplementary information in order to titrate dosages of stimulant medication to therapeutic levels. A diagnosis of APD should not be made without first ruling out the possibility that the child's poor performance on central auditory testing may be secondary to the inattention and impulsivity associated with ADHD.

Considerable effort needs to be placed into being able to better determine when APD is really ADD, when ADD is really APD, and when APD and ADD are coexisting. Being sensitive to the existence of both disorders certainly provides a good start.

For a practicing psychologist, being able to make a differential diagnosis between ADHD and APD might be analogous to differentiating ADHD from a depressive disorder. In order to make this differential diagnosis, one would utilize the various tests and measures known to be effective in distinguishing these two groups, such as standardized personality measures, measures of impulsivity, objective measures of attention, behavioral assessment, and developmental history. It has yet to be demonstrated what tools might be available to the clinician that can most accurately differentiate children with ADHD, APD or both disorders. For example, one might hypothesize that children with ADHD will as a group perform poorly on measures of auditory memory secondary to inattention, but that only children with APD will perform poorly on an auditory closure task secondary to their central auditory processing deficits. While the relationship between APD and ADHD has yet to be described, I will leave the researchers among us to consider the following:

1. Can it be shown that children with ADHD will show difficulties with tasks such as the Auditory Figure Ground test on the *SCAN* or the Noise subtest on the *Test of Auditory Discrimination* secondary to their inattention and distractibility while performing well on other auditory perceptual tasks?

2. Can ADHD children be differentiated from children with primary auditory perceptual difficulties based upon progressive deterioration performance owing to difficulties with *sustained* attention and concentration?

3. Are there differences in the types of learning difficulties that may occur with ADHD or APD?

4. Can it be shown that children with APD will perform well on objective measures of attention as compared with children with ADHD? Will children with APD perform poorly on central auditory tests but perform adequately on a measure of auditory vigilance such as proposed by Keith?[21]

5. Do children with APD differ from children with ADHD with respect to their performance on measures of auditory attention as opposed to measures of visual attention? Can ADHD children be differentiated from those with APD based upon their performance on such measures as a visual continuous performance test vs. an auditory continuous performance test?

6. Do children with APD show any specific profiles on intellectual evaluation or can they be differentiated based upon suppressed verbal scores relative to performance scores?

7. Will ADHD children show a greater complex of symptoms, such as minor physical anomalies, impulsivity, enuresis and encopresis, and greater socioemotional difficulties?

8. Do children with APD present with

greater speech articulation difficulties, spelling difficulties, and suppressed language functioning than those with ADHD?

9. Do children with ADHD present with more severe behavioral difficulties as opposed to children with APD?

10. Should audiologists screen for ADHD using such items as the *Conner's Scales,* the *Child Behavior Checklist,* or the *Personality Inventory for Children,* which are helpful in identifying children with ADHD?

11. Should psychologists and psychiatrists be including auditory problems checklists in their assessments of "hyperactive" children in order to help rule out auditory processing problems?

12. Can it be demonstrated that measures of auditory vigilance and/or auditory distractibility are sensitive to the effects of stimulant medication?

13. How can we identify children whose poor performance on measures of auditory processing capabilities can be significantly improved with stimulant medication?

14. Is the group of children whom we describe as having an ADD without hyperactivity largely composed of children who might be experiencing APD?

## REFERENCES

1. American Psychiatric Association: *Diagnostic and Statistical Manual of Mental Disorders,* ed 3, rev. Washington, DC, 1987.
2. Baker L, Cantwell DP: A prospective psychiatric follow-up of children with speech and language disorders. *J Am Acad Child Psychiatr* 1987; 26:546–553.
3. Barkley RA: *Hyperactive Children: A Handbook for Diagnosis and Treatment.* New York, Guilford Press, 1981.
4. Barkley R: An alert to a national campaign of disinformation! *Clin Child Psych Newslett* 1988; 3:1–2.
5. Barkley R: *Attention Deficit Hyperactivity Disorder: A Handbook for Diagnosis and Treatment.* New York, Guilford Press, 1990.
6. Burd L, Fisher W: Central auditory processing disorder or attention deficit disorder? *Dev Behav Pediatr* 1986; 7:215.
7. Conners CK: *Feeding the Brain: How Foods Affect Children.* New York, Plenum Press, 1989.
8. Gascon GG, Johnson R, Burd L: Central auditory processing and attention deficit disorders. *J Child Neurol* 1986; 1:27–33.
9. Gittelman R, Mannuzza A, Shenker R, et al: Hyperactive boys almost grown up. I. Psychiatric status. *Arch Gen Psychiatr* 1985; 42:937–947.
10. Goldstein S, Goldstein M: *Managing Attention Disorders in Children: A Guide for Practitioners.* New York, John Wiley and Sons, 1990.
11. Gordon M: *ADHD/Hyperactivity: A Consumer's Guide.* DeWitt, NY, GSI Publications, 1991.
12. Hagerman RJ, Falkenstein AR: An association between recurrent otitis media in infancy and later hyperactivity. *Clin Pediatr* 1987; 5:253–257.
13. Halperin JM, Gittelman R, Klein DF, et al: Reading-disabled hyperactive children: A district subgroup of attention deficit disorder with hyperactivity? *J Abnorm Child Psychol* 1984; 12:1–14.
14. Ingersoll B: *Your Hyperactive Child.* New York, Doubleday, 1988.
15. Keith RW: SCAN: A screening test for auditory processing disorders. San Antonio, Texas, The Psychological Corporation, 1986.
16. Love AJ, Thompson NGG: Language disorders and attention deficit disorders in young children referred for psychiatric services: Analysis of prevalence and a conceptual synthesis. *Am J Orthopsychiatry* 1988; 58:52–64.
17. Lou HC, Henriksen L, Bruhn P: Focal cerebral hypoperfusion in children with dysphasia and/or attention deficit disorder. *Arch Neurol* 1984; 41:825–829.
18. Matkin ND: *Research Issues and Future Directions, personal communication,* 1992.
19. Pelham WE, Bender ME: Peer relationships and hyperactive children: Description and treatment, in Gadow K, Bailer I (eds): *Advances in Learning and Behavioral Disabilities,* vol 1. Greenwich, Conn, JAI Press, 1982.
20. Pomeroy JC, Sprafkin J, Gadow KD: Minor physical anomalies as a biologic marker for behavioral disorders. *J Am Acad Child Adolesc Psychiatr* 1988; 27:466–473.
21. Quinn P, Rapoport J: Minor physical anomalies and neurologic status in hyperactive boys. *Pediatrics* 1974; 53:742–747.
22. Safer DJ, Allen RP: *Hyperactive Children: Diagnosis and Management.* Baltimore, University Park Press, 1976.
23. Wender E: The food additive-free diet in the treatment of behavior disorders: A review. *J Dev Behav Pediatr* 1986; 7:35–42.
24. Zametkin AJ, Nordahl TE, Gross M, et al: Cerebral glucose metabolism in adults with hyperactivity of childhood onset. *N Engl J Med* 1990; 323:1361–1367.

*PART* ***IV***

# AUDIOLOGIC CONSIDERATIONS AND APPROACHES

*Chapter* **9**

# Central Auditory Processing: Implications in Audiology

**Nancy A. Stecker, Ph.D.**

Audiologists have been involved in central auditory testing for over 30 years. Bocca[5] and his colleagues were the first to use special tests to evaluate problems at various levels of the central auditory nervous system (CANS).

This chapter will discuss the audiologist's role in the evaluation of central auditory processing disorders (CAPDs). Various behavioral measures used by audiologists to assess peripheral and central auditory function will be presented. This discussion is not meant to review all known measurement techniques but to provide the reader with information on the most widely used and studied procedures.

Audiologists have some unique abilities to offer in the evaluation of CAPD. The functioning of the entire auditory system can be assessed in a controlled environment using carefully controlled stimuli. Also, the audiologist can assess auditory function to provide the best management strategies.

## PERIPHERAL ASSESSMENT

Assessment of peripheral auditory function is essential in a CAPD evaluation. Pure-tone air-and bone-conduction thresholds must be obtained to rule out conductive and sensorineural hearing losses, which have been shown to influence central auditory test results.[1] The thresholds are also used for calculating the presentation levels of suprathreshold tests. Word discrimination scores in quiet are used for comparison with speech-in-noise test results and are needed for the corrected Staggered Spondaic Word (SSW) test score.

Immittance testing should be carried out to rule out middle-ear pathology. Contralateral and ipsilateral acoustic reflex thresholds can be used to assess lower brain-stem functioning.

There has been some evidence to suggest that persons with CAPD have an abnormal audiometric contour.[19] The thresholds are often within defined normal limits of hearing sensitivity yet display a rising audiogram. Jerger[19] in 1988 compared three groups of children: those with known auditory brain lesions, those with known nonauditory brain lesions, and those with suspected CAPD. Average thresholds were within normal limits bilaterally for all groups: better than 20 dB HL. Children with confirmed auditory brain lesions and suspected CAPD had thresholds significantly poorer in the low frequencies relative to those in the nonauditory lesion group.

Pure-tone thresholds for 75 clients evaluated at the University at Buffalo Speech, Language, and Hearing Clinic over a 2-year period were studied. These clients with known CAPDs showed similar results to Jerger's findings.[19] Although pure-tone thresholds were within defined normal limits, a rising audiometric slope was evident.

Hasbrouck[13] in 1989 reported on a study of 22 patients who presented with nonorganic hearing loss. They were evaluated using a battery of tests that examined eight areas of auditory function. The test results demonstrated that all 22 patients with nonorganic hearing loss had significant auditory processing disorders. Hasbrouck suggested that these results indicate a specific CAPD could adversely affect a patient's hearing ability.[13]

The value of the peripheral evaluation cannot be underestimated. Frank Musiek, in Chapter 2, states that the connection between the peripheral and central auditory systems is not fully understood, nor is the role the periphery plays in auditory perception. Typically, persons are referred for auditory assessment because of difficulty hearing or listening. The complaints of those with CAPD are often similar to those with peripheral hearing loss. It is our responsibility as audiologists to investigate to the best of our abilities the auditory complaints our clients present. We must continue our evaluation by broadening the tests we use or using new procedures to define the specific auditory problem.

## CENTRAL AUDITORY PROCESSING ASSESSMENT

The original use of most CAP tests was for the detection of CANS lesions. Over the past 20 years, many or these tests have been adapted for use in the evaluation of CAPD. These tests include both adult tests for site-of-lesion that have adjusted norms for individuals with suspected CAPD and tests that were developed to conform to children's interests to describe auditory function.[1]

A study reported by Jerger et al[19] in 1988 compared 3- to 8-year-old children with confirmed lesions with those with suspected CAPD. Test results were compared for the groups on pure-tone thresholds, acoustic-reflex thresholds (ART), and the Pediatric Speech Intelligibility (PSI) test. Children with confirmed lesions in auditory areas and those with suspected CAPD had normal hearing sensitivity with an abnormal rising contour, normal ART, and abnormal speech perception for both monotic and dichotic materials. These results were consistent with patterns found in previous adult studies supporting the usefulness of central auditory tests in evaluating CAPD.

The discussion of available CAP tests in this chapter is not exhaustive but presents the evaluation tools most widely researched and those used most frequently in clinical settings. The tests are grouped into monotic speech and tone tests, dichotic tests, binaural tests, and other tests that do not fit into the previous categories.

### Monotic Speech Tests

**Low-Pass Filtered Speech.**—Bocca and his colleagues[5] were the first to use low-pass filtered speech to measure central auditory functioning. Since that time many authors have reported on the use of LPFS testing.[11, 15, 34] Willeford's LPFS subtest is probably the most commonly used form of the Colorado State University Battery.[48] His test uses consonant-nucleus-consonant stimuli low-passed at 500 Hz with an 18 dB/octave rejection rate. The words are presented monaurally at 50 dB SL. The scores are compared with age norms and ear asymmetry is examined. The norms suggest a maturation effect with minimal ear difference.

The SCAN test by Keith[25] also has a Filtered Words subtest. Twenty monosyllabic words are presented monaurally. They are low-passed at 1,000 Hz with a 32 dB/octave rejection rate. The scores are compared to norms by age. The SCAN and Willeford tests are described in more detail in Chapter 10.

**Time-Altered Speech.**—Time-or rate-altered speech tests evaluate temporal auditory processing, an area that is not often tapped in other central auditory tests. In these tests speech stimuli are accelerated or expanded monosyllables, spondees, or sentences that are presented monaurally. Beasley and Maki[3] in 1976 used NU-6 word lists compressed at different ratios (0%, 30%, 40%, 50%, 60%, and 70%). In normal listeners 60% compression ratio has been shown to be the cutoff level for normal performance. Data has also shown that there is a significant difference in performance at the 60% rate between normals and persons with CAPD.[27, 31]

The Wichita Auditory Processing Test (WAPT) by McCroskey[30] uses time-altered sentences at four different ratios presented in this order: 100%, 200%, 70%, and 130%. Ten sentences are presented at each rate with a picture-pointing response required. The scores are compared with norms by age and scores are compared among the four ratio levels.

**Speech-in-Noise Tests.**—One of the most common complaints of individuals with CAPD is the inability to process speech in a background of noise. The ability to process speech in the presence of noise is tested in a variety of ways. Baran and Musiek[1] reported that the most common speech-in-noise tests use monosyllables presented at 40 dB SL with a background of white or speech noise at a 0 to +10 signal-to-noise ratio. There is no one standard way of conducting speech-in-noise tests and several variables need to be standardized before using these tests clinically. The audiologist may choose from several types of speech stimuli (monosyllables or sentences), different types of noises (white, speech, cafeteria, multitalker, or running discourse), various signal-to-noise ratios (ranges from −10 to +20), and presentation types (ipsilateral or contralateral under phones or in the sound field). Therefore it is imperative that each clinic standardize its test conditions and establish norms for various age groups for their speech-in-noise tests to be valid.

There are some commercially available speech-in-noise tests. The Goldman-Fristoe-Woodcock Test of Auditory Discrimination includes a quiet and noise subtest. Monosyllabic words are presented binaurally using cafeteria noise at a +9 signal-to-noise ratio. Scores are compared with norms by age.

The Selective Auditory Attention Test (SAAT) by Cherry[7] is a binaural speech-in-noise test that uses white noise at a 0 dB signal-to-noise ratio. This test is described in greater detail in Chapter 10.

The Auditory Figure Ground subtest of the SCAN test by Keith[25] uses monosyllablic words presented monaurally in a babble noise at a +8 dB signal-to-noise ratio. Scores are compared with norms by age.

The Speech Perception in Noise Test (SPIN) was reported by Bilger.[4] This test uses sentences as the speech stimuli and the final word is the target response. The final word in half of the sentences is either easily predicted based on the context of the sentence or not predictable. Babble noise is presented at the signal-to-noise ratio of +8 dB.

The Ipsilateral Competing Message (ICM) portion of the Synthetic Sentence Identification Test (SSI) by Jerger et al[17] can be used as a speech-in-noise test. Ten nonsense sentences, printed on a response card, are used as the speech stimuli. The subject is required to only give the number of the sentence heard. The noise is a continuous discourse and the signal-to-noise ratio is varied in order to complete a performance-intensity function. The authors provide a normal performance range for ear scores and suggest comparing ear asymmetries. Subjects must be able to read the sentences for this task. The Pediatric Speech Intelligibility Test (PSI)[16] is a children's version of the SSI and does not require the individual to read. This test is described in greater detail in Chapter 10.

A few recent studies have been reported that employ speech-in-noise tests in CAPD evaluation. Chermak et al[6] in 1989 reported on a study that compared word identification performance in noise in learning-disabled adults. Eight learning-disabled and eight normal control adults were tested using NU-6 word lists presented in speech spectrum noise and three different linguistic maskers: grammatic linguistic strings, semantic anomolous strings, and ungrammatic strings. These maskers were chosen to evaluate the strength of the linguistic content of the noise. A +12.5 dB signal-to-noise ratio was used. The results showed that the learning-disabled group performed significantly more poorly on all measures than the control group. Both groups scored worst with the speech noise masker. There was no difference between groups using the three linguistic maskers. The result suggested that the speech spectrum noise was the more effective masker and that the linguistic content of the speech maskers was not important.

### Monotic Tone Tests

**Pitch Pattern Sequence (PPS) Test.**—This test is an example of a monaurally presented central auditory test using tones as stimuli. The test was reported by Pinheiro[38] in 1977 to assess pattern perception and temporal sequencing skills. The stimuli include low (880 Hz) and high (1,430

Hz) tones of 500 ms duration with a 300-ms interval between tones. The tones are presented in groups of three with six possible sequences. Thirty stimuli are presented monaurally to each ear at a comfortable listening level. Three response modes are used: hummed, verbal, or point. Normal listeners can respond well in all three modes. Musiek et al[35] in 1982 reported that learning-disabled individuals could hum the correct response but did poorly on verbal and pointing tasks. This test can be used with all ages, but there is wide scatter in performance seen under age 7 years. In 1978, Pinheiro[39] compared normal and dyslexic children using the PPS test and found significant differences in performance for two age groups.

**Duration Pattern Test.**—Baran and coauthors[2] in 1987 reported on the Duration Pattern Test (DPT). The design of the test is similar to the PPS test but uses short (250 ms) and long (500 ms.) stimuli. The test stimuli are in sets of three with six possible patterns. Responses are either verbal or pointing. A 70% correct score has been suggested as the normal performance cutoff score. In 1990, Musiek et al[33] reported on a study evaluating learning-disabled college students on several CAP measures and found the DPT to be one of the most sensitive tests for this age group. Because this test uses tonal stimuli rather than linguistic stimuli, it is more challenging.[2] In 1991, Jerger et al[18] used the DPT as one of many CAP measures to evaluate an 18-year-old college student with suspected CAPD. Although the student scored within normal limits overall, she had an abnormally low score on the short-long-short sequence in the left ear. Therefore, careful examination of each pattern may provide useful information regarding the processing skills of an individual.

**Wichita Auditory Fusion Test.**—In 1984, McCrosky[29] devised the Wichita Auditory Fusion Test (WAFT) to evaluate temporal functioning. The test uses pairs of tonal stimuli that are gradually separated in time by millisecond intervals, called interpulse intervals. The response required is to report if one or two tones are heard. There is a screening version, short, and expanded versions of the test. An auditory fusion threshold is calculated for each ear at each frequency. There is an age effect but no frequency or ear effect. The younger the subject, the longer it takes to hear two tones. More information on temporal processing can be found in Chapter 7.

Monotic speech and tonal tests can be an important addition to a central auditory test battery. Overall, the tests show improved performance with increasing age. There appears to be no ear effect for normal subjects on these tests. Considerable variability is generally found at each age level but severely depressed scores can be considered abnormal and ear asymmetries can provide useful information.

### Dichotic Speech Tests

Kimura[26] in 1961 developed a model to explain how the CANS handles dichotically presented stimuli—that is, different signals to each ear. Her model states that contralateral pathways are more numerous and stronger than ipsilateral pathways. In monaural presentations either pathway is capable of initiating an appropriate response. In dichotic presentations the stronger contralateral pathway will take precedence over the weaker ipsilateral ones and may even cause suppression of the ipsilateral pathway. Several dichotic tests have been developed to evaluate central auditory function based on this model.

**Dichotic Digits Test.**—Several investigators have used digits as stimuli in dichotic testing including Kimura,[26] Sparks,[43] and Musiek.[32] Musiek used two digits presented to each ear simultaneously. The test is reportedly sensitive to brainstem and cortical lesions. He suggests that because the response is easier than words for some and the test takes only four minutes to administer, it may be a useful screening test for CANS disorders.[32]

**Staggered Spondaic Word Test.**—In 1962 Katz[20] reported on the SSW as a measure of central auditory function. The test stimuli are spondees presented dichotically in a staggered manner resulting in four conditions: right noncompeting (RNC), right competing (RC), left competing (LC), and left noncompeting (LNC). Figure 9–1 presents an example of the pattern of presentation. Although the test was originally developed as a site-of-lesion test, it is now used for evaluating children and adults with suspected CAPD. The test is scored

| | RNC | RC | |
|---|---|---|---|
| RE: | UP | STAIRS | |
| LE: | | DOWN | TOWN |
| | | LC | LNC |

**FIG 9–1.**
Staggered Spondaic Word (SSW) Test stimuli.

quantitatively and qualitatively (see Chapter 6 for more details on scoring and test results). Several studies have shown this test to be a very useful measure of CAP function.[22, 24, 25]

**Competing Environmental Sounds (CES) Test.**—The CES test was developed by Katz[23] to be used in conjunction with the SSW test. The CES test uses familiar everyday sounds as stimuli that are presented dichotically, one to each ear simultaneously. Four pictures are displayed per test item and the individual either points or verbalizes which two of the four were heard. Scoring is in percent error and is compared to the SSW test results to better delineate site-of-lesion.

**Contralateral Competing Message (CCM).**—The SSI-CCM developed by Jerger[17] in 1974 is part of the same test reported earlier in this chapter (SSI-ICM). The stimuli are the same ten sentences on a response plate and the competing message is continuous running speech. The competing message in this part of the test is presented in the ear contralateral to the sentence stimuli at varied signal-to-noise ratios (−40 to 0 dB). A comparison of performance between the two ears and the overall score are calculated. Also, the SSI-CCM results are compared to the SSI-ICM results in order to determine site-of-lesion.

**Dichotic Sentence Identification (DSI) Test.**—The DSI test was reported in 1983 by Fifer et al[10] as a dichotic test that could be administered to individuals with hearing loss. The test uses six of the ten SSI sentences as stimuli. As with the SSI, the sentences are written on a response plate and the individual reports the number of the sentences heard, one presented to each ear simultaneously. Normal performance is a score of 75% or better for each ear. There are also norms provided for individuals with hearing loss.

**Competing Sentences (CS).**—The CS subtest of the Willeford test battery[48] uses a primary sentence presented at 30 dB SL and a competing sentence presented contralaterally at 50 dB SL. The subject is expected to repeat the primary sentence. A variation of the test has been used in which the sentences are presented at the same level binaurally and both sentences must be repeated. Age norms are provided for the test and it is best used at age seven and above.

**Competing Words (CW).**—The CW subtest of the SCAN test by Keith et al[25] uses familiar monosyllabic words presented dichotically as stimuli. The child is instructed to repeat both words presented but is asked to focus on and say the word from the right ear first. Then the child is instructed to do the same for the left ear. Norms are provided by age and a comparison is made between the performance of the two ears. More detail of this test is provided in Chapter 10.

Overall, dichotic tests have been very popular and quite useful in the evaluation of CAPD. There are a few important variables to consider when using dichotic tests. There is a right-ear advantage in younger children and there is a maturational effect especially in the left ear. In cases with CAPD, test results often show the left ear scores to be depressed compared with age-appropriate norms.[1]

### Binaural Integration/Interaction Tests

Binaural integration/interaction tests include measures in which both ears are stimulated, but unlike dichotic tests, the stimuli is the same for both ears. These binaural tests evaluate the integration between the two ears and tests functions thought to be carried out at the brain-stem level of the CANS.

**Masking Level Difference (MLD) Test.**—The MLD test has been reported to be useful as a clinical tool to assess lower brain-stem function.[14, 46] The MLD depends on the ability of the auditory system to process subtle interaural time and amplitude differences. The stimulus most often used is a 500-Hz pure tone or spondaic words.

The masker is narrowband noise centered around 500 Hz or speech noise. The stimulus and masker are presented binaurally for two conditions. In the first condition the stimulus and masker are both in phase between the earphones. In the second condition the stimulus is out of phase and the masker is in phase. A threshold for the stimulus in the noise is obtained for each condition. The MLD test score is the difference between the two thresholds. The norms reported for this test have varied considerably, probably owing to differences in equipment and the test variables chosen. Therefore it is essential to develop norms for individual equipment, populations served, and for different age groups.

Hall and Grose[12] in 1990 reported on the effect of age on the MLD score for a 500-Hz pure-tone signal. Subjects were 4- to 9-year-old children and adult controls. The mean MLD score was 15 dB for the adult subjects and 13 dB for the children. Test results showed that the MLD score increased as a function of age up to 5 to 6 years old. This might suggest that the auditory processing of interaural difference cues that account for the MLD are not developmentally mature until age 5 to 6 years. The authors suggested that reduced MLD scores in children above age 6 may be related to reduced ability of the CANS to interpret information from binaural difference cues that are available in the auditory brainstem.

**Binaural Fusion (BF) Tests.**—The first BF test was reported by Matzker[28] in 1959 as a test of lower auditory brain-stem functioning. Robert Ivey's BF subtest 8 of the Colorado State University or Willeford's battery is probably the most commonly used BF test today.[2] The stimuli are spondaic words that are filtered into two bands: 500 to 700 Hz and 1,900 to 2,100 Hz. A dichotic presentation, in which one ear receives the low-pass words and the opposite ear receives the high-pass words, is compared with a diotic presentation, in which both ears receive both band-passes. The score recorded is the percent of words repeated correctly for the ear receiving the low-pass filtered words. This test is normed by age from 6 years to adult.

**Rapid Alternating Speech Perception (RASP) Test.**—The RASP test is another subtest of the Colorado State University or Willeford battery.[48] Sentence stimuli are presented in alternating bursts of 300 ms duration between the ears. The entire sentence must be repeated as the response and a percent correct score is compared with norms by age. This test has been reported to be the least sensitive of the Willeford test battery.[1]

**Speech-in-Noise Tests.**—Speech-in-noise tests were discussed earlier in this chapter as a monotic procedure but can also be presented in a binaural manner. Either under earphones or in the sound field, both the speech stimuli and the noise can be presented to both ears. The binaural score may yield important functional information concerning auditory processing ability, especially when compared to monotic scores. For example, a person who scores more poorly on one ear but has binaural score as good as the better ear would be managed differently from someone who has a binaural score that is similar to the poorer ear. This comparison may assist in planning a successful management program.

Papso and Blood[37] in 1989 reported on a study that compared the word recognition performance of 4- to 6-year-old children and adults on the Word Intelligibility by Picture Index (WIPI) test presented at 0° azimuth in the sound field in quiet and noise. Both pink noise and a multitalker noise were employed at a +6 dB signal-to-noise ratio. Results showed that adults were not affected by either noise. Children performed significantly more poorly on both noise conditions than adults. The multitalker noise was more adverse than the pink noise. The authors suggested that speech-in-noise data collected on adults cannot be applied to children, therefore separate norms should be developed for testing children.

Binaural tests can be used to assess binaural integration skills. These tests seem most sensitive to lower brain-stem functioning. The BF test seems to be the most sensitive and the most popular clinical binaural test administered.[1]

**Other Central Auditory Processing**

**Phonemic Synthesis (PS) Test.**—The PS test by Katz[21] is an example of a test that does not fit into the previously described categories of CAP tests, yet can be very useful as part of a CAP test battery. The PS test uses speech sounds of monosyllabic words presented at least 1 second apart as stimuli. Saying the correct word is the expected response. The test is normed by grade level. This test is described in greater detail in Chapter 6.

In 1984, Stecker[44] compared normal children and those with CAPD on several tasks designed to tap efferent auditory system functioning. In studies where sectioning of the olivocochlear bundle was carried out to study the effect on audition, reports of behavioral changes were quite similar to those of individuals with CAPD (normal hearing sensitivity yet abnormal suprathreshold skills and limited auditory attention).[8, 41, 47] Therefore tasks were developed based on research tests used in animal and human studies of efferent auditory system functioning to determine if children with CAPDs had poorer performance than controls. Several masking paradigms were used and are summarized in Table 9–1. Results showed significant differences between groups on all measures except for one of the experimental procedures. There were no significant differences for the control procedures that were similar to the experimental tests but had been shown to be insensitive to olivocochlear damage. Efron[9] suggested that activation of the efferent pathways may enhance our ability to perceive a stimulus on the contralateral side of auditory space. In addition, interaction between the ears, speech-in-noise skills, binaural integration, and frequency, intensity, and time perception may all be influenced by efferent auditory system functioning. Therefore, further study is needed in this area in order for audiologists to better understand efferent influence on CAP and to identify its influence in clinical cases.

Another assessment tool that could be included in the CAP test battery is a self-assessment scale. It was reported previously that those with CAPD often complain of difficulty hearing in the presence of normal peripheral hearing. Therefore, a self-assessment scale might better specify those symptoms and yield a better understanding of the auditory functioning of the individual. Jerger et al[18] in 1991 reported on the use of a self-assessment scale as part of an extensive CAP battery administered to an 18-year-old college student with auditory complaints. Although her hearing sensitivity was within normal limits, her score on the self-assessment scale was associated with a mild auditory handicap. Further testing concluded a specific CAPD was present. In this case, the scale provided valuable information in the overall test battery.

Saunders and Haggard[40] in 1989 used the British Hearing Questionnaire in their study comparing CAPD subjects with normal controls. Their experimental group reported significant disability on the scale and their score was not diminished when anxiety level, performance disability, hearing levels, and otologic history were taken into account.

In 1987, Smoski[42] reported on a Children's Auditory Processing Performance Scale (CHAPPS) to be completed by parents, teachers, or the subjects themselves. The scale assesses listening abilities in six categories: noise, quiet, ideal, multiple inputs, auditory memory/sequencing, and auditory attention span. Six questions in each category are ranked and a total score is calculated. The author suggests using the CHAPPS as a pretherapy and posttherapy measure.

Other tests to be used in CAP evaluation include several tests devised by Jerger et al[18] in 1991 to evaluate the 18-year-old college student mentioned previously. They used speech-in-noise tasks in the sound field with three different stimuli (500 Hz pure tone, monosyllabic words, SSI sentences) and three different noises (speech noise, babble noise, and discourse). The results showed a specific deficit when the left ear received the

**TABLE 9–1.**
Masking Paradigms[44]

| Test | Stimulus | Masker Level | Masker |
|---|---|---|---|
| Pure tone masker | 2,000 Hz tone | 40 dB | 2,000 Hz |
| Narrowband masker | 2,000 Hz tone | 40 dB | 2,000 Hz NBN |
| Contralateral narrowband masker | 500, 1,000 4,000 Hz | 20,40,70 dB | 500, 1,000, 4,000 Hz NBN |
| Vowel discrimination difference | /i/,/u/ | Varied | LPN, HPN |

primary message and the right ear the competition. Through use of several measures, her subtle auditory disability was defined. This would not have been possible if not for the persistance of the evaluators and the use of numerous types of tests to search for the auditory disorder reported by the patient. Lauter, in Chapter 5, also stresses the importance of considering individual differences and for assessing ear asymmetries.

## TEST-BATTERY APPROACH

It is suggested that a test-battery approach be used in every CAP evaluation. Audiologists need to choose tests that will evaluate various levels of the CANS and may need to be flexible in order to account for individual auditory complaints. Although only behavioral tests were discussed in this chapter, electrophysiologic measures reported in Chapter 12 may also be included when warranted. Furthermore, a multidisciplinary team approach to assessment of CAPD is desirable in most cases.

Oliver[36] in 1987 reported on the current trends in CAP testing. She surveyed 726 audiologic clinics and had a 54% return rate. Fifty-two percent reported using a total of 33 different CAP tests. Table 9–2 summarizes her results on measures used for children and Table 9–3 for adults. These results do not suggest that these measures are the best or most sensitive tests but they are the most popular, which may indicate ease of administration, presentation, and scoring, availability, and usefulness in planning management strategies.

**TABLE 9–2.**
Most Common Central Auditory Tests Used With Children[36]

| Test | Mean % |
|---|---|
| Staggered Spondaic Word test | 63 |
| Willeford Competing Sentence test | 55 |
| Willeford Filtered Speech test | 46 |
| Willeford Binaural Fusion test | 45 |
| Willeford Rapid Alternating Speech Perception | 44 |
| Speech-in-noise ipsilateral | 42 |
| ABR | 36 |
| Speech-in-noise contralateral | 24 |
| Pitch pattern sequence test | 18 |
| SSI-ICM | 16 |
| SSI-CCM | 13 |
| Time-compressed Speech tests | 11 |
| Dichotic Digits | 7 |
| Phonemic Synthesis Test | 4 |
| Masking level difference | 3 |

**TABLE 9–3.**
Most Common Central Auditory Tests Used With Adults[36]

| Test | Mean % |
|---|---|
| Staggered Spondaic Word test | 59 |
| ABR | 48 |
| Speech-in-noise ipsilateral | 41 |
| Willeford Competing Sentences | 32 |
| SSI-ICM | 29 |
| Willeford Filtered Speech test | 26 |
| SSI-CCM | 24 |
| Willeford Binaural Fusion test | 24 |
| Speech-in-noise contralateral | 23 |
| Willeford RASP | 22 |
| Pitch Pattern Sequence test | 11 |
| Time-Compressed Speech test | 10 |
| Dichotic CVs | 7 |
| Masking level difference | 5 |
| Dichotic Digits | 4 |
| Phonemic Synthesis test | 2 |
| Wichita Auditory Processing test | 1 |

In summary, audiologists should choose a battery of tests that assess all levels and functions of the CANS. CAPD is not a homogeneous problem and therefore selection of tests may vary for each individual. Katz, in Chapter 6, suggests looking for patterns of weaknesses and Lauter, in Chapter 5, stresses being sensitive to individual differences. Norms need to be carefully developed for some tests in individual settings and for different age groups. A self-assessment scale may be a beneficial addition to the test battery. Most importantly, tests should be chosen that can be easily translated into an operational, feasible management plan for each person tested.

It is suggested that a test-battery approach be used in every CAP evaluation. Audiologists need to choose tests that will evaluate various levels of the CANS and may need to be flexible in order to account for individual auditory complaints. Although only behavioral tests were discussed in this chapter, electrophysiologic measures reported in Chapter 12 may also be included when warranted. Furthermore, a multidisciplinary team approach to assessment of CAPD is desirable in most cases.

## REFERENCES


1. Baran J, Musiek F: Behavioral assessment of the central auditory nervous system, in Rintelman W (ed): *Hearing Assessment.* Austin, Texas, Pro-Ed, 1990.
2. Baran J, Musiek F, Gollegly K, et al: Auditory duration pattern sequences in the assessment of CANS pathology. Paper presented at the American Speech-Language-Hearing Association annual meeting, New Orleans, Nov 15, 1987.
3. Beasley D, Maki J: Time- and frequency-altered speech, in Lass N (ed): *Contemporary Issues in Experimental Phonetics. New York,* Academic Press, 1976.
4. Bilger R, Nuetzel J, Rabinowitz W, et al: Standardization of the test of speech perception in noise. *Speech Hear Res* 1983; 27:32–48.
5. Bocca E, Calearo C, Cassinari V: A new method for testing hearing in temporal lobe tumors. *Acta Otolaryngol* 1954; 44:219-221.
6. Chermak G, Vonhof M, Bendel R: Word identification performance in the presence of competing speech and noise in learning disabled adults. *Ear Hear* 1989; 10:90–93.
7. Cherry R, Kruger B: Selective auditory attention abilities of learning disabled and normal achieving children. *J Learn Disabil* 1983; 16:202–205.
8. Dewson J III: Efferent olivo-cochlear bundle: Relationships to stimulus discrimination in noise. *J Neurophysiologica* 1968; 31:122.
9. Efron R, Crandall P: Central auditory processing: Effects of anterior temporal lobectomy. *Brain Lang* 1983; 19:237–253.
10. Fifer R, Jerger J, Berlin C, et al: Development of a dichotic sentence identification test for hearing impaired adults. *Ear Hear* 1983; 4:300–305.
11. Gilroy J, Lynn G: Reversability of abnormal auditory findings in central hemisphere lesions. *J Neurol Sci* 1974; 21:117–131.
12. Hall J, Grose J: The masking-level difference in children. *J Am Acad Audiol* 1990; 2:81–88.
13. Hasbrouck J: Auditory perceptual problems in non-organic hearing disorders. *Laryngoscope* 99:855–860.
14. Hirsh I: The influence of interaural phase on interaural summation and inhibition. *J Acoust Soc Am* 1948; 20:536–544.
15. Jerger J: Audiological manifestations of lesions in the auditory nervous system. *Laryngoscope* 1960; 70:417–425.
16. Jerger S: Validation of the pediatric speech intelligibility test in children with central auditory system lesions. *Audiology* 1987; 26:298–311.
17. Jerger J, Jerger S: Auditory findings in brainstem disorders. *Arch Otolaryngol* 1974; 99:342–349.
18. Jerger J, Johnson K, Jerger S, et al: Central auditory processing disorder: A case study. *J Am. Acad Audiol* 1991; 2:36–54.
19. Jerger J, Johnson K, Loiselle L: Pediatric central auditory dysfunction: Comparison of children with confirmed lesions versus suspected processing disorders. *Am J Audiol* 1988; 9(supp).
20. Katz J: The use of staggered spondaic words for assessing the integrity of the central auditory system. *J Audit Res* 1962; 2:327–337.
21. Katz J: Phonemic Synthesis, in Lasky E, Katz J (eds): *Central Auditory Processing Disorders: Problems of Speech, Language, and Learning.* Baltimore, University Park Press, 1983, pp 269–295.
22. Katz J, Illmer R. Auditory perception in children with learning disabilities, in Katz J (ed): *Handbook of Clinical Audiology.* Baltimore, Williams and Wilkins, 1972, pp 540–563.
23. Katz J, Kushner D, Pack G: The use of competing speech (SSW) and environmental sounds (CES) tests for localizing brain lesions. Poster session at American Speech and Hearing Association annual meeting, Washington, DC, 1975.
24. Keith R: Interpretation of the staggered spondaic word (SSW) test. *Ear Hear* 1983; 4:287–292.
25. Keith R, Rudy J, Donahue P, et al: Comparison of SCAN results with other auditory and language measures in a clinical population. *Ear Hear* 1989; 10:382–393.
26. Kimura D: Some effects of temporal lobe damage on auditory perception. *Can J Psychol* 1961; 15:157–165.
27. Kurdziel S, Noffsinger D, Olsen W: Performance by cortical lesion patients on 40% and 60% time-compression materials. *J Am Audiol Soc* 1976; 2:3–7.
28. Matzker J: Two methods for the assessment of central auditory functions in cases of brain disease. *Ann Otol Rhinol Laryngol* 1959; 68:1155–1197.
29. McCroskey R: *Wichita Auditory Fusion Test: User's Manual.* Tulsa, Okla, Modern Education Corp, 1984.
30. McCroskey R: *Wichita Auditory Processing Test: User's Manual.* Tulsa, Okla, Modern Education Corp, 1984.
31. Mueller G, Beck G, Sedge R: Comparison of the efficiency of cortical level speech tests. *Semin Hear* 1987; 8:279–298.
32. Musiek F: Assessment of central auditory dysfunction: The dichotic digits test revisited. *Ear Hear* 1983; 4:79–83.

33. Musiek F, Baran J, Pinheiro M: Duration pattern recognition in normal subjects and patients with cerebal and cochlear lesions. *Audiology* 1990; 29:304–313.
34. Musiek F, Geurkink N: Auditory brainstem response and central auditory findings for patients with brainstem lesions: A preliminary report. *Laryngoscope* 1982; 92:891–900.
35. Musiek F, Geurkink N, Keitel S: Test battery assessment of auditory perceptual dysfunction in children. *Laryngoscope* 1982; 92:251–257.
36. Oliver S: Current trends in central auditory processing testing. Paper presented at the California Speech-Language-Hearing Association meeting, Los Angeles, 1987.
37. Papso C, Blood I: Word recognition skills of children and adults in background noise. *Ear Hear* 1989; 10:235–236.
38. Pinheiro M: Tests of central auditory function in children with learning disabilities, in Keith R, (ed): *Central Auditory Dysfunction*. New York, Grune and Stratton, 1977, pp 223–256.
39. Pinheiro M: Central auditory test profile in children with learning disabilities, in Bradford L (ed): *Communication Disorders: An Audio Journal for Continuing Education,* vol 3. New York, Grune and Stratton, 1978.
40. Saunders G, Haggard M: The clinical assessment of obscure auditory dysfunction. I. Auditory and psychological factors. *Ear Hear* 1989; 10:200–208.
41. Schwartz M: The effects of efferent auditory pathology on difference limens and critical bandwidths in chronic alcoholics. Unpublished doctoral dissertation, State University of New York at Buffalo, 1979.
42. Smoski W: The Children's Auditory Processing Performance Scale (CHAPPS): A preliminary report. Paper presented at the American Speech-Language-Hearing Association annual meeting, New Orleans, Nov 14, 1987.
43. Sparks R, Goodglass H, Nichel D: Ipsilateral versus contralateral extinction in dichotic listening resulting from hemisphere lesions. *Cortex* 1970; 6:249–260.
44. Stecker N: A comparison of efferent auditory system functioning in three groups of children. Unpublished dissertation, 1984.
45. Stubblefield J, Young C: Central auditory dysfunction in learning disabled children. *J Learn Disabil* 1975; 8:32–37.
46. Sweetow R, Reddell R: The use of masking level differences in the identification of children with perceptual problems. *J Am Audiol Soc* 1978; 4:52–56.
47. Trahiotis C, Elliott D: Behavioral investigation of some possible effects of sectioning the crossed olivocochlear bundle. *J Acoust Soc Am* 1970; 47:592.
48. Willeford J: Assessing central auditory behavior in children: A test battery approach, in Keith R (ed): *Central Auditory Dysfunction*. New York, Grune and Stratton, 1977, pp 43–72.


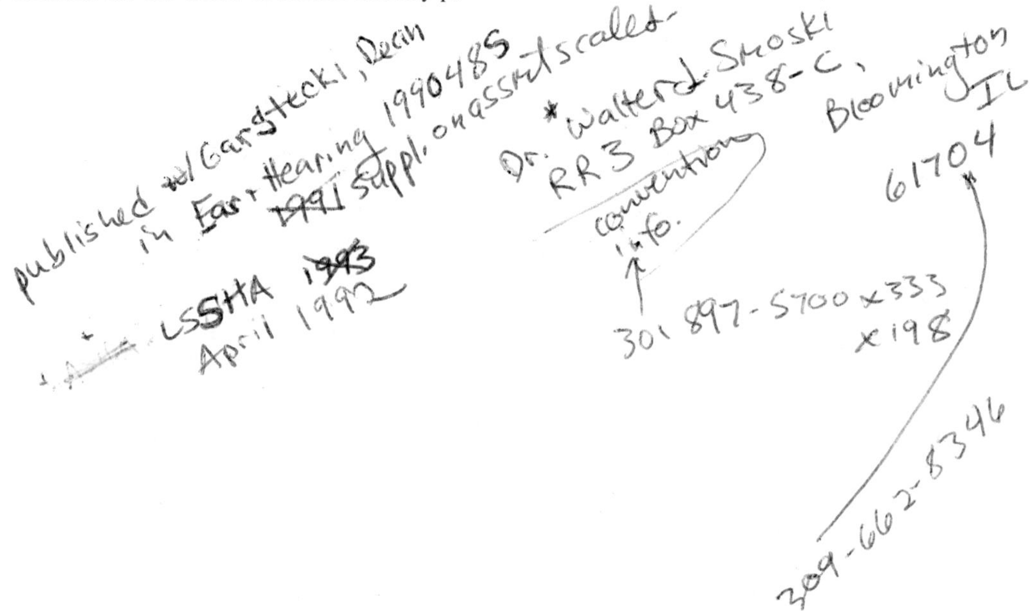

## APPENDIX 9–1

### Test Suppliers

1. American Guidance Service
   4201 Woodland Rd.
   PO Box 99
   Circle Pines, MN 55014-1796
   1-800-328-2560

   G-F-W Test of Auditory Discrimination
   G-F-W Auditory Skills Test Battery

2. Auditec of St. Louis
   330 Selma Ave.
   St. Louis, MO 63119
   1-314-962-5890

   SSI-ICM, SSI-CCM
   Time Compressed Tests
   Binaural Fusion Tests
   SAAT, PPS Tests

3. Robert C. Bilger, Ph.D.
   901 South Sixth St.
   Dept. of Speech & Hearing Science
   University of Illinois
   Champaign, IL 61820

   SPIN Test

4. Developmental Learning Materials
   1 DLM Park
   Allen, TX 75002
   1-800-527-4747

   Phonemic Synthesis Test

5. Modern Education Corp.
   PO Box 721
   Tulsa, OK 74101
   1-800-331-3762

   Wichita Auditory Fusion Test
   Wichita Auditory Perception Test

6. Precision Acoustics
   411 NE 87th St., Ste. B
   Vancouver, WA 98664
   1-206-892-9367

   SSW Test

7. The Psychological Corp.
   Harcourt, Brace, Jovanovich
   555 Academic Ct.
   San Antonio, TX 78204-2498
   1-800-228-0752

   Scan Test

8. Western Psychological Services
   12031 Wilshire Blvd.
   Los Angeles, CA 90025
   1-800-648-8857

   Wepman Auditory Discrimination Test

9. Jack A. Willeford, Ph.D.
   Colorado State University
   Dept. of Communication Disorders
   Ft. Collins, CO 80523

   Willeford Central Auditory Test Battery

*Chapter* **10**

# Screening and Evaluation of Central Auditory Processing Disorders in Young Children

**Rochelle Cherry, Ed.D.**

The need for early identification of children with central auditory processing disorders (CAPDs) has been stressed repeatedly in the literature.[5, 32, 47] CAPD has been linked to communication problems and failure in school, as well as problems with social development.[24]

Identification of CAPD can lead to a better understanding of the child's behavior or poor performance, which can help generate more positive attitudes toward that child. Parents and teachers no longer blame the victim since disruptive behavior or poor performance is not under her or his control. This better understanding can enable professionals to neutralize the antisocial behavior found in many of these children. Identification should also lead to remediation to minimize the educational deficits so often seen in these children by controlling the environment (room acoustics), use of amplification (FM units), auditory training, developing compensatory strategies, and appropriate educational placement[6, 7, 26, 40] (see Chapter 13 for more information). This chapter will describe the most widely used tests currently available for the screening and diagnosis of CAPD in young children and report on the available research that evaluates and compares these tests.

## SCREENING ISSUES

The criteria used to determine the appropriateness of CAPD screening are listed in Table 10–1. The screening process involves a series of decisions: which populations are appropriate for screening; choice of test to be used; criteria used to determine if follow-up testing is necessary; selection and training of personnel; and monitoring the screening program results.[33]

There are several populations that could be screened for CAPD. The broadest group would include a mass screening of all young children in a particular educational placement to identify children at risk for auditory-based learning disabilities before problems emerge. A narrower population would be to screen all children demonstrating behavior typical of CAPD.[10] These children are generally identified as a result of parental or teacher concerns and are often referred for audiological evaluations. Many of these children behave as though they have a peripheral hearing loss, demonstrating attention problems such as difficulty listening in noise.

Audiologists typically rule out peripheral hearing loss, as well as middle-ear pathology.

**TABLE 10–1.**

Criteria for Selecting Conditions for Screening and Application to Screening for CAPD in Children*

| | |
|---|---|
| Condition should be prevalent. | 6.5% of children 3–17 years old have learning disabilities[51]; a high proportion of these have CAPD. |
| Condition is serious. | Academic achievement and social development can be adversely affected.[24] |
| Screening decreases time to diagnosis. | In the absence of screening, diagnosis of CAPD is often delayed until child begins to fail in school.[4] |
| Diagnostic tests are available to confirm problem. | Comprehensive diagnosis is available. |
| Condition is treatable and progress is improved with early identification. | Management is available and should begin as soon as possible—educational placement, auditory training, compensatory strategies, etc.[40] |
| Screening should not be harmful. | Screening procedure is noninvasive. |
| Cost of screening, diagnosis, and treatment is reasonable. | Cost of screening can be minimized by eliminating unnecessary follow-ups. |

*Adapted from Hayes D, Pashley N: Assessment of infants for hearing impairment, in Jacobson J, Northern J (eds): *Diagnostic Audiology*. Austin, Texas, Pro-Ed, 1991, pp 251–266.

However, the currently used standard audiological evaluation does not focus on the more subtle problems found in children with CAPD. Thus, parents and teachers are often told that there is no "hearing problem."[31] Many of these children should be evaluated further. A screening test could help to determine whether or not a potential CAPD exists in order to address more appropriately the specific child's needs.[33] Several questionnaires have been proposed to help identify children at risk for CAPD.[10, 11, 35, 41] Clinicians should be encouraged to incorporate some of the ideas suggested in these questionnaires in their routine case history forms.

The screening test procedure used should yield preliminary data enabling the clinician to determine which children require further and more specific testing and which children do not. Screening procedures must be relatively quick and inexpensive since they are generally applied to large numbers.[27] Therefore, before choosing a test, the following issues should be considered: length of time necessary for administration and scoring, equipment and personnel requirements, validity and reliability, and appropriateness for population (age and linguistic background).

There are currently two audiological tests marketed as screening tools for CAPD: the Selective Auditory Attention Test (SAAT) and the Screening Test for Auditory Processing Disorders (SCAN). Both the SAAT[4] and the SCAN[23] were developed to be used for both mass and individual screening. The SAAT has been normed for children ages 4 to 9 years old, whereas the SCAN has been normed for children ages 3 to 11 years old. Caution is advised in the interpretation of results for both tests when younger children are tested since the normative data for these children are based on small samples with large variability. The large variability of test scores for children under the age of 5 years old is a problem for most CAPD tests.[33] Both tests require a prior pure-tone sweep screening to rule out peripheral hearing loss since CAPD test results can be contaminated by a peripheral loss.[21, 30] When English is the child's second language, both tests should be used with caution.

Both tests can be administered by personnel other than audiologists, specifically speech-language pathologists and learning specialists. Both tests can be administered using a portable cassette tape recorder, although headphones are necessary only for the SCAN. Both tests include a 1,000 Hz calibration tone but they can be administered at a comfortable loudness level in a quiet room. As with all tests, the examiner should observe the child and note any behavior that might aid in interpretation, such as very slow responses or a low frustration level. The SAAT takes 8 minutes to administer whereas the SCAN takes 20 minutes.

On the one hand, scoring and interpretation are less complicated with the SAAT; on the other hand, the SCAN comprises three subtests, assessing several central auditory processing abilities.

### The Selective Auditory Attention Test (SAAT)

The SAAT has two parts: (1) a list of 25 monosyllabic words prerecorded in quiet, providing a speech recognition score in percentage correct, and (2) an equivalent list prerecorded with a semantic distractor providing a selective listening score, also in percentage correct. The selective listening list should not be administered unless a score of at least 88 percent is obtained in the quiet condition to establish the child's ability to perform the task (point to the appropriate picture). Two matched forms are available that have high interlist equivalence.[3, 4]

The Word Intelligibility by Picture Identification Test[36] lists and test plates were chosen as stimuli because: (1) the words are within the receptive vocabulary of young children; (2) it is a closed-response task; (3) it does not require the ability to read; (4) it does not require a verbal response, eliminating the problem of misarticulation; and (5) it has been demonstrated to be a valid test of speech recognition for young children.[37]

A diotic mode of presentation—same stimuli to both ears simultaneously—was chosen because it tends to be more difficult than a dichotic mode.[45] An interesting semantic distractor was chosen because such distractors were found to be more efficient in differentiating between normal-achieving and learning-disabled children than either broadband noise or speech played backwards.[5] Level of difficulty is manipulated by using a 0 dB signal-to-noise ratio[13] and by having both the stimulus words and the story prerecorded by the same speaker, eliminating voice cues.[44]

Normative data for the SAAT was obtained from 325 children, prekindergarten through second grade (ages 4 to 9 years old). These children were divided into three groups: normal-achieving, learning-disabled, and teacher concerned with school progress. Linear regression and analysis of variance results indicated that selective listening skills improve with age for each of the three groups. While there was no significant difference between the three groups when tested in quiet, significant differences appeared when children were tested under the distractor condition. At each age level, learning-disabled children scored significantly lower than "teacher-concerned" children who scored significantly lower than normal-achieving children (Table 10–2 and Fig 10–1).

Most important, the SAAT appears to be efficient at identifying those children who may be at risk for learning problems as measured by teacher concern. Table 10–3 is a distribution of percentile ranking based on age and performance score. Only 13% of normal-achieving children but 40% of teacher-concerned children and over 90% of learning-disabled children scored at risk (their scores falling into the lower 25th percentile of all children tested). These findings have clinical implications. Specifically, it appears that the SAAT is an efficient screening device to help identify children with learning difficulties resulting from a CAPD. Thus, this test can be used as a screening tool for deciding when to administer a lengthy battery of central auditory processing tests.

**Case Presentation.**—DW, a 4-year and 2-month-old girl, was referred for a complete audi-

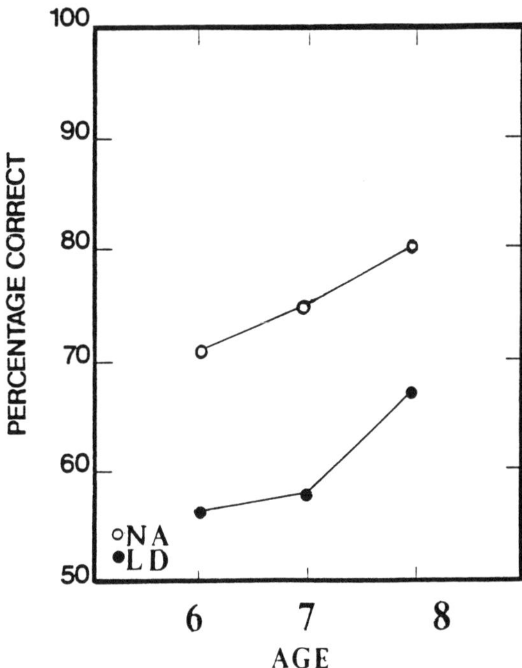


**FIG 10–1.**
Mean test scores for normal-achieving (NA) and learning-disabled (LD) children on the Selective Auditory Attention Test.

**TABLE 10–2.**
Mean Performance Scores in Percentage Correct by Age and by Subject Group Under the Competing Message Condition

| | Normal Achievers | | Learning Disabled | | Teacher Concerned | | All Subjects | |
|---|---|---|---|---|---|---|---|---|
| Age (Years) | % Correct | Number | % Correct | Number | % Correct | Number | % Correct | Number |
| 4 | 62.80 | 10 | — | — | 50.00 | 2 | 60.67 | 18* |
| 5 | 66.42 | 38 | 60.00 | 1 | 58.07 | 27 | 63.84 | 77 |
| 6 | 70.61 | 66 | 56.00 | 1 | 67.28 | 39 | 69.25 | 106 |
| 7 | 74.57 | 67 | 57.17 | 17 | 69.87 | 15 | 72.63 | 99 |
| 8 | 79.40 | 20 | 66.79 | 17 | 76.00 | 5 | 76.52 | 42 |

*There were six 4-year-olds and eleven 5-year-olds who were unclassified and are only included in "All Subjects."

ological evaluation because of unclear speech and a possible hearing loss. Ms. W described her child as "bright, talkative, delightful. . . , however, she sometimes ignores or does not hear me." DW had a history of occasional ear infections and asthma. Her developmental milestones were within expected age levels. She had recently been enrolled in a prekindergarten program.

Pure-tone thresholds, using play audiometric techniques under headphones, revealed hearing within normal limits bilaterally (Fig 10–2). Speech recognition thresholds of 5 dB HL for each ear corroborated the three-frequency pure-tone averages of 0 dB HL for the right ear and 3 dB HL for the left ear. Immittance pressure function revealed normal middle ear peak pressure point (peaking at −10 daPa in the right ear and −25 daPa in the left ear) and normal static admittance bilaterally. Acoustic reflex thresholds were consistent with normal auditory function through the eighth nerve.

The SAAT was administered in a sound-treated booth in the sound field at 50 dB HL (normal conversational level), first in a noncompeting mode, followed by a competing mode presentation. DW obtained a score of 88 percent in the noncompeting condition and 12 percent in the competing condition, placing her at risk (below the 25th percentile) for auditory-based learning problems. Observation of her behavior during the competing condition indicated that DW became agitated and found it difficult to sit still. She appeared to be aware of her difficulty and indicated that she was glad when the test was over.

DW was referred for a speech and language evaluation. Results of both formal and informal assessment revealed receptive and expressive linguistic delays, characterized by her inability to follow complex directions, relate events in a logical sequence, maintain a topic, or problem solve. When tasks became too difficult, a breakdown in behavior (rocking, extraneous movements) occurred. Several misarticulations were noted that were felt to indicate a phonological processing disorder. DW was accepted for speech and language

**TABLE 10–3.**
Distribution of Percentile Ranking by Age and by Classification

| | Normal Achieving | | Teacher Concerned | | Learning Disabled | |
|---|---|---|---|---|---|---|
| Age (Years) | Passing | At Risk* | Passing | At Risk* | Passing† | At Risk* |
| 4 | 9 | 1 | 0 | 2 | — | — |
| 5 | 33 | 5 | 14 | 13 | 1 | 0 |
| 6 | 56 | 10 | 26 | 13 | 0 | 1 |
| 7 | 57 | 10 | 9 | 6 | 1 | 16 |
| 8 | 20 | 0 | 4 | 1 | 1 | 16 |

*All children whose percentile ranking was 25% or less.
†Of these three learning-disabled children, one 5-year-old was classified solely on the basis of visual and motor problems, and the 7- and 8-year-olds were in the process of being unclassified and mainstreamed by their respective schools.

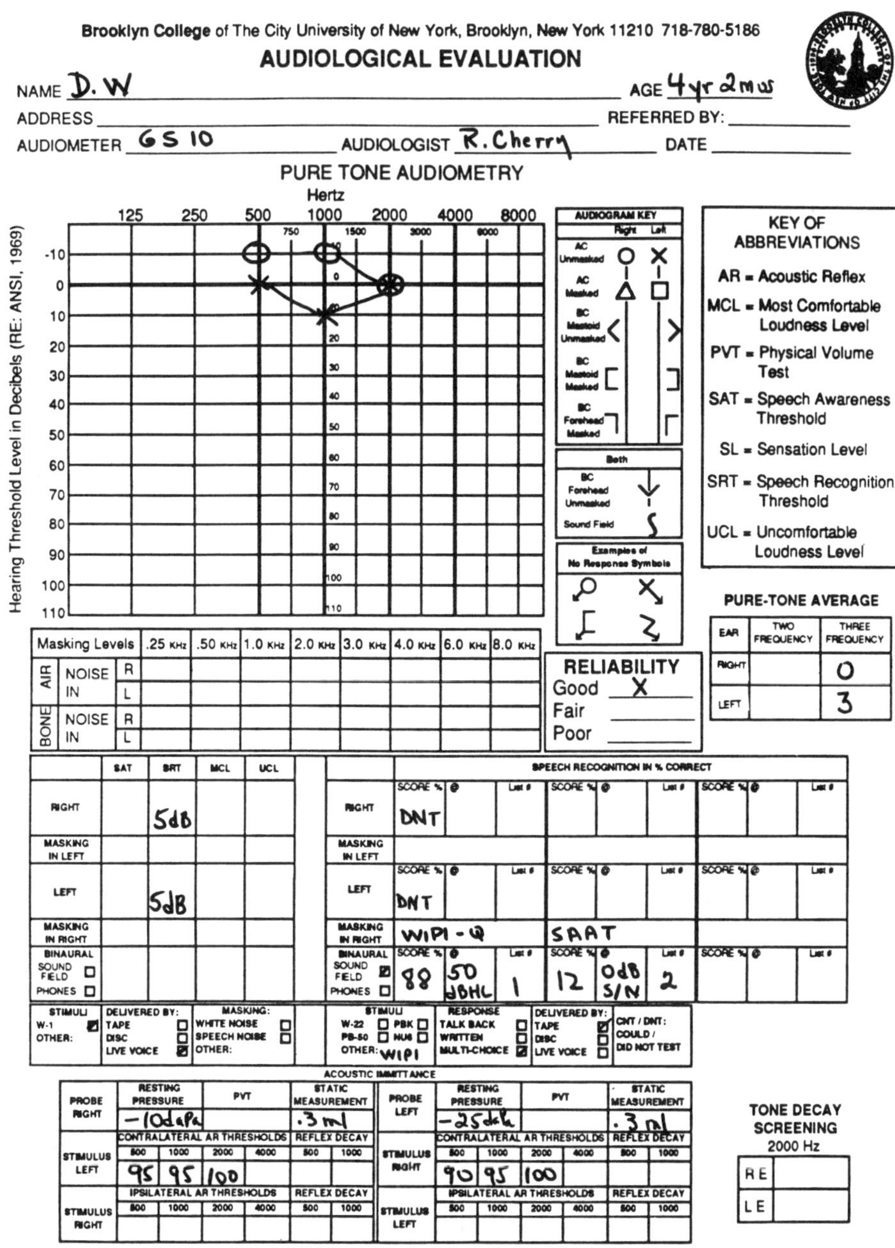

**Brooklyn College** of The City University of New York, Brooklyn, New York 11210 718-780-5186

**AUDIOLOGICAL EVALUATION**

NAME D. W  AGE 4 yr 2 mos

ADDRESS  REFERRED BY:

AUDIOMETER GS 10  AUDIOLOGIST R. Cherry  DATE

**PURE TONE AUDIOMETRY**



**KEY OF ABBREVIATIONS**

- AR = Acoustic Reflex
- MCL = Most Comfortable Loudness Level
- PVT = Physical Volume Test
- SAT = Speech Awareness Threshold
- SL = Sensation Level
- SRT = Speech Recognition Threshold
- UCL = Uncomfortable Loudness Level

| Masking Levels | | | .25 KHz | .50 KHz | 1.0 KHz | 2.0 KHz | 3.0 KHz | 4.0 KHz | 6.0 KHz | 8.0 KHz |
|---|---|---|---|---|---|---|---|---|---|---|
| AIR | NOISE IN | R | | | | | | | | |
| | | L | | | | | | | | |
| BONE | NOISE IN | R | | | | | | | | |
| | | L | | | | | | | | |

**RELIABILITY**

Good X
Fair
Poor

**PURE-TONE AVERAGE**

| EAR | TWO FREQUENCY | THREE FREQUENCY |
|---|---|---|
| RIGHT | | 0 |
| LEFT | | 3 |

| | SAT | SRT | MCL | UCL |
|---|---|---|---|---|
| RIGHT | | 5dB | | |
| MASKING IN LEFT | | | | |
| LEFT | | 5dB | | |
| MASKING IN RIGHT | | | | |
| BINAURAL SOUND FIELD ☐ PHONES ☐ | | | | |

**SPEECH RECOGNITION IN % CORRECT**

| | SCORE % | @ | List # | SCORE % | @ | List # | SCORE % | @ | List # |
|---|---|---|---|---|---|---|---|---|---|
| RIGHT | DNT | | | | | | | | |
| MASKING IN LEFT | | | | | | | | | |
| LEFT | DNT | | | | | | | | |
| MASKING IN RIGHT | WIPI - Q | | | SAAT | | | | | |
| BINAURAL SOUND FIELD ☒ PHONES ☐ | 88 | 50 dBHL | 1 | 12 | 0dB S/N | 2 | | | |

STIMULI: W-1 ☒ OTHER: — DELIVERED BY: TAPE ☐ DISC ☐ LIVE VOICE ☒ — MASKING: WHITE NOISE ☐ SPEECH NOISE ☐ OTHER:

STIMULI: W-22 ☐ PBK ☐ PB-50 ☐ NU6 ☐ OTHER: WIPI — RESPONSE: TALK BACK ☐ WRITTEN ☐ MULTI-CHOICE ☒ — DELIVERED BY: TAPE ☒ DISC ☐ LIVE VOICE ☐ — CNT / DNT: COULD / DID NOT TEST

**ACOUSTIC IMMITTANCE**

| PROBE RIGHT | RESTING PRESSURE | PVT | STATIC MEASUREMENT |
|---|---|---|---|
| | −10daPa | | .3 ml |

| STIMULUS LEFT | Contralateral AR Thresholds 500 | 1000 | 2000 | 4000 | Reflex Decay 500 | 1000 |
|---|---|---|---|---|---|---|
| | 95 | 95 | 100 | | | |

| STIMULUS RIGHT | Ipsilateral AR Thresholds 500 | 1000 | 2000 | 4000 | Reflex Decay 500 | 1000 |
|---|---|---|---|---|---|---|
| | | | | | | |

| PROBE LEFT | RESTING PRESSURE | PVT | STATIC MEASUREMENT |
|---|---|---|---|
| | −25daPa | | .3 ml |

| STIMULUS RIGHT | Contralateral AR Thresholds 500 | 1000 | 2000 | 4000 | Reflex Decay 500 | 1000 |
|---|---|---|---|---|---|---|
| | 90 | 95 | 100 | | | |

| STIMULUS LEFT | Ipsilateral AR Thresholds 500 | 1000 | 2000 | 4000 | Reflex Decay 500 | 1000 |
|---|---|---|---|---|---|---|
| | | | | | | |

**TONE DECAY SCREENING**
2000 Hz

| RE | |
|---|---|
| LE | |

**FIG 10–2.**
Audiological evaluation form from the Brooklyn College of The City University of New York, with test results of DW (case presentation).

therapy. Her parents and teacher were counseled about her CAPD.

### The Screening Test for Auditory Processing Disorders (SCAN)

The SCAN comprises three subtests: a test of low-pass filtered words, an auditory figure-ground test, and a competing word test. The filtered word subtest (FW) is composed of two 20-word lists of 1,000 Hz low-pass filtered monosyllabic words (with a filter rolloff of 32 dB/octave) presented monotically (to each ear separately). The auditory figure-ground subtest (AFG) also consists of two 20-word lists presented one to each ear with a multitalker babble background recorded at a +8 dB signal-to-noise ratio. The child is requested to repeat the monosyllabic word heard in both of these subtests. The competing word subtest (CW) consists of two lists of 25 paired monosyllabic words presented dichotically (one word to each ear with simultaneous onset times). The child is now requested to repeat the word heard in the right ear first (list 1) and then the left ear first (list 2). Total score and ear advantage score are computed for this subtest. A composite score is obtained for all subtests, as well as individual subtest scores.

The SCAN was standardized on 1,034 normal-achieving children attending regular classrooms across the United States.[23] The SCAN yields a total test raw score or composite scores that can be converted to standard scores (mean=100 and SD=15), percentile ranks, and age equivalents, using a series of tables found in the manual. In addition, for each subtest a standard score (mean=10, SD=3) and a percentile ranking are also available. Examiners are encouraged to use the standard error of measurement to establish confidence intervals around the child's standard score for each subtest and composite score.

The SCAN was subsequently administered to 155 children, ages 6 to 15 years, who were referred for assessment of CAPD.[25] In addition to the SCAN, the CAPD assessment included two dichotic tests: the Staggered Spondaic Word (SSW) test list EC[1] and the Competing Sentence Test (CST) of the Willeford battery.[47] There was a significant correlation between the CW subtest of the SCAN and the other dichotic tests. The FW and AFG subtests showed low correlations with the dichotic tests, indicating that they were assessing different functions. In addition, children with histories of attention-deficit disorder (ADD) had lower SCAN scores than children with no histories of ADD, especially on the AFG and FW subtests. (See Chapter 8 for a discussion of ADD.) In fact, a discriminant analysis showed that the AFG alone was best at classifying children with ADD.[25]

### Summary

The SAAT may be more useful than the SCAN as a screening device, particularly when a large population is surveyed, because it is quicker and easier to score whereas the SCAN may be more appropriate as part of a more in-depth CAPD evaluation. Keith[23] indicates that in addition to screening, the SCAN can be used to obtain data on auditory maturation and auditory processing, as well as to document usefulness of intervention. Regardless of the screening device used, a follow-up diagnostic evaluation is warranted whenever a child scores at risk for CAPD so that appropriate treatment can begin.

## DIAGNOSTIC PROCEDURES

Once a decision is made to evaluate a child for CAPD, the first step is to rule out a peripheral hearing problem, using pure tone thresholds, speech audiometry, and immittance measures. Behavioral tests that distort the signal (generally speech) have been shown to be useful in evaluating problems in the central auditory pathway by reducing the normal level of redundancy present in that signal. The methods used to degrade the signal have included low-pass filtering, altering temporal aspects through interruption or compression, introducing a competing signal in the same or opposite ear, and through binaural stimulation requiring integration of stimuli from both ears. These tests can be presented monotically (a stimulus to one ear at a time), diotically (the same stimulus to both ears), dichotically (a different stimulus to each ear presented simultaneously), or through binaural integration (incomplete messages presented simultaneously to each ear). A more thorough coverage of these tests can be found in Chapter 9.

Most of the available tests have been shown to be useful in detecting specific lesions in the central auditory nervous system of adults. The assumption made by some clinicians is that children with CAPD either have developmental delay or an abnormality of the CANS and will, therefore, function as though a lesion exists. Caution must be exercised, however, in generalizing test results found in adults with confirmed lesions with children suspected of CAPD since these groups may differ in both severity and specificity of deficit.[16] Vocabulary level and level of difficulty of stimuli may also be inappropriate for young children.[14]

It is generally accepted that no one test is sufficiently sensitive to evaluate CAP problems.[14 24]

In addition, many of the tests used have wide variability, especially when testing young children.[14] Therefore, a battery of well-chosen tests is recommended.[32, 48] The decision to include a test within a CAPD battery should be based on its efficiency, reliability, and validity with a similar population, as well as the specific auditory skills assessed, the child's age, and linguistic background.

Musiek and Geurkink[31] have identified five distinct areas in which processing disorders could occur: (1) selective listening or the ability to focus attention on one auditory signal while tuning out others; (2) binaural separation or the ability to integrate acoustic information presented to one ear while tuning out information presented to the other ear; (3) binaural integration or the ability to combine different information which is presented to each ear into one comprehensible signal; (4) temporal sequencing or the ability to recognize and report the appropriate sequence of acoustic events; and (5) interhemispheric interaction or the ability for both hemispheres to communicate.

They further note the types of tests that may assess processing capabilities in each of these areas. For example, selective listening can be assessed using a speech-in-noise, dichotic, or filtered speech test; binaural separation can be assessed using a competing message test; binaural integration can be assessed through binaural fusion; temporal sequencing can be assessed through the PPS test; and interhemispheric interaction can be assessed through dichotic tests. Other researchers have proposed different sets of skills with other tests required to evaluate them.[7, 24]

Now let us turn to an assessment of some prerecorded commercially available tests used in CAPD evaluations. Only tests with normative data for young children (ages 3 to 7 years old) will be discussed. See Chapter 9 for a further discussion of CAPD tests. These tests should be administered by an audiologist in a sound-treated room using calibrated equipment.

Jerger and Jerger[15] developed the Pediatric Speech Intelligibility (PSI) Test, based upon research using the Synthetic Sentence Identification (SSI) Test[42] with adults. It is the only CAPD test developed specifically for use with children 3 to 6 years old. The PSI uses performance-intensity functions in quiet and in noise. The test includes 20 monosyllabic words, grouped into four lists of five words and two types of sentence materials based on receptive language ability (10 for each level). Test materials were generated by normal children (3 to 6 years old), depicted on response cards, and normed on 40 normal-achieving children. The noise or competition was also composed of sentences generated by these young children. The noise is presented either to the ear under test, which is a monotic task and is referred to as the ipsilateral competing message (ICM) condition, or to the opposite ear, which is a dichotic task or the contralateral competing message (CCM) condition.

When evaluating either noise condition, testing must be performed using headphones. The child is required to point to the appropriate picture. The performance-intensity functions are obtained at various intensity levels in quiet. The message-to-competition ratio (MCR) functions are obtained for the sentence material for ICM and CCM conditions only when there is no peripheral hearing loss. The stimulus items are presented at 30 dB HL and the competing sentences are varied to produce MCRs of +10 dB and 0 dB for the ICM condition and 0 dB and −20 dB for the CCM condition. Guidelines for interpretation of PSI and illustrative cases are outlined in the manual. Normative data are presented for four indices from the PI function: threshold, steepness, rollover, and the relationship between intelligibility scores for quiet and competing conditions and the ICM and CCM conditions. Scores falling outside the 95 percent confidence interval are considered suspect.[15]

Using the PSI, Jerger, Johnson, and Loiselle[16] compared results of four groups of children (3 to 8 years old): those with (1) nonauditory central nervous system (CNS) lesions, (2) auditory CNS lesions of the brain stem, (3) auditory CNS lesions of the temporal lobe, and (4) 11 children suspected of CAPD specifically referred for audiological evaluation. The children with confirmed lesions outside of the auditory CNS performed like the normal children. However, the performance of children with confirmed brain-stem lesions was typically abnormal for the ICM and normal for the CCM. In contrast, the children with temporal lobe lesions showed either normal ICM and abnormal CCM or abnormality on both measures. Similar results have been noted using the SSI in adults with confirmed lesions. Children with suspected CAPD had normal results for the ICM but abnormal results for the CCM condition with greater deficits on the left ear. Only one of the children tested performed within the normal range on all measures. Based on these results, it appears that the PSI is useful in the identification of young children with CAPD.

Willeford[47] published one of the first papers describing a battery of tests to be used in evaluating CAPD in children. The battery included two tests useful in evaluating cortical function, a dichotically competing sentence (CS) test and a filtered speech (FS) test, and two tests that assessed brain stem integrity, a binaural fusion (BF) test and a rapidly alternating speech (RASP) test. This group of tests had been used successfully to identify localized CNS lesions in adults.[28]

The CS test involves a series of paired sentences related in content. The primary sentence is presented at 35 dB SL (re: pure tone average [PTA] for the speech frequencies) and the competing sentence is presented at 50 dB SL (re:PTA). The child is asked to repeat the softer (primary) sentence and ignore the other one. Twenty pairs of sentences are presented first with the right ear receiving the primary sentence and then with the left ear receiving the primary sentence.

Normative data reveal improvement in the "weak-ear" CS score as age increased from 5 to 10 years old. There were high "strong-ear" scores for all children, even those 5 years old. In general, the strong ear was the right ear. Inspection of ranges of scores reveals large intersubject variability in the weak-ear score, which limits its usefulness with younger children. For example, 5-year-olds are expected to obtain 20 percent for the weak ear with a range of 0 to 80% noted; for the strong-ear score, both the expected result and the range are 90% to 100%.[48]

The FS test is a monotic test comprising two lists of monosyllabic words low-pass filtered at 500 Hz, with a rejection characteristic of 18 dB per octave, presented at 50 dB SL (re:PTA). Normative data are available for children 6 to 10 years old, with insufficient data presented for 5-year-olds. Scores also improve with age, with large intersubject variability plaguing this test as well, especially for younger children. To illustrate, for 6-year-olds the mean score for each ear is approximately 60% with a possible range of 42% to 84%. Willeford[48] suggests that a CAPD should be suspected when a score falls outside of the normal range or when an ear asymmetry of greater than 10% is obtained.

The BF test requires binaural integration of two incomplete signals. Low-pass filtered (500 to 700 Hz) spondee words are presented to one ear while the same word, which has been high-pass filtered (1,900 to 2,100 Hz) is presented to the other ear. Willeford suggests that this test be presented at 30 to 40 dB SL (re: threshold for 500 Hz for the low-pass words and 2,000 Hz for the high-pass word). For scoring, the ear receiving the low-pass filtered band is considered the test ear. Normative data are available for children ages 5 to 9 years old. Again a maturational effect can be observed with significant variability for the youngest children.

The fourth test of the Willeford battery is the RASP, which uses simple sentences switched alternately between the two ears every 300 ms. It is presented at 30 dB SL (re:PTA) and scored in terms of the lead ear. Normative data for children ages 5 to 9 years old reveal that even the youngest are able to do this test as well as adults.

Willeford[47] administered this battery of tests to seven children with learning disabilities. He reported abnormally reduced scores on at least one of these tests in all of the children, with different children failing different tests. Subsequently, this battery was administered to 150 learning-disabled children with more than 90% failing at least one test.[49] Although some investigators have proposed a failure criterion of 1 SD below the mean,[9] Willeford requires a score below any normal-achieving child within the same age group to minimize false-positive results.[50]

Both the BF and RASP tests have been criticized in the literature. For example, Martin and Clark[29] did not find the BF test to be effective in identifying children with suspected CAPD. In an attempt to explain this discrepancy, Shea and Raffin[38] evaluated several Willeford battery test tapes and found significant intertape differences, with the largest differences found on the BF test. They suggested that the tape differences might account for the large range of results reported. The RASP test was the least sensitive test in the battery, with positive results found in only a small percentage of LD children.[32, 48, 49] As a result, the RASP is rarely used in CAPD test batteries. The CS and FS tests continue to be used as part of a CAPD battery, although the BF test is used to a lesser extent because of a high false-positive rate. In addition to the PSI and the Willeford battery, several other tests have been used to evaluate CAPD in children. Most of the studies found in the literature focus on the ability of a particular test to differentiate between normal achievers and children with CAPD.

The Pitch Pattern Sequence (PPS) test[34] is a monotic test that does not use speech stimuli but instead, uses sets of three tone bursts, varied in frequency, and permits the evaluation of both pattern perception and temporal sequencing. The child can respond to the pattern presented by humming, by describing it verbally (high, low, etc.), or manually. Children with learning disabilities are generally able to hum patterns but demonstrate difficulty when they are required to respond manually or verbally.[31, 32, 34] This test is normed for three age groups: 6- to 7-year-olds, 7- to 8-year-olds, and 8- to 9-year-olds.

Several dichotic tests using speech stimuli have included nonsense syllables,[2] digits,[32] and spondee words,[18, 20] in addition to the CS previously discussed.[47] A nonlinguistic dichotic test, the Competing Environmental Sounds (CES) test,[19] has been used in conjunction with the SSW to provide a broader picture of auditory processing problems in learning-disabled children.[17] As with monotic tests, dichotic test results show improvement with increasing age, as well as a wide range of scores, especially in the weak ear. It is not necessary to administer all of these dichotic tests since they should be tapping similar skills. There is no consensus in the literature as to which dichotic test should be used.[9, 32]

The ultimate goal of a CAPD evaluation is to identify children with auditory processing problems as early as possible. There are several problems in determining the optimal test battery for young children. First is the issue of prior assignment to groups (children with vs. without CAPD) on which the basis of test(s) will be validated. This is especially a problem with younger children, in whom learning problems are generally not identified. Comparison of results from one study to another is also difficult because of differences in methodology used. In addition, few studies have compared the results of a battery of tests on the same population. Two exceptions are studies by Musiek et al[32] and Ferre and Wilber.[9] Both of these studies, however, evaluated children who were at least 8 years old. Furthermore, no consensus can be found between these studies regarding the optimal test battery to be used.

Musiek et al[32] evaluated a test battery on 22 children (ages 8 to 10 years) with CAPD. The battery included RASP, BF, LPFS, CS,[47] SSW,[18] Dichotic Digits,[31] and the PPS.[34] Test results revealed that the PPS and CS tests were the most sensitive, followed by dichotic digits and the SSW. The LPFS was similar in sensitivity to the dichotic digit and SSW with the least number of errors found on the BF and then the RASP. It should be noted that in this study the BF test was administered at 50 dB SL rather than the levels recommended by Willeford[47,48] (30 or 40 dB SL). If the test were administered at either of the lower SL levels, the BF may have demonstrated greater sensitivity. The authors concluded that the detection sensitivity of the entire battery was better than the best individual test. All children who failed either the RASP, BF, or LPFS also failed at least one other test, making these tests less valuable.[32] An attempt should be made to replace less sensitive tests.

Ferre and Wilber[9] evaluated an experimental CAPD test battery on a group of normal-achieving and learning-disabled children, ages 8 to 12 years. They used two groups of learning-disabled children: one group with assumed CAPD and the other with normal auditory processing abilities, grouped on the basis of a pretest consisting of auditory language tests. All experimental tests were new recordings of the NU-CHIPS[8] in order to keep the test material consistent. The test battery included an LPFS test, BF, Time-Compressed (TC) with a 60% compression ratio, and a dichotic monosyllable (DM) test. Test results for each procedure revealed that the LPFS test was the most sensitive, BF the next most sensitive, and TC and DM equally sensitive. The sensitivity of the entire battery was also evaluated with results again suggesting better sensitivity of the entire battery than of any single test. In addition, Ferre and Wilber[9] examined false-positive rates of specific tests and found that the TC test misclassified 62% of the children. In contrast, the LPFS test was the most useful; it correctly identified 92% of the children and only misclassified 23%. Ferre and Wilber[9] also discuss the importance of establishing a pass-fail criterion for the entire test battery. They report that if failure on any single test in the battery is used, all learning-disabled children with CAPD would have been identified; however, this criterion would have misdiagnosed 85% of the children who did not have a CAPD. On the other hand, if failure on all five tests was the criterion, no child without a CAPD would have been misdiagnosed but only 23% of the learning-disabled children with a CAPD would have been identified. In this study, the best criterion was felt to be failure on three or more conditions, with an across-test failure of 1 SD or more below the normal mean. It should be noted that their conclusions are based on the assumption that some of the learning-disabled children did not have CAPD. If that assumption was not correct, the sensitivity of each test, as well as the entire battery, would not be valid.

## SUMMARY

In summary, it appears as though there are tests available that may be useful in identifying children with CAPD. Currently, the only tests that have sufficient normative data on young children are the SAAT, SCAN, and PSI, with several other tests available for use beginning at ages 5 to 7. More research is needed regarding specific tests and test batteries to be used. The test battery should challenge the integrity of the central auditory nervous system in an efficient manner, tapping several different abilities without overly fatiguing the child. There is a need for standardization of tests and scoring techniques, more normative data especially on younger children, and data on sensitivity and specificity of procedures.[39, 46] There are no reported longitudinal studies that follow large groups of children (pass vs. fail) over time to validate test results. There is also the need for publishing individual cases, in addition to group data, in an attempt to correlate classroom behavior with specific test failures. Patterns of strengths and weaknesses on tests should be used as a guide to management.[6, 22] In addition, children with CAPD should be referred to other professionals within a team approach (i.e., neurologists, speech-language pathologists, and psychologists) to best understand and meet each child's individual needs.

## REFERENCES


1. Arnst D, Katz J: *Central Auditory Assessment. The SSW Test: Development and Clinical Use.* Boston, College Hill Press, 1982.
2. Berlin C, Hughes L, Lowe-Bell S, et al: Dichotic right ear advantage in children 5 to 13. *Cortex* 1973; 9:393–401.
3. Chermak G, Montgomery J: Interlist equivalence of the Selective Auditory Attention Test. Paper presented at the American Academy of Audiology conference, Denver, April 1991.
4. Cherry R: *Selective Auditory Attention Test (SAAT).* St Louis, Auditec of St Louis, 1980.
5. Cherry R, Kruger B: Selective auditory attention abilities of learning disabled and normal achieving children. *J Learn Disabil* 1983; 16:202–205.
6. Cline J: Auditory processing deficits: Assessment and remediation by the elementary school speech and language pathologist. *Semin Speech Lang* 1988; 9:367–382.
7. Dempsey C: Selecting tests of auditory function in children, in Lasky E, Katz J (eds): *Central Auditory Processing Disorders.* Baltimore, University Park Press, 1983, pp 203–221.
8. Elliot L, Katz D: *Development of Northwestern University Children's Perception of Speech (NU-CHIPS) Test.* St Louis, Auditec of St Louis, 1979.
9. Ferre J, Wilber L: Normal and learning disabled children's central auditory processing skills: An experimental test battery. *Ear Hear* 1986; 7:336–343.
10. Fisher L: *Fisher's Auditory Problems Checklist.* Cedar Rapids, Iowa, Grant Wood, 1980.
11. Glass M, Franks J, Potter R: A comparison of two tests of auditory selective attention. *Lang Speech Hear Serv Sch* 1986; 17:300–306.
12. Hayes D, Pashley N: Assessment of infants for hearing impairment, in Jacobson J, Northern J (eds): *Diagnostic Audiology.* Austin, Texas, Pro-Ed, 1991, pp 251–266.
13. Hedrick D, Kunze L: Diotic listening in young children. *Percept Mot Skills* 1974; 6:243–250.
14. Hood L, Berlin C: Central auditory function and disorders, in Boller F, Grafman J (eds): *Handbook of Neuropsychology.* Amsterdam, Elsevier Science Publishers, in press.
15. Jerger S, Jerger J: *The Pediatric Speech Intelligibility Test (PSI).* St Louis, Auditec of St Louis, 1984.
16. Jerger S, Johnson K, Louiselle L: Pediatric central auditory dysfunction: Comparison of children with confirmed lesions versus suspected process-

ing disorders. *Am J Otolaryngol* 1988; 9(suppl):63–71.

17. Johnson D, Enfield M, Sherman R: The use of the Staggered Spondaic Word Test and the Competing Environmental Sounds Test in the evaluation of central auditory function in hearing disabled children. *Ear Hear* 1981; 2:70–77.
18. Katz J: The SSW test: An interim report. *J Speech Hear Disord* 1968; 33:132–146.
19. Katz J: The Staggered Spondaic Word Test, in Keith R (ed): *Central Auditory Dysfunction*. New York, Grune and Stratton, 1977, pp 103–127.
20. Katz J: Clinical use of central auditory tests, in Katz J (ed): *Handbook of Clinical Audiology*. Baltimore, Williams and Wilkins, 1978, pp 233–243.
21. Katz J: The effects of conductive hearing loss on auditory function. *ASHA* 1978; 20:879–886.
22. Katz J, Wilde L: Auditory perceptual disorders in children, in Katz J (ed): *Handbook of Clinical Audiology*. Baltimore, Williams and Wilkins, 1985, pp 664–688.
23. Keith R: *SCAN: A Screening Test for Auditory Processing Disorders*. San Diego, The Psychology Corp, 1986.
24. Keith R: Central auditory tests, in Lass N, McReynolds J, Yoder D, (eds): *Handbook of Speech-Language Pathology and Audiology*. Toronto, BC Decker, 1988, pp 1215–1236.
25. Keith R, Ruby J, Donahue P, et al: Comparison of SCAN results with other auditory and language measures in a clinical population. *Ear Hear* 1989; 10:382–386.
26. Lasky E, Cox L: Auditory processing and language interaction: Evaluation and interaction strategies, in Lasky E, Katz J (eds): *Central Auditory Processing Disorders*. Baltimore, University Park Press, 1983, pp 243–268.
27. Lessler K: Screening, screening programs, and the pediatrician. *Pediatrics* 1974; 54:608–611.
28. Lynn G, Gilroy J: Evaluation of central auditory dysfunction in patients with neurological disorders, in Keith R (ed): *Central Auditory Dysfunction*. New York, Grune and Stratton, 1977, pp 177–222.
29. Martin F, Clark J: Audiologic detection of auditory processing disorders in children. *J Am Audiol Soc* 1977; 3:140–146.
30. Mittenberger G, Dawson G, Raica A: Central auditory testing with peripheral hearing loss. *Arch Otolaryngol* 1978; 104:11–15.
31. Musiek F, Geurkink N: Auditory perceptual problems in children: Considerations for otolaryngologists and audiologists. *Laryngoscope* 1980; 90:962–971.
32. Musiek F, Geurkink N, Kietel S: Test battery assessment of auditory perceptual dysfunction in children. *Laryngoscope* 1982; 92:251–257.
33. Musiek F, Gollogly K, Lamb L et al: Selected issues in screening for central auditory processing dysfunction. *Semin Hear* 1990; 4:372–384.
34. Pinherio M: Tests of central auditory function in children with learning disabilities, in Keith R (ed): *Central Auditory Dysfunction*. New York, Grune and Stratton, 1977, pp 223–256.
35. Priotti E, Young M, Byrne P: The evaluation of a child with auditory perceptual difficulties: An interdisciplinary approach. *Semin Speech Lang Hear* 1980; 1:167–179.
36. Ross M, Lerman J: A picture identification test for hearing impaired children. *J Speech Hear Res* 1970; 13:44–53.
37. Sanderson-Leepa M, Rintelman N: Articulation functions and test-retest performance of normal-hearing children on three speech discrimination tests: WIPI, PB-50, and NU Auditory test, No. 6. *J Speech Hear Disord* 1976; 41:503–519.
38. Shea S, Raffin M: Assessment of electromagnetic characteristics of the Willeford Central Auditory Processing Test Battery. *J Speech Hear Res* 1983; 26:18–21.
39. Silman S, Silverman C: Central auditory speech tests, in Silman S, Silverman C (ed): *Auditory Diagnosis: Principles and Application*. New York, Academic Press, 1991, pp 215–248.
40. Sloan C: *Treating Auditory Processing Difficulties in Children*. San Diego, College Hill Press, 1986.
41. Smoski W: Use of CHAPPS in a children's audiology clinic. *Ear Hear* 1990; 11(Suppl):53–56.
42. Speaks C, Jerger J: Method for measurement of speech identification. *J Speech Hear Res* 1965; 8:185–194.
43. Spritzer J: A central auditory evaluation protocol: A guide for training and diagnosis of lesions of the central system. *Ear Hear* 1983; 4:221–228.
44. Triesman A: Verbal cues, language and meaning in selective attention. *Am J Psychol* 1964; 77:206–219.
45. Triesman A: The effect of irrelevant material on the efficiency of selective listening. *Am J Psychol* 1964; 77:533–546.
46. White E: Children's performance on the SSW Test and the Willeford battery: Interim clinical data, in Keith R (ed): *Central Auditory Dysfunction*. New York, Grune and Stratton, 1977, pp 319–340.
47. Willeford J: Assessing central auditory behavior in children: A test battery approach, in Keith R (ed): *Central Auditory Dysfunction*. New York, Grune and Stratton, 1977, pp 43–72.

48. Willeford J: Assessment of central auditory disorders in children, in Pinhiero M, Musiek F (eds): *Assessment of Central Auditory Dysfunction: Foundation and Clinical Correlates*. Baltimore, Williams & Wilkins, 1985, pp 404–420.
49. Willeford J, Bilger J: Auditory perception in children with learning disabilities, in Katz J (ed): *Handbook of Clinical Audiology*. Baltimore, Williams & Wilkins, 1978, pp 410–425.
50. Willeford J, Burleigh J: *Handbook of Central Auditory Processing Disorders in Children*. New York, Grune and Stratton, 1985.
51. Zill N, Schoenborn C: *Health of Our Nation's Children, United States, 1988*. Bethesda, Md, National Center for Health Statistics, 1990.

## Chapter 11

# Central Auditory Processing Disorders in the Elderly: Fact or Fiction?

**Larry Humes, Ph.D.**
**Laurel Christopherson, M.A.**
**Carol Cokely, M.A.**

Many people older than 65 years have considerable difficulty understanding speech. This may be expected given the prevalence of sensorineural hearing loss among this population. In many cases, however, the difficulty experienced by the hearing-impaired elderly appears to be greater than expected given the amount of hearing loss. Although few would challenge the existence of large individual differences in speech understanding among the elderly population, there is considerable debate as to the factors underlying these individual differences.

A recent review of the progress in this area provided three alternative hypotheses as explanations for the individual differences in performance among the elderly listeners[6]: (1) the peripheral or multiple-distortion hypothesis, (2) the cognitive hypothesis, and (3) the central auditory nervous system (CAPD) hypothesis.

The peripheral hypothesis maintains that individual differences in speech-understanding performance result from individual differences in the peripheral encoding of sound by the outer, middle, and inner ears. The most obvious peripheral deficit in many elderly people is the presence of a bilateral high-frequency hearing loss of cochlear origin.[4, 13] In its simplest form, the peripheral hypothesis maintains that most of the individual variability in speech-understanding performance can be explained by individual variations in hearing loss. This simple rule has proven to be quite appropriate for hearing-impaired young adults[16] and under the peripheral hypothesis would simply be extended to the older population. A more complex version of the peripheral hypothesis maintains that individual variations in other peripheral encoding mechanisms, such as spectral and temporal resolution, underlie the individual differences in performance among the elderly. Individual differences in the filtering of sound by the mechanical portion of the inner ear would be one example of a peripheral function that could affect the encoding of speech signals.

The cognitive hypothesis, on the other hand, maintains that much of the individual variability in speech-understanding performance observed in the elderly is a result of individual variations in cognitive abilities. Cortical functions such as information processing, labeling, storage (memory), and retrieval are all cognitive processes that might underlie individual differences in speech understanding in elderly people. A key feature of the cognitive hypothesis is that these deficits are not specific to the auditory modality. Individual differences in working (short-term) memory, for example, can be measured equally well for either auditory or visual presentation of stimuli.

Finally, the central auditory nervous system

hypothesis maintains that individual differences in speech-understanding performance are a result of dysfunction of the auditory pathways within the brain stem or brain. In this hypothesis, impairments in processes, such as neural transmission, feature extraction, or information processing, labeling, or storage are limited to the auditory system. This impairment is generally referred to as a central auditory processing disorder (CAPD). According to this hypothesis, elderly individuals who perform poorly on speech-recognition tasks are believed to have CAPD, whereas those who perform well do not.

Which of these three hypotheses is correct? In the remainder of this chapter the evidence supporting each hypothesis will be reviewed, beginning with the CAPD hypothesis.

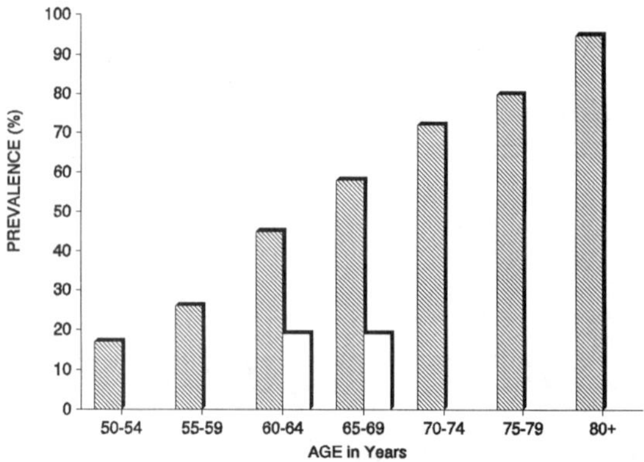


**FIG 11–1.**
Estimates for prevalence of CAPD among the elderly from Stach et al[30] *(striped bars)* and Jerger et al[22] *(unfilled bars)*. Identical test protocols were employed in each study. All 53 of the subjects in the group from the study by Jerger et al,[22] however, had pure-tone averages less than 20 dB HL. The amount of peripheral hearing loss was not controlled in the study by Stach et al.[30]

## CAPD HYPOTHESIS

In several recent investigations CAPD has been found to be very prevalent among the elderly.[20, 22, 27, 30] In general, these studies report a prevalence of CAPD of 50% to 70% among those 65 years of age and older. Moreover, as shown by the striped bars in Figure 11–1, Stach et al[30] found that the prevalence of CAPD increased steadily with age from approximately 20% in people aged 50 to 54 years to 95% in people 80 years of age and older.

The prevalence estimates obtained in these recent studies, however, are questionable. These estimates most likely overestimate the "true" prevalence of CAPD in the elderly population for three reasons. First, the battery of tests used in each study included tests that may have been unreliable. Second, in each study, the presence or absence of CAPD was determined by using tests in a battery administered in parallel with a loose criterion for abnormality. Third, performance on the speech-recognition measures comprising the CAPD test battery was most likely affected by peripheral hearing loss.

Let us first consider the confounding influence of peripheral hearing loss on the estimates of CAPD prevalence. The two unfilled bars in Figure 11–1 represent CAPD prevalence estimates derived from a study by Jerger et al[22] for a group of 53 listeners ranging in age from about 60 to 70 years. Note that the prevalence estimates from this sample are much lower than those obtained by Stach et al[30] over a similar age range. Unlike the group studied by Stach et al[30] *all* of the listeners in this particular elderly group evaluated by Jerger et al[22] *had normal hearing* (midfrequency pure-tone averages less than 20 dB HL). It is clear that elimination of the confounding influence of peripheral hearing loss in the 60- to 70-year-old age range resulted in a dramatic decline in the estimated prevalence of CAPD.

Let us now consider the issue of test reliability. Although the composition of the test battery varied slightly from study to study, all four studies made use of the Synthetic Sentence Identification (SSI) test.[23] Typically, performance-intensity functions were obtained both for the 10-item SSI and for 25-item lists of monosyllabic words. Presence of CAPD was indicated if the maximum score for PB words (PBmax) exceeded the maximum score for the SSI (SSImax) by more than 20% or the SSI score declined to a score more than 20% below SSImax as intensity was increased beyond the level corresponding to maximum performance. The latter measurement is referred to as rollover and was often also determined for the PB words.

The focus here, however, is on the reliability of the SSI. Because the SSI is a test in which each item is judged as correct or incorrect and performance is reflected in the proportion or percentage of correct responses, the distribution of scores has characteristics consistent with the binomial distribution.[31] Because the SSI score is based on only 10 items, considerable variability is expected across repeated test sessions for a given individual. Consider the following example. The SSI is administered to a listener and a score of 60% is obtained. Then we administer the test again to the same listener after increasing the intensity by 20 dB. What score at this higher intensity would correspond to a significant decrease in performance? According to the criteria used in recent studies of CAPD in the elderly, we would consider a score of 30% to be low enough to indicate significant rollover for this patient. According to Thornton and Raffin,[31] however, only scores of 0 or 10% should be considered as being significantly ($P<.05$) lower than the first score of 60% when a 10-item list is used. In other words, if the intensity of the SSI materials was never changed for this hypothetical listener with a "true" score of 60% and the test was simply readministered at the same intensity 100 times, 95 of the scores would fall between 20% and 90%. Given the small number of items in the SSI, a 20% criterion for a significant amount of rollover is too small to yield reliable results.

The same can be said, moreover, for other uses of SSI scores, such as the difference between PBmax and SSImax. If the PBmax score is stable at 80% and the SSImax score fluctuates moment to moment from 20% to 90% for a true score of 60% (as in the previous example for rollover), then the difference between PBmax and SSImax will also vary over a wide range (60% to −10%). In other words, for a given test session, our hypothetical elderly listener might have a PBmax-SSImax difference of 20% (80% to 60%), but have a difference ranging from −10% to 60% on an immediate retest. In this example, moreover, we have assumed that the PB score itself is stable over time. However, based on lists of 25 items, PB scores are themselves quite variable. Furthermore, the variance of difference scores, such as PBmax-SSImax, is greater than the variance of either score alone. Consequently, if we had also considered the variability of the PB score in the preceding example, the range of possible PBmax-SSImax differences may have been even greater.

In addition to theoretical problems with scores from the SSI, there is direct evidence regarding the poor reliability of this test. Several previous investigators, for example, have observed large improvements in performance of the SSI simply by repeating the measurements (practice effects).[2, 9, 28, 29] In a detailed study of SSI reliability, moreover, Dubno and Dirks[10] measured performance on the SSI in 33 listeners with sloping sensorineural hearing loss (not unlike that in presbycusis) across 12 repetitions of the test. They reported significant effects of trial on SSI score and between-trial correlations less than 0.45 across the 12 trials. Both of these results from the study by Dubno & Dirks[10] indicate that the SSI may not be a reliable test when administered in typical clinical fashion.

We have examined the reliability of two of the other tests used to establish high prevalence of CAPD in the elderly: the revised Speech Perception in Noise (SPIN) test[3] and the Dichotic Sentence Identification (DSI) test.[12] In this study[7] each of 17 elderly listeners received the SPIN and DSI tests at three presentation levels on each of three occasions. The results of this study revealed significant effects of trial on DSI and SPIN scores. Moreover, the individual data revealed extreme variability such that 40% to 60% of the subjects demonstrated significant ($P<.05$) test-retest differences when comparing scores on the first trial to scores obtained on either an immediate retest or a retest 1 to 2 weeks later. The significant effects of trial for the group data and the high percentage of individual subjects evidencing significant fluctuations in performance over time both suggest that the DSI and SPIN tests may not be reliable measures of performance in the elderly.

Cokely and Humes[7] also noted that SPIN and DSI scores were strongly and significantly correlated with degree of hearing loss. Correlations of DSI and SPIN scores with pure-tone average ranged from −0.7 to −0.85 for the 17 elderly listeners in that study. Jerger, Jerger, and Pirozzolo[21] have also recently reported that performance on the SPIN, SSI, and DSI tests is strongly affected by the amount of peripheral hearing loss. As mentioned previously, measures of "central" auditory processing should be unconfounded by the degree of peripheral impairment if they are to be interpreted appropriately when applied to the hearing-impaired elderly population. This does not appear to be the case for the DSI and SPIN tests, even when administered at relatively high presentation levels in an attempt to minimize the effects of the peripheral impairment.

Another factor influencing estimates of CAPD prevalence among the elderly in the studies cited previously concerns the design of the test battery itself. In every study, a parallel test battery was employed with a "loose" criterion. A parallel test battery is one in which all of the listeners receive all of the tests in the battery. Given three tests in a parallel test battery for CAPD, the researcher is free to establish the criterion for presence or absence of CAPD. A strict criterion would require failure on all three tests before identifying the listener as having CAPD, whereas a loose criterion would accept failure on any single test as evidence for the presence of CAPD. In each of the recent studies of the prevalence of CAPD among the elderly, a loose criterion for presence of CAPD was adopted.

A parallel test battery with loose criterion frequently overestimates the number of members of the population with the disorder.[32] Consider three tests for CAPD, tests A, B, and C, with corresponding hit rates (HR) and false-alarm rates (FAR) of 0.74/0.04 (HR/FAR), 0.80/0.20, and 0.60/0.30. The latter two sets of hit rates and false-alarm rates are best guesses for representative CAPD tests based on the limited data available[24, 25] whereas the first set of rates is one established previously for PI-PB functions by Turner et al.[33] Assuming no correlation among the three tests, administering these tests in a parallel fashion, and applying a loose criterion ("fail" = failure on *any one* of the three tests), results in a hit rate and false-alarm rate for the protocol of 0.98 and 0.46, respectively. What do these numbers mean? Consider the following example. A group of 100 elderly persons, 10 of whom actually have CAPD, are given this test battery. This parallel test battery with loose criterion will correctly identify all 10 as having CAPD, *but will also indicate that 41 of the listeners without CAPD have CAPD*. Thus, the "true" CAPD prevalence of 10% will be estimated to be 51% [(41+10)/100] with this protocol, reflecting a marked overestimation of the prevalence of the disorder. Application of this approach to the identification of CAPD in the elderly appears to be no exception.

The protocol hit rates and false-alarm rates described in the previous paragraph were calculated assuming that the individual tests in the battery were uncorrelated. The correlation among tests in a battery will affect the performance of the test protocol.[32] Unfortunately, none of the studies of CAPD prevalence in the elderly have reported the correlation among tests in their test battery. Recent results from Cokely and Humes,[7] however, indicate that it would be more accurate to assume a mid-positive correlation among the tests in the CAPD test battery. Correlation coefficients between DSI scores and SPIN scores in the study by Cokely and Humes,[7] for example, ranged from about 0.45 to 0.95 with an average correlation of 0.77. Under a more realistic assumption of a mid-positive correlation among tests in the test battery, the protocol hit rate and false-alarm rate in the preceding example would decrease slightly to 0.89 and 0.38, respectively. Under this more realistic set of assumptions, the prevalence of CAPD among our hypothetical sample of 100 elderly individuals would be 43%. Although better than the estimated prevalence of 51% under the assumption of zero correlation among tests in the battery, the prevalence estimated with this protocol remains much greater than the "true" prevalence of 10%.

Of course, the size of the overestimation error made with our hypothetical parallel test protocol with loose criterion depends on the estimated "true" prevalence. If, for example, the true prevalence of CAPD among the elderly is actually 50%, then our hypothetical test protocol with assumed midpositive correlations among the tests in the battery would estimate the prevalence to be 63.5%. In this case, the overestimate of CAPD prevalence is obviously much smaller than when a "true" prevalence of 10% was assumed.

If such batteries tend to overestimate the prevalence of a disorder, how large is the error? This is difficult to determine regarding the prevalence of CAPD among the elderly because there is no "gold standard" available to confirm the accuracy of the diagnosis. When the tests comprising the CAPD test battery used with the elderly were originally validated it was with a completely different test population. The tests of the CAPD test battery were validated in cases of surgically or radiologically confirmed lesions in the auditory portions of the central nervous system. Interestingly, in these validating applications parallel test batteries have always been employed with strict criteria, rather than loose ones.[1, 19, 26] The reasons behind the change to a loose criterion for applications to the elderly are unclear. In addition, the validating studies of CAPD were usually conducted on persons with normal or near-normal hearing so that the confounding influence of peripheral hearing loss was avoided. This is seldom possible in the elderly. Finally, the reasoning behind the extension of test-battery profiles validated on young normal-hearing adults with known central auditory pathology to the elderly population is weak. The reasoning is essentially as follows: (1) young normal-hearing adults with confirmed lesions in the auditory portions of the central nervous system yield a certain pattern of results on a battery of tests; (2) elderly hearing-impaired adults show a similar result on any one of the tests in the battery; (3) we conclude that the elderly hearing-impaired listeners performing in this manner have dysfunction in the auditory portion of their central nervous system. This reasoning is not very compelling and fails to validate a causal relation between the speech-recognition difficulties of the hearing-impaired elderly and the presence of CAPD.

To summarize briefly: CAPD prevalence estimates reported in several recent studies are most likely inflated owing to the confounding influence of peripheral hearing loss, the use of unreliable speech-recognition measures to establish the presence of CAPD, and the use of a parallel test battery with a loose criterion for failure. Gates[13] has provided other direct evidence that CAPD prevalence estimates, such as those shown previously in Figure 11–1, are very high. Gates[14] reported the results from a sample of 1,026 elderly subjects from the famous Framingham cohort. Using the norms established by Yellin, Jerger, and Fifer[38] for word-recognition performance disproportionately poorer than predicted by pure-tone hearing thresholds, Gates found only three subjects who had greater-than-expected speech-recognition difficulty. This is a prevalence rate of less than 0.3%! Using PI-PB rollover measures, PBmax-SSImax differences, and the Staggered Spondaic Word (SSW) test, performance was found to be consistent with the presence of CAPD in 0.75%, 9%, and 14.6% of the subjects for each test, respectively. Moreover, only 5% of the 1,026 subjects had abnormal scores on both the SSI and the SSW and *none* of the subjects failed all three tests. Thus, these CAPD prevalence estimates from a large random sample of the general population are much lower than those summarized previously in Figure 11–1.

## PERIPHERAL HYPOTHESIS

Given the weak support for the widespread existence of CAPD among the elderly, let us consider the alternative hypotheses described previously. Consider first the simplest form of the peripheral hypothesis. The most obvious and well-documented change in the auditory system with advancing age is the development of a bilateral high-frequency sensorineural hearing loss.[5, 8, 14] How well does this hearing loss itself account for individual variations in speech understanding? Several recent studies have examined this question.[15, 17, 18, 34–36] In each of these studies, speech-recognition tests having reliability coefficients varying from approximately 0.8 to 0.9 were used to measure speech understanding. These reliability coefficients suggest that roughly 64% to 81% of the variance in speech-recognition performance was systematic variance reflecting true individual differences, with the balance (19% to 36%) consisting of error variance. Figure 11–2 reveals the percentage of systematic variance in speech-recognition scores that was accounted for by the peripheral hearing loss of the elderly lis-

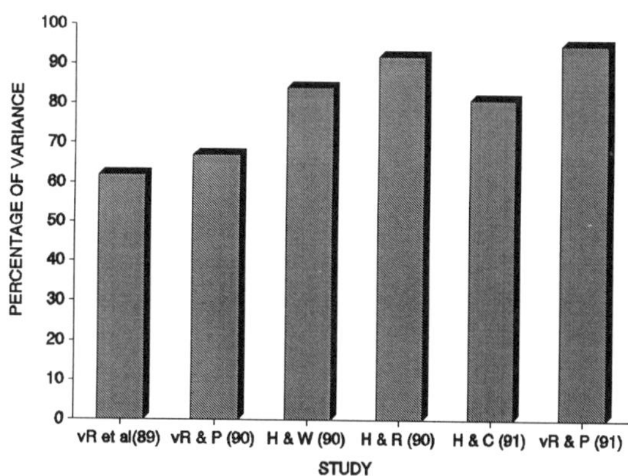


**FIG 11–2.**
The percentage of systematic variance in speech-recognition score accounted for by peripheral hearing loss in six recent studies. Studies, from *left* to *right:* van Rooij et al,[36] Helfer and Wilber,[15] Humes and Roberts,[18] van Rooij and Plomp,[34] Humes and Christopherson,[17] and van Rooij and Plomp.[35]

teners in each of the six studies. These percentages were calculated from the correlation coefficients reported in each study between pure-tone average and speech-recognition score. These correlations were squared to determine the proportion of total variance accounted for by the hearing loss and then divided by the proportion of total variance that was systematic variance. Figure 11–2 indicates that roughly 70% to 95% of the systematic variance in speech-recognition performance was associated with individual differences in hearing loss. It should be noted, moreover, that these high percentages of systematic variance associated with variations in hearing loss were observed for quiet test conditions, as well as conditions employing speech that was degraded. Forms of degradation investigated in the various studies included background noise, reverberation, filtering, and various combinations of these factors.

The results of these recent studies indicate that peripheral hearing loss is the major contributor to the speech-understanding problems of the elderly, accounting for most of the systematic variation in measured performance. Only a small percentage of variance remains to be accounted for by other factors. Jerger and co-workers[21] have reached a similar conclusion in a recent study of 200 elderly people.

## OTHER HYPOTHESES

Ideally, we would like to be able to account for *all* of the systematic variance in speech-recognition performance. Can additional variability across subjects be accounted for by factors other than peripheral hearing loss? Specifically, can the cognitive hypothesis or more complex forms of the peripheral hypothesis (those invoking deficits in peripheral encoding beyond simple loss of hearing sensitivity) account for some of the variance unaccounted for by hearing loss? Several recent studies provide some insight into the answers to these questions.[17, 21, 34–36]

In the studies by Van Rooij and co-workers,[34–36] in addition to measures of hearing loss for pure tones and speech, a variety of other measurements, both psychoacoustic and cognitive, were performed. Both auditory and visual tasks were used to measure various aspects of cognitive function. As mentioned previously, these investigators found that the majority of systematic variance in speech-recognition performance could be explained by the hearing loss. Their results indicated, moreover, that the balance of the systematic variance could be attributed to individual differences in cognitive function. It made no difference whether cognitive function was measured for visual or auditory tasks, indicating that it was not a modality-specific processing disorder, as is CAPD. Finally, they noted that the role of cognitive factors in speech understanding did not vary with age. That is, cognitive factors accounted for 5% to 30% of the variance in speech-recognition performance for young and old adults alike.

More recently, Humes and Christopherson[17] measured speech-recognition and auditory-processing abilities in young and elderly listeners. Measures of speech-recognition consisted of identification scores for nonsense syllables presented in three listening conditions: (1) undistorted in quiet; (2) band-pass filtered (500 to 2,000 Hz) in quiet; and (3) band-pass filtered and reverberation-processed ($T_{60}$ = 0.8 sec) in quiet.

Measures of auditory processing consisted of a series of eight discrimination tasks comprising the Test of Basic Auditory Capabilities (TBAC)[37] This battery of tests consists of measures of: (1) intensity discrimination for a 1-kHz tone; (2) frequency discrimination for a 1-kHz tone; (3) duration discrimination for a 1-kHz tone; (4) jitter or rhythm discrimination for a series of 1-kHz tone pulses; (5) intensity discrimination for a single pure-tone component in the middle of a ten-tone sequence (referred to as the embedded test-tone task); (6) temporal-order discrimination for midfrequency tones differing in pitch; (7) temporal-order discrimination for consonant-vowel syllables, or syllable sequence; and (8) closed-set consonant-vowel syllable identification.

The TBAC has several characteristics that make it particularly desirable for application to hearing-impaired elderly individuals. First, research in our laboratory has demonstrated that the tests comprising the TBAC are reliable with no significant effects of trial found across six repetitions of the TBAC for normal-hearing young adults or across three repetitions of the TBAC for hearing-impaired elderly listeners. Second, most of the tests make use of midfrequency (500 to 2,000 Hz) stimuli which minimizes the potential effect of high-frequency sensorineural hearing loss on the tests. Third, previous studies of the TBAC with hearing-impaired listeners indicated that the test results are unaffected by peripheral hearing loss as long as sensation levels of at least 25 dB are used.[11] Fourth, many of the TBAC tests are temporally based discrimination tasks and make use of complex stimuli. It has been suggested previously that elderly listeners may be particularly vulnerable to temporal-processing problems and more complex listening tasks.[6]

In the study by Humes and Christopherson,[17] regression analyses performed on the data from the elderly listeners revealed that the hearing loss was the main factor underlying speech-recognition performance for all three measures of speech recognition (unfiltered, filtered, and filtered + reverberation-processed). Figure 11–3 shows the results of the regression analyses, with each panel depicting the results for a different set of speech materials. Although a high-frequency pure-tone average (1,000, 2,000, and 4,000 Hz) accounted for most of the total variance in speech-recognition performance for all three sets of speech materials, other variables entered in the regression analyses accounted for significant additional proportions of the variance. As indicated in this figure, various measures of auditory processing from the TBAC accounted for significant proportions of variance for the unfiltered and filtered speech materials, whereas the age of the listener entered the regression equation for speech that was both filtered and reverberation-processed.

The results in Figure 11–3 indicate that the peripheral hearing loss is the most important determiner of speech-recognition performance in the elderly. This is support for the simplest form of the peripheral hypothesis. The results also indicate, however, that significant additional proportions of variance can be accounted for by factors other than the hearing loss, especially for unfiltered speech presented in quiet. Thus, speech-recognition predictions made by the simplest form of the peripheral hypothesis *can* be improved upon by including scores from various tests of the TBAC. Until the processes underlying performance on the TBAC tests are better delineated, however, it is not possible to determine which of the competing alternative hypotheses might be supported by these results. Although we have referred to the TBAC tests as measures of auditory

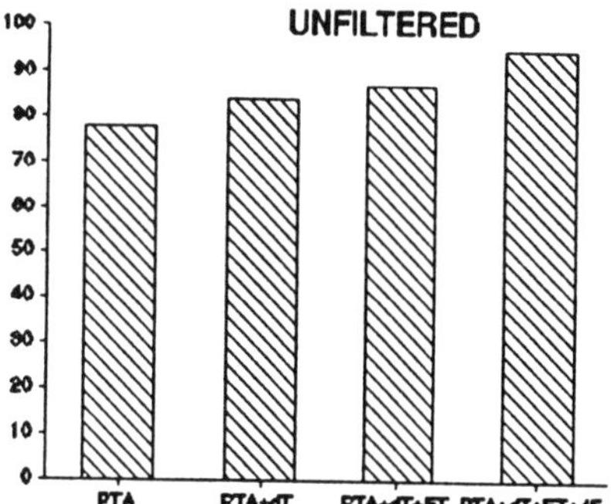


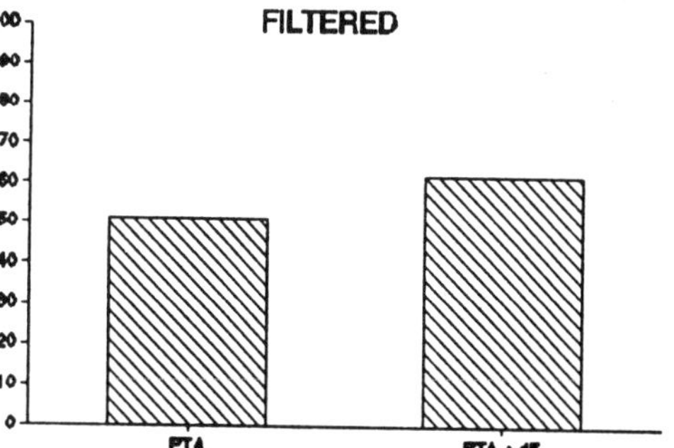


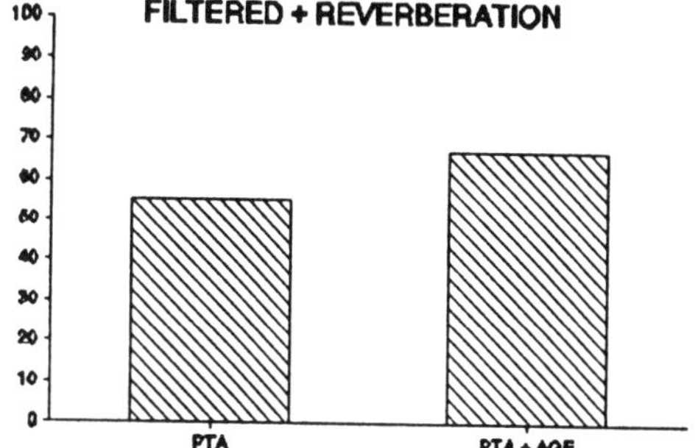


**FIG 11–3.**
Summary of the regression analyses from the study by Humes & Christopherson.[17] Each panel illustrates the percentage of total variance accounted for by each variable listed along the x axis. The listening condition for the speech-recognition task varies across panels (*top,* unfiltered speech in quiet; *middle,* bandpass-filtered (500–2,000 Hz) speech in quiet; *bottom,* bandpass-filtered and reverberation-processed speech in quiet). Note that the high-frequency pure-tone average (PTA) is the variable that accounts for the largest proportion of the variance in each panel. The *top two panels,* however, also indicate that additional proportions of variance in speech-recognition score can be accounted for by including measures of "auditory" processing from the TBAC.

processing because they make use of acoustic stimuli, individual differences in performance on some tasks may reflect differences in cognitive processing, rather than auditory processing. This possibility could be examined by evaluating performance of the same group of subjects on auditory, visual, and tactile versions of various tests comprising the TBAC.

## SUMMARY

In summary, peripheral hearing loss is the primary factor underlying the speech-recognition difficulties of the elderly. Approximately 70% to 95% of the variability in speech-recognition performance among the elderly can be attributed to individual variations in hearing loss. This supports the simplest form of the peripheral hypothesis. At present, it appears that most of the remaining variability can be accounted for by individual differences in cognitive processing. The prevalence of modality-specific CAPDs among the elderly appears to have been grossly overestimated in the recent literature and appears to play a relatively minor role in determining the individual variations in speech recognition among the elderly.

## REFERENCES

1. Baran JA, Musiek FE: Behavioral assessment of the central auditory nervous system, in Rintelmann WF (ed): *Hearing Assessment*. Austin, Tex, Pro-Ed, 1991.
2. Beattie RC, Clark N: Practice effects of a four-talker babble on the Synthetic Sentence Identification test. *Ear Hear* 1982; 3:202–206.
3. Bilger RC, Nuetzel JM, Rabinowitz WM, et al: Standardization of a test of speech perception in noise. *J Speech Hear Res* 1984; 27:32–48.
4. Bohne BA, Gruner MM, Harding GW: Morphological correlates of aging in the chinchilla cochlea. *Hear Res* 1990; 48:79–92.
5. Bunch C: Age variations in auditory acuity. *Arch Otolaryngol* 1929; 9:625–636.
6. CHABA (Committee on Hearing, Bioacoustics and Biomechanics): Speech understanding and aging. *J Acoust Soc Am* 1988; 83:859–893.
7. Cokely CG, Humes LE: Reliability of two measures of speech recognition in the elderly. *J Speech Hear Res* 1992; in press.
8. Corso J: Aging and auditory thresholds in men and women. *Arch Environ* 1963; 77:385–405.
9. Dirks DD, Bower DR: Masking effects of speech competing messages. *J Speech Hear Res* 1969; 12:229–245.
10. Dubno JR, Dirks DD: Suggestions for optimizing the reliability of the synthetic sentence identification test. *J Speech Hear Disord* 1983; 48:98–103.
11. Espinoza-Varas B, Watson CS: Temporal-processing abilities of hearing-impaired listeners. *J Acoust Soc Am* 1986; 80:S12.
12. Fifer R, Jerger J, Berlin C, et al: Development of a dichotic sentence identification test for hearing-impaired adults. *Ear Hear* 1983; 4:300–305.
13. Gates G: Presbycusis: An overview. Paper presented at the Symposium on Presbycusis: A Broad Overview. National Academy of Sciences, Washington, DC, October, 1990.
14. Gates GA, Cooper JC Jr, Kannel WB, et al: Hearing in the elderly: The Framingham cohort, 1983–1985. *Ear Hear* 1990; 11:247–256.
15. Helfer KS, Wilber LA: Hearing loss, aging, and speech perception in reverberation and noise. *J Speech Hear Res* 1990; 33:149–155.
16. Humes LE: Understanding the speech-understanding problems of the hearing impaired. *J Am Acad Audiol* 1991; 2:59–70.
17. Humes LE, Christopherson L: Speech identification difficulties of hearing-impaired elderly persons: The contributions of auditory-processing deficits. *J Speech Hear Res* 1991; 34:686–693.
18. Humes LE, Roberts L: Speech-recognition difficulties of the hearing-impaired elderly: The contributions of audibility. *J Speech Hear Res* 1990; 33:726–735.
19. Jerger J: Diagnostic audiology, in Jerger J (ed): *Modern Developments in Audiology*. New York, Academic Press, 1973.
20. Jerger J, Jerger S, Oliver T, et al: Speech-understanding in the elderly. *Ear Hear* 1989; 10:79–89.
21. Jerger J, Jerger S, Pirozzolo F: Correlational analysis of speech audiometric scores, hearing loss, age and cognitive abilities in the elderly. *Ear Hear* 1991; 12:103–109.
22. Jerger J, Oliver TA, Pirozzolo F: Impact of central auditory processing disorder and cognitive deficit on the self-assessment of hearing handicap in the elderly. *J Am Acad Audiol* 1990; 1:75–80.
23. Jerger J, Speaks C, Trammell J: A new approach to speech audiometry. *J Speech Hear Disord* 1968; 33:318–328.

24. Lynn GE, Gilroy J: Evaluation of central auditory dysfunction in patients with neurological disorders, in Keith RW (ed): *Central Auditory Dysfunction*. New York, Grune & Stratton, 1977.
25. Mueller H, Sedge R, Salazar A: Auditory assessment of neural trauma, in Miner M, Wagner K (eds): *Neurotrauma: Treatment, Rehabilitation and Related Issues*. Boston, Butterworths, 1986.
26. Musiek FE: Application of central auditory tests: An overview, in Katz J (ed): *Handbook of Clinical Audiology*. Baltimore, Williams & Wilkins, 1985.
27. Rodriguez GP, DiSarno NJ, Hardiman CJ: Central auditory processing in normal-hearing elderly adults. *Audiology* 1990; 29:85–92.
28. Speaks C, Jerger J: Method for measurement of speech identification. *J Speech Hear Res* 1965; 8:185–194.
29. Speaks C, Karmen JL, Benitez L: Effect of a competing message on synthetic sentence identification. *J Speech Hear Res* 1967; 10:390–395.
30. Stach BA, Spretnjak ML, Jerger J: The prevalence of central presbycusis in a clinical population. *J Am Acad Audiol* 1990; 1:109–115.
31. Thornton A, Raffin MJM: Speech discrimination scores modeled as a binomial variable. *J Speech Hear Res* 1978; 2:507–518.
32. Turner RG: Making clinical decisions, in Rintelmann WF (ed): *Hearing Assessment*. Austin, Tex, Pro-Ed, 1991.
33. Turner RG, Shepard NT, Frazer GJ: Clinical performance of audiological and related diagnostic tests. *Ear Hear* 1984; 5:187–194.
34. van Rooij JCGM, Plomp R: Auditive and cognitive factors in speech perception by elderly listeners. II. Multivariate analyses. *J Acoust Soc Am* 1990: 88:2611–2624.
35. van Rooij JCGM, Plomp R: Auditive and cognitive factors in speech perception by elderly listeners. III. *J Acoust Soc Am* 1991; 91:1028–1033.
36. van Rooij JCGM, Plomp R, Orlebeke JF: Auditive and cognitive factors in speech perception by elderly listeners. I. Development of test battery. *J Acoust Soc Am* 1989; 86:1294–1309.
37. Watson CS, Johnson DM, Lehman JR, et al: An auditory discrimination test battery. *J Acoust Soc Am* 1982; 71:S73.
38. Yellin MW, Jerger J, Fifer RC: Norms for disproportionate loss in speech intelligibility. *Ear Hear* 1989; 10:231–234.

*Chapter* **12**

# Auditory Event-Related Potentials in Central Auditory Disorders

**Frank Musiek, Ph.D.**
**Steve Bornstein, Ph.D.**

The late auditory event-related potential identified as the P300 wave is related to the broad category of late auditory evoked potentials extending from approximately 90 ms through 700 ms. The N1 and P2 late potentials normally occur at around 100 and 200 ms, respectively, in response to tone bursts or clicks. They are commonly called exogenous potentials because they are dependent on stimulus properties and are essentially unrelated to internal cognitive processes but can be generated as long as a listener is in a conscious, alert state. However, considerable evidence suggests that the amplitudes of N1 and P2 are affected to some degree by attention.[7, 44] The P300 is called an endogenous potential because it is generated by a listener making a cognitive decision regarding a stimulus and involves processes such as attention, recognition, and categorization.[54] Although the exogenous potentials may be affected by cortical and subcortical dysfunction,[26, 36, 42, 51] the P300 may be more useful than the exogenous potential for providing information about deficits involving auditory processing at higher levels. Because the listener is actively involved in a cognitive behavior that causes the averaged neural activity, the P300 measure could be viewed as a correlate between neural substrates and behavior.

The most common way of obtaining the P300 is by the "oddball" paradigm. In this paradigm, the same stimulus is presented repeatedly; at random intervals, a rare or "odd" stimulus is substituted. Generally, two different sounds are presented, such as 1,000- to 2,000-Hz tone bursts, and the listener is asked to count the number of rare tones. Several hundred averaged trials are used to derive a waveform and the frequent stimulus occurs in a high proportion of the trials (80% to 85%). The "rare" stimulus can also be omitted; the subject is asked to count the number of times there is a "gap" or missing stimulus. This omitted paradigm can also result in a P300.[53] It has been shown that the P300 can be obtained in a passive condition, without the subject attending to the target (rare) stimuli.[47] The P300s obtained in a passive condition are smaller in amplitude and often are greater in latency than the conventionally obtained P300s. The use of "novel" stimuli also can evoke a P300. These are target stimuli that differ dramatically from the nontarget or frequent stimuli, thus alerting the subjects.[4] An important deviation from the above procedure is the use of various types of speech as stimuli. Using linguistic stimuli can provide indications of speech discrimination, recognition, or language abilities.

If a person can attend to the "odd" stimulus, a large positive peak (about 7 to 25 μV in normal individuals) in averaged brain electrical activity occurring approximately 300 ms after the initiation stimulation is detected by scalp electrodes. Although several electrode montages may be used, commonly noninverting electrodes are placed at the vertex (Cz), midline frontal (Fz), and parietal-occipital region (Pz), inverting, linked electrodes are placed at left and right earlobes, and a ground electrode is placed at the forehead.

Although there are considerably more data published on the various parametric measures of P300, a comprehensive review is beyond the scope of this paper. For those interested in further basic aspects of the P300, suggested reviews include Squires and Hecox[54] and Hillyard and Picton.[20]

## NEURAL GENERATORS OF THE P300

The auditory P300 wave has been studied in normal and disordered populations, including children and adults with brain and cognitive disorders. However, its exact neural generators are not known. Propagation of the P300 may involve the amygdala and hippocampal areas deep within the temporal lobes, as well as the posterior hippocampus, since the P300 has been shown to be unaffected with anterior hippocampal resection.[12, 18, 23, 37, 59] Support for the contribution of these generators comes from studies on Alzheimer's patients, in whom deficits in acetylcholine input to the hippocampus have been found that may account for the memory loss found in this disease. Dysfunction of inferior parietotemporal areas has also been implicated in Alzheimer's patients, as well as involvement of prefrontal cortex as seen by positron emission tomography.[23] The frequent occurrence of a bipeaked P300 (labeled P3a and P3b) under the oddball paradigm may reflect contributions of both frontal and parietal generator sites. Latency prolongation and amplitude reduction have been found in patients with Alzheimer's disease.[55] However, studies of focal brain lesions suggest that P300 is not generated by superior parietal or rostral inferior parietal regions, but is critically mediated in the temporoparietal junction area.[24, 25] Midline thalamic and midbrain structures have also been implicated as contributing to the P300, although electrophysiological evidence of this is not compelling.[56] These regions have been shown to be important for orientation and attention, both critical components needed for generation of a scalp-recorded P300. In essence, complex neural networks from thalamic to temporoparietal to hippocampal or back to thalamic nuclei, prefrontal cortex, and limbic regions probably are some of the mechanisms responsible for P300 generation.[32, 33, 60]

These studies suggest that multiple loci in the brain may be generators of the P300. This is consistent with the fact that several processes are necessary to obtain the P300, including the involvement of the auditory cortex (for detection, sensation, and discrimination of the acoustic stimuli), and the complex neural network of the reticular formation (for arousal and attention). In addition, memory functions are tapped in the oddball paradigm and it is likely that the hippocampus and amygdala are involved. The parallel and sequential interaction of these processes requires intrahemispheric function, which, in turn, is dependent on association areas of the brain. There may be several interhemispheric interactions that contribute to the P300 (as will be discussed later). Electrophysiological factors such as dipole orientation and timing of neural activity are also critical to P300 generation. Thus, multiple brain loci as a basis for the generation of P300 is highly probable.

## P300 IN SELECTED BRAIN PATHOLOGIES

Our focus in this chapter is a discussion of the P300 as it relates to central auditory dysfunction, especially for pathologies encountered by the specialists in communication disorders.

It is known that the P300 increases in amplitude and decreases in latency throughout childhood and adolescence,[4, 49] and thereafter progressively diminishes in amplitude and increases in latency[50] (Fig 12–1). Furthermore, increased amplitude and decreased latency have been correlated with better short-term memory skills.[21, 48] The P300 may be one of the last evoked potentials to reach maturation.[38] Because of the ability required to perform the task, conventional P300 information usually cannot be obtained in children under 5 years of age. However, children younger than 5 years have been tested using the novel stimulus paradigm to obtain the P300.[4]

The most widespread use of the P300 has

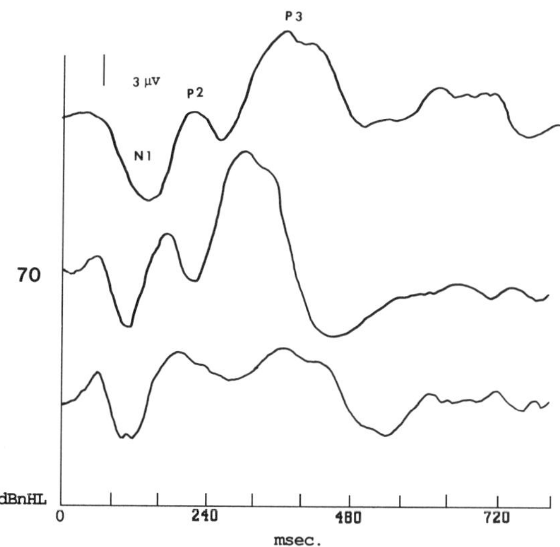


**FIG 12–1.**
Three P300s from normal subjects: *top,* 9-year-old girl; *middle,* young adult man; *bottom,* 73-year-old woman.

been for documenting abnormal prolongation of latency and decreased amplitude in patients with dementia—primarily Alzheimer's disease.[15, 55] Knight[23] presented evidence that P300 abnormalities early in the progression of Alzheimer's disease may reflect an acetylcholine deficit in hippocampal and parietotemporal cerebral regions, although this may be only one factor that can influence P300 generation. Abnormalities in P300 in other forms of dementia resulting from other metabolic, genetic, and structural factors have also been found.[3, 13, 16]

Nevertheless, the memory deficits presented by patients with Alzheimer's disease, and the abnormalities in parietotemporal areas suggest that auditory association areas are involved in P300 generation. It has been argued that use of P300 may differentiate true organic dementia from other psychiatric disorders. For example, Squires et al[53] and Gordon et al[17] found that P300 latency was abnormally prolonged in a high percentage of patients with dementia, but was found in a low percentage of patients with other psychiatric disturbances. These findings have been disputed by other investigators.[9, 43] The sensitivity of the measure probably is a result of stimulus and task complexity and the severity of dementia.

Goodin et al[14] investigated P300s in 55 men infected with human immunodeficiency virus. They found that decreased amplitude and prolonged latency were more sensitive in detecting cerebral dysfunction (often in asymptomatic individuals) than were magnetic resonance imaging, computed tomography scans, and electroencephalograms. These findings demonstrate the importance of auditory electrophysiologic tests because they assess function and not necessarily structure.

## FOCAL BRAIN LESIONS AND TRAUMA

There have been several reports of abnormal P300 waves in patients with brain lesions. These studies help explain the localization of brain functions and possible generators of the P300; they are a basis for clinical use of the P300 in detecting central dysfunction and are fundamental to the application of P300 in monitoring changes in central nervous system function in the same patient.

Knight[23] reported on six patients with unilateral lesions of superior parietal cortex and rostral sections of the inferior parietal cortex, including parts of the supramarginal and angular gyri. Three patients had left-hemisphere lesions and three had right-hemisphere lesions. In response to monaural stimulation from either the contralateral or ipsilateral ear, no amplitude or latency differences in the P300 generated by the rare or other novel stimuli were seen across various recording sites. However, an absent N200 event-related potential (ERP) to rare stimuli to which patients were instructed to attend, and a reduced amplitude N200 to various kinds of interpersonal novel acoustic stimuli, were found regardless of ear of stimulation. The N200 ERP is seen as a negative peak in response to selective attention.

In contrast, P300s were absent or markedly reduced for six patients in this study who had discrete, unilateral lesions of the temporal junction (i.e., the posterior superior temporal plane). Five patients had left-hemisphere lesions and one had a right-hemisphere lesion. In this group, the N200 latency and amplitude to both rare and novel stimuli were equivalent to those of the control group. However, the P300 to the rare sound (P3a) was absent and was significantly reduced in amplitude to the novel stimuli (P3b), despite the fact that the task was easily performed and the patients had similar reaction times to the stimuli as compared with the control group. These electrophysiological differences existed regardless of which ear was stimulated and regardless of the recording site (central-frontal, vertex, or central-parietal). These results suggest that N200 and P300 potentials reflect different and parallel stages of processing, each having corresponding neural substrates.

The N200 generation probably reflects integration of sensorimotor processes mediated in the parietal lobe, whereas P300 generation is not due to a sensorimotor integration or to a detection process, but rather to later stages of processing.[53]

Michalewski, Rosenberg, and Starr[34] also reported prolonged P300 latencies in patients with cerebrovascular lesions and brain tumors. It is possible that the reduced neural substrate needed to generate the P300 causes an increase in P300 latency and an increased decision-processing time. The task became more difficult for the patients with brain lesions. This is consistent with research showing that when the task within the oddball paradigm is made more difficult in the normal population, the P300 latency is increased.[45]

Olbrich et al[41] measured P300s in 21 patients with brain tumors and 21 patients with severe head injuries. They found abnormally prolonged latencies in both groups, but primarily in patients who met a criterion of cognitive disability as measured by a psychiatric rating scale. They concluded that P300 abnormalities did not necessarily reflect dysfunction of specific neural pathways, but reflected a more generalized cognitive deficit resulting from dysfunction of several areas, including primary auditory cortex of both hemispheres and deep temporal structures such as the hippocampus and amygdala.

Similarly, Ebner et al[8] recorded P300s and administered neuropsychological tests to 16 patients with chronic focal brain lesions. Their results supported the view that P300 abnormalities reflect impairment of cognitive abilities, rather than being direct effects of focal frontal or retrorolandic brain lesions. In their study, patients with abnormal P300s performed poorly on neuropsychological tests while patients with normal P300s performed normally on the same tests.

Obert and Cranford[40] examined P300 waveforms in ten patients with neocortical lesions of various sites. Several experimental conditions were presented to patients. Two patients did not produce a P300 to any condition, while the remaining patients demonstrated either absent or delayed waveforms to 53% of the experimental conditions. Obert and Cranford were unable to find a relationship between site or extent of lesion and P300 abnormalities.[40] They also noted that in some conditions where P300 was absent, a waveform appeared to develop during early averages, but then disappeared. They postulated that some form of neurological "jitter" might have canceled the averaged waveform.[40] This deserves further investigation, and may be an interesting phenomenon in itself. Obert and Cranford[40] also demonstrated that by increasing task difficulty in the auditory domain (i.e., reducing stimulus duration or presenting competing sound) greater information may be obtained regarding auditory-cognitive processing.

A few investigations have examined P300 as a function of recovery from various forms of head injury.[2, 6, 19, 28] In these investigations, the amount of P300 abnormality generally correlated with the extent of injury, and improvements in P300 latency and amplitude occurred with cognitive and behavioral recovery, although abnormalities generally remained. Harris and Hall[19] did not find a correlation between the P300 and other auditory evoked potentials, standard audiometric results, the Staggered Spondaic Word test or the Willeford Competing Sentence test. This points out a possible disassociation between behaviorally measured auditory abilities and auditory ERPs. The relationship between auditory behavior and P300 is an important area that requires more study.

Musiek et al.[36a] controlled for age and hearing loss in a group of 20 patients having focal brain lesions and in a group of 20 normal controls. Patients had lesions affecting (but not limited to) auditory areas of the brain as defined by Galaburda and Sanides.[11] As a group, the patients with brain lesions showed significantly prolonged latencies and decreased amplitudes for the P300 but not for the exogenous potentials (N1 and P2) (Fig 12–2). The decreased amplitude may have been the result of a smaller number of functioning neurons or diminished intensity of neural firing, possibly because of neurotransmitter-synaptic compromise. The fact that the P2 was relatively unimpaired in the brain-lesion group suggests that the auditory processing deficits may have been more cognitive than sensory in nature. As a group, laterality effects were not found either in

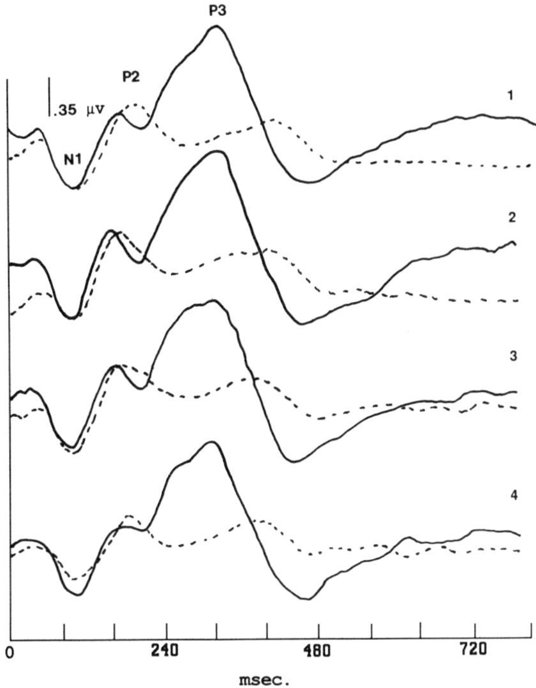


**FIG 12–2.**
Grand mean averages (N1, P2, P3) from a group of normal control subjects (*solid* lines) and a group of patients with brain lesions of the auditory regions (*dotted* lines). The stimuli were 1,000-Hz (frequent) and 2,000-Hz (rare) tone bursts (10 ms rise/fall, 20 ms plateau) presented monaurally at 75 dB SPL. *1* = left ear, C3 recording site; *2* = left ear, C4 recording site; *3* = right ear, C4 recording site; *4* = right ear, C3 recording site.

the recording electrode site (C3 and C4, left and right lateral parietal, respectively), or the ear being stimulated, similar to the findings of Knight[23] (Fig 12–3). However, in the group with pathology there were more absent P300s than in the control group (Table 12–1). When P300 waves were present, it made no difference whether the electrode was over the damaged hemisphere, or which ear was stimulated. However, there were cases where the electrode over the same hemi-

**TABLE 12–1.**

P300 Presence/Absence in Controls and Patients With Central Nervous System Lesions*

| Condition (Ear and Recording Site) | LE C3 | LE C4 | RE C3 | RE C4 |
|---|---|---|---|---|
| Patients | 15/5 | 16/4 | 16/4 | 16/4 |
| Controls | 20/0 | 20/0 | 20/0 | 20/0 |

*Expressed as present/absent.

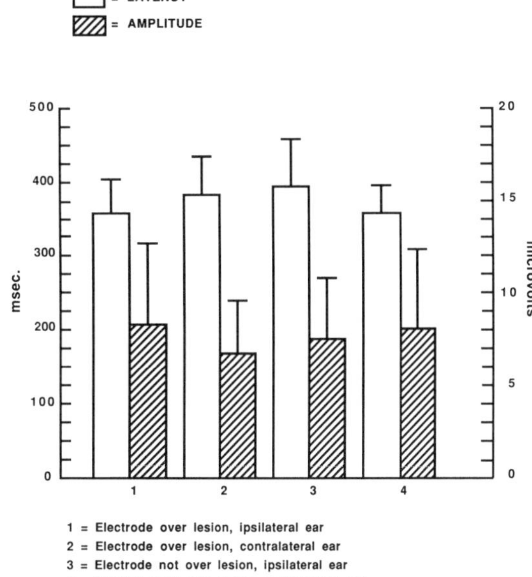


**FIG 12–3.**
Latency *(clear bars)* and amplitude *(striped bars)* for patients with lesions or auditory areas of the cerebrum (N = 13) limited to one hemisphere. The four conditions shown are for the electrode ipsilateral and contralateral to the side with the lesion and the ear stimulated ipsilateral or contralateral to the side with the lesion. Statistical analysis indicated no significant difference for latency or amplitude among conditions 1, 2, 3, and 4. (From Musiek FE, Baran J, Pinheiro M: *J Am Acad Audiol* 1992; 3:5–15. Used by permission.)

sphere as the lesion yielded poorer responses than when over the normal hemisphere. These findings and those of Knight et al[24] suggest that both hemispheres may participate via the corpus callosum in the cognitive processes generating P300.

A recent study by Kutus et al[27] on split-brain patients may indicate that the corpus callosum is not required for generation of the P300. These researchers obtained P300s on five split-brain patients showing a larger response over the right hemisphere than over the left hemisphere. Since a P300 was generated (though smaller on the left), Kutus et al suggest that the corpus callosum is not needed for P300 generation.[27] It would seem that the Kutus study cannot rule out some contribution of the corpus callosum to the P300 because of the asymmetry of the P300 in the patients who have had commissurotomy. This asymmetry could have a variety of other causes in this population, as the authors acknowledge.[27] Pre- and post-P300 measures on these patients would provide the best insight into an association between corpus callosum function and the ERP.

It appears that the neural networks involved in the P300 are diffuse. If cells in a damaged hemisphere cannot send or receive impulses and the normal hemisphere is dependent on these impulses to complete the cognitive process, abnormalities would be recorded from both hemispheres. The P300 may reflect an integration of information from various areas of the brain. Areas that may be involved include auditory cortical association areas,[24] the hippocampus and amygdala,[58] and the right hemisphere.[29] If these different areas are involved, then intrahemispheric and interhemispheric neural networks must be present (e.g., subcortical white matter and the corpus callosum). Extensive and deep brain lesions, such as those found in the patients in the Musiek et al.[36a] (submitted for publication) study, affected the subcortical neural substrate. In this study, most of the patients with deep brain lesions yielded absent P300s; however, these patients demonstrated near-perfect psychophysical performance (e.g., counting). This may indicate a dissociation of P300 and certain aspects of behavior, such as detection and other simple processes. Similar findings were reported by Obert and Cranford.[40] This interpretation is consistent with that of Knight,[23] who found a similar dissociation between P300 and behavior and concluded that processes such as memory and orientation were important to generation of a P300.

Related to the P300 is a negative wave (N2) occurring just before the P300. Selinger et al[52] reported that in patients with aphasia, P2 and N2 values were elicited by tones when listening to tasks requiring either right- or left-hemisphere processing. The study found larger right-hemisphere responses in the aphasic group that listened to speech. These trends in responses were not present in the control group, suggesting that right-hemisphere function had taken over some of the language functions from the damaged left hemisphere. Interestingly, the increased right-hemisphere amplitude was negatively correlated with performance on the Porch Index of Communicative Abilities and the Boston Diagnostic Aphasia Examination test, suggesting that increased right-hemisphere involvement in language reflects greater left-hemisphere damage. Although this was not a study of the P300, the N2 response is also an internally generated or endogenous potential and it suggests the potential for using the P300 and other endogenous potentials to monitor the effects of aphasia, treatment efficacy, and brain organization.

## CHILDREN AND SPECIAL POPULATIONS

Jirsa and Clontz[22] investigated P300 in 18 children ranging in age from 9.0 to 11.5 years, and who were identified as having central auditory processing disorders (CAPD). The tests used to identify CAPD disorders were the Selective Auditory Attention test, Willeford's Competing Sentence test, and the Pitch Patterns Sequence test. Fourteen children with CAPD demonstrated abnormally delayed P300 latencies and nine showed reduced P300 amplitudes; no control subject had prolonged latencies. There were significant differences in mean P300 latency, but not mean amplitude between a control group and the CAPD group. There was no direct relationship between behavioral and electrophysiological measures.

Squires and Hecox[54] reported that they had monitored several pediatric patients with normal speech and language development who experienced a sudden deterioration in expressive and receptive language. In these patients, P300 responses to tone burst stimuli were absent and in many of these patients bilateral temporal lobe electroencephalographic abnormalities were found; this is consistent with involvement of hippocampal and other temporal lobe structures.

The potential use of P300 to document subtle auditory dysfunction was also shown by Squires and Hecox[54] in their report of a patient with speech-discrimination difficulties who presented normal auditory brain-stem response, middle latency, long-latency exogenous potential, and P300 results in quiet. However, long-latency exogenous potential abnormalities were found and P300 was absent when the task was presented with background noise, thereby electrophysiologically substantiating the patient's symptoms.

Finley et al[10] found an 11% prevalence of prolonged P300 latency in 282 children with various psychiatric, learning, and medical problems.

Delayed P300 responses occurred in 85% of the cases in which an organic etiology was suggested by abnormal performance on the Halstead-Reitan test battery. Thus, if the Halstead-Reitan is taken as a valid measure of organicity, the P300 had an 85% accuracy rate. Also, in all cases where P300 latency was abnormal, abnormality on the Halstead-Reitan was present. These results support the presence of an organic basis in many children diagnosed as having functional problems and that the P300 may be sensitive to detecting these organic deficits.

Loiselle et al[31] reported on P300s in 11 boys classified as hyperactive, defined as "a disorder of selective attention to certain stimuli, but not, or to a lesser degree, a disorder of concurrent attention to all stimuli."[31] In their paradigm, tone-pip stimuli were presented dichotically and P300s were recorded, with attention focused on one ear. There was no difference in P300 latencies between the hyperactive group and a control group for the nonattended stimuli, but the P300 latency was longer in the control group for the attended stimuli. Although P300 amplitudes did not differ between groups for the nonattended stimuli, the control group showed significantly greater amplitudes for the attended stimuli. These results may be interpreted as indicating that the control group required a longer processing time to detect and process the attended stimulus because they were cognitively listening for the stimulus, while the hyperactive boys were listening to each stimulus concurrently owing to selective attention deficits. The increased amplitude of the control group, as compared with the hyperactive boys, also is consistent with the hypothesis that increased neural activity occurred when they were listening to the target ear.

Courchesne et al[5] examined ERPs in ten autistic persons, ages 13 to 25 years, who had intelligence in the "average" range. Their oddball paradigm consisted of linguistic frequent and rare target stimuli, as well as a variety of vocal and nonvocal novel sounds. When subjects passively listened to the stimuli, no differences were found in several different types of ERP's, including P300, as compared with a matched control group. When subjects were instructed to indicate when they heard the rare target "you," significant amplitude differences were found for all the different types of ERPs, whereas P300 latency differences were insignificant. An additional positive ERP wave following the P300, the slow wave, was significantly delayed in the autistic group. These results suggest that in the population studied, autism was the result of an information-processing disorder, rather than a disorder of either oversensitivity to auditory stimuli or an inability to recognize auditory information as novel. Furthermore, they noted different visual ERP abnormalities, which appeared to be less impaired than auditory ERPs.

Using P300 measures, Lincoln et al[30] presented evidence that children with Down's syndrome showed deficits in information processing and motor organization owing to differences in brain function and organization, rather than to maturational delay. Although children with Down's syndrome showed prolonged latencies for most endogenous waves as compared with a chronological age-matched group, latencies were shorter in the Down's syndrome group as compared with a group matched for mental age when using simple linguistic targets as the "odd" stimulus. However, latencies were longer in the Down's syndrome group than in the group matched for mental age when using novel probe stimuli as the "odd" stimulus.

Blackwood et al[1] examined the relationship between Alzheimer's dementia and P300 in 89 subjects with Down's syndrome ranging in age from 16 to 66. They found a significant increase in P300 latency and a decrease in amplitude in the older Down's syndrome group, which was due to a significant number of subjects developing dementia beginning at age 37. A high incidence of Alzheimer's disease occurs in patients with Down's syndrome. Many of these patients cannot perform neuropsychological tests to monitor cognitive changes. Because neuropathological changes in Down's syndrome are similar to those in Alzheimer's disease,[57] monitoring cognitive function electrophysiologically may be a useful measure in the Down's syndrome population. In a two-year follow-up study, Muir et al[35] found a progression of Alzheimer's disease in patients that was correlated with P300-latency increases and amplitude decreases. Also, onset of dementia was found in other patients who demonstrated significant latency shifts and amplitude decrements who initially had ERPs within normal limits.

## FUTURE DIRECTIONS

The use of the auditory P300 holds promise as a diagnostic and rehabilitative tool, though further research is needed before definitive interpretations can be made. Although not discussed in this paper, ERPs are not modality-specific, (i.e., the P300 can also be generated by visual and somatosensory stimuli). Future research may delineate between auditory-cognitive and generalized deficits by using ERPs evoked by different sensory stimuli. Nevertheless, there are several potential applications for ERPs: they may provide an objective electrophysiologic basis for central processing in speech and language disorders, aphasia, and head injury. The ERPs may aid in planning therapeutic strategies in aphasia and learning disabilities, or monitoring recovery from pathologic conditions due to behavioral or pharmacologic treatment. The ERPs may also help to better define the relationship between CAPD and attention-deficit disorders in children. Finally, future applications of the P300 should use linguistic stimuli because they may provide an objective measure of speech sound discrimination ability or the ability to make semantic and syntactic categorizations. Presently, ERPs are still in the clinical investigative stage, and cautious clinical use is limited to those experienced with the procedure.

## REFERENCES


1. Blackwood DHR, St. Clair DM, Muir WJ, et al: The development of Alzheimer's disease in Down's syndrome assessed by auditory event-related potentials. *J Ment Defic Res* 1988; 32:439–453.
2. Campbell K, Houle S, Lorrain D, et al: Event-related potentials as an index of cognitive functioning in head-injured outpatients, in McCallum WC, Zappoli R, Denoth F (eds): *Cerebral Psychophysiology: Studies in Event-Related Potentials*. Amsterdam, Elsevier, 1986, pp 486–488.
3. Cohen SN, Syndulko K, Rever B, et al: Visual evoked potentials and long latency event-related potentials in chronic renal failure. *Neurology* 1983; 33:1219–1222.
4. Courchesne E: Neurophysiological correlates of cognitive development: Changes in long-latency event-related potentials from childhood to adulthood. *Electroencephalogr Clin Neurophysiol* 1978; 45:468–482.
5. Courchesne E, Lincoln AJ, Kilman BA, et al: Event-related brain potential correlates of the processing of novel visual and auditory information in autism. *J Autism Dev Disord* 1985; 15:55–75.
6. Curry SH: Event-related potentials as indicants of structural and functional damage in closed head injury, in Kornhuber HH, Deecke L (eds): *Progress in Brain Research Motivation, Motor and Sensory Processes of the Brain: Electric Potentials, Behavior and Clinical Use,* vol 54. Amsterdam, Elsevier, 1980, pp 507–515.
7. Davis H: Principles of electric response audiometry. *Ann Otol Rhinol Otolaryngol* 1976; 85(Suppl 28):1–96.
8. Ebner A, Haas JC, Lucking CH, et al: Event-related brain potentials (P300) and neuropsychological deficit in patients with focal brain lesions. *Neurosci Lett* 1986; 64:330–334.
9. Erwin RJ, Edwards R, Tanguay PE: Abnormal P300 responses in schizophrenic children. *J Am Acad Child Psychiatry* 1986; 25:615–622.
10. Finley WW, Faux SF, Hutcheson J, et al: Long-latency event-related potentials in the evaluation of cognitive function in children. *Neurology* 1985; 35:323–327.
11. Galaburda AM, Sanides F: Cytoarchitectonic organization of the human auditory cortex. *J Comp Neurol* 1980; 190:597–610.
12. Goff WR, Allison T, Vaughan HG: The functional anatomy of event-related potentials, in Callaway E Tueting P, Koslow SH (eds): *Event-Related Brain Potentials in Man*. New York, Academic Press, 1978, pp 1–80.
13. Goodin D, Aminoff MJ: Electrophysiological differences between subtypes of dementia. *Brain* 1986; 109:1103–1113.
14. Goodin D, Aminoff M, Chernoff C, et al: Long latency event-related potentials in patients infected with human immunodeficiency virus. *Ann Neurol* 1990; 27:414–420.
15. Goodin D, Squires K, Starr A: Long latency event-related components of the auditory evoked potential. *Brain* 1978; 101:635–648.
16. Goodin D, Starr A, Chippendale T, et al: Sequential changes in the P3 of the auditory evoked potential in confusional states and dementing illnesses. *Neurology* 1983; 33:215–218.
17. Gordon E, Kraiuhin C, Harris A, et al: The differential diagnosis of dementia using P300 latency. *Biol Psychiatry* 1986; 21:1123–1132.
18. Halgren E, Squires NK, Wilson CL, et al: Endegenous potentials generated in the human

hippocampal formation and amygdala by infrequent events. *Science* 1980; 210:803–805.
19. Harris DF, Hall JW: Feasibility of auditory event-related potential measurement in brain injury rehabilitation. *Ear Hear* 1990; 11:340–350.
20. Hillyard S, Picton T: Electrophysiology of cognition, in Plum F (ed): *Handbook of Physiology. V. The Nervous System.* Baltimore, American Physiology Society, pp 519–584.
21. Howard L, Polich J: P300 latency and memory span development. *Dev Psychol* 1985; 21:283–289.
22. Jirsa RE, Clontz KB: Long latency auditory event-related potentials from children with auditory processing disorders. *Ear Hear* 1990; 11:222–232.
23. Knight RT: Neural mechanisms of event-related potentials: Evidence from human lesion studies, in Rohrbaugh JW, Parasuraman R, Johnson R (eds): *Event-Related Brain Potentials: Basic Issues and Applications.* New York, Oxford University Press, 1990, pp 3–18.
24. Knight RT, Scabini D, Woods DL, et al: Contributions of temporal-parietal junction to the human auditory P3. *Brain Res* 1989; 502:109–116.
25. Knight RT, Scabini D, Woods DL, et al: The effects of lesions of superior temporal gyrus and inferior parietal lobe on temporal and vertex components on the human AEP. *Electroencephalogr Clin Neurophysiol* 1988; 70:499–509.
26. Kraus N, Ozdaman O, Hier D et al: Auditory middle latency responses (MLR) in patients with cortical lesions. *Electroencephalogr Clin Neurophysiol* 1982; 54:275–287.
27. Kutus M, Hillyard S, Volpe B, et al: Late positive event-related potentials after commissural section in humans. *J Cognit Neurosci* 1990; 2:258–271.
28. Levin HD: Neurobehavioral recovery, in Becker DP, Povlishock JT (eds): *Central Nervous System Trauma Status Report,* part II. Bethesda, Md, National Institute of Neurological and Communicative Disorders and Stroke, National Institutes of Health, 1985, pp 281–299.
29. Levy-Agresti, J, Sperry RW: Differential perceptual capacities in major and minor hemispheres. *Proc Nat Acad Sci USA* 1968; 61:1151.
30. Lincoln AJ, Courchesne E, Kilman BA, Neuropsychological correlates of information-processing by children with Down's syndrome. *Am J Ment Defic* 1985; 89:403–414.
31. Loiselle DL, Stamm JS, Maitinsky S, et al: Evoked potential and behavioral signs of attentive dysfunctions in hyperactive boys. *Psychophysiology* 1980; 17:193–201.
32. Mesulam MM, Hoesen GWV, Pandya DN, et al: Limbic and sensory connections of the inferior parietal lobule (area PG) in the rhesus monkey: A study with a new method for horseradish peroxidase histochemistry. *Brain Res* 1977; 136:393–414.
33. Metter E, Jackson C, Kemper D, et al: Left hemisphere intracerebral hemorrhages studied by (F-18)-fluorodeoxyglucose PET. *Neurology* 1986; 36:1155–1162.
34. Michalewski H, Rosenberg C, Starr A: Event related potentials in demential, in Cracco R, Bodis-Wollner I (eds): *Evoked Potentials.* New York, Alan R Liss, 1986, pp 521–528.
35. Muir WJ, Squire I, Blackwood DHR, et al: Auditory P300 response in the assessment of Alzheimer's disease in Down's syndrome: A two-year follow-up study. *Jo Ment Defic Res* 1988; 32:455–463.
36. Musiek FE: Neuroanatomy, neurophysiology, and central auditory assessment. II. The cerebrum. *Ear Hear* 1986; 7:283–293.
36a. Musiek F, Baran J, Pinheiro M: p300 results in patients with lesions of the auditory areas of the cerebrum. *J Am Acad Audiol* 1992; 3:5–15.
37. Musiek F, Bromley M, Roberts D, et al: Improvement of central auditory function after partial temporal lobectomy in a patient with seizure disorder. *J Am Acad Audiol* 1990; 1:146–150.
38. Musiek FE, Gollegly K: Maturational considerations in the neuroauditory evaluation of children, in Bess FH (ed): *Hearing Impairment in Children.* Parkton, Md, York Press, 1988, pp 231–252.
39. Musiek FE, Gollegly K, Baran J: Myelination of the corpus callosum and auditory processing problems in children: Theoretical and clinical correlates. *Semin Hear* 1984; 5:219–229.
40. Obert AD, Cranford JL: Effects of neocortical lesions on the P300 component of the auditory evoked response. *Am J Otol* 1990; 11:447–453.
41. Olbrich HM, Nau HE, Zerbin D, et al: Clinical application of event related potential patients with brain tumors and traumatic head injuries. *Acta Neurochirurg* 1986; 80:116–122.
42. Peronnet F, Michel F: The asymmetry of auditory evoked potentials in normal man and patients with brain lesions, in Desmedt J (ed): *Auditory Evoked Potentials in Man: Psychopharmacology Correlates of EPs.* Basel, Switzerland, Karger, 1977, pp 130–141.
43. Pfefferbaum A, Ford JM, Kraemer HC: Clinical utility of long latency "cognitive" event-related potentials (P3): The cons. *Electroencephalogr Clin Neurophysiol* 1990; 76:6–12.

44. Picton TW, Hillyard SA: Human auditory evoked potentials. II. Effects of attention. *Electroencephalogr Clin Neurophysiol* 1974; 36: 312–320.
45. Polich J; Task difficulty, probability, and interstimulus interval as determinants of P300 from auditory stimuli. *Electroencephalogr Clin Neurophysiol* 1987; 68:311–320.
46. Polich J: Frequency, intensity and duration as determinants of P300 from auditory stimuli. *J Clin Neurophysiol* 1989; 6:277–286.
47. Polich J: P300 from a passive auditory paradigm. *Electroencephalogr Clin Neurophysiol* 1989; 74:312–320.
48. Polich J, Howard L, Starr A: P300 latency correlates with digit span. *Psychophysiology* 1983; 20:665–669.
49. Polich J, Howard L, Starr A: Effects of age on the P300 component of the event-related potential from auditory stimuli: Peak definition, variation and measurement. *J Gerontol* 1985; 40:721–726.
50. Polich J, Starr A: Evoked potentials in aging, in Alpert ML (ed): *Clinical Neurology of Aging*. New York, Oxford University Press, 1984, pp 149–177.
51. Scherg M, von Cramon D: Psychoacoustic and electrophysiologic correlates of central hearing disorders in man. *Psychiatr Neurol Sci* 1986; 236:56–60.
52. Selinger M, Prescott TE, Shucard DW: Auditory event-related potential probes and behavioral measures of aphasia. *Brain Lang* 1989; 36:377–390.
53. Squires KC, Chippendale T, Wrege K, et al: Electrophysiological assessment of mental function in aging and dementia, in Curski GE (ed): *Determining the effects of aging on the central nervous system*. Berlin, Free University of Berlin, 1980, pp 93–104.
54. Squires K, Hecox K: Electrophysiological evaluation of higher level auditory processing. *Semin Hear* 1983; 4:415–432.
55. Syndulko K, Hansch EC, Cohen SN, et al: Long latency event-related potentials in normal aging and dementia, in Courjon J, Maugiere F, Revol M (eds): *Clinical Applications of Evoked Potentials in Neurology*. New York, Raven Press, pp 279–285.
56. Velasco M, Velasco F, Velasco AL, et al: Subcortical correlates of the P300 potential complex in man to auditory stimuli. *Electroencephalogr Clin Neurophysiol* 1986; 64:199–210.
57. Wisniewski KE, Wisniewski HM, Wen GY: Occurrence of neuropathological changes and dementia of Alzheimer's disease in Down's syndrome. *Ann Neurol* 1985; 17:278–282.
58. Wood CC, Allison T, Goff WR, et al: On the neural origin of P300 in man. *Prog Brain Res* 1980; 54:51–56.
59. Wood CC, McCarthy G, Squires NK, et al: Anatomical and physiological substrates of event-related potentials. Two case studies. *Ann NY Acad Sci* 1984; 425:681–721.
60. Yetterian EH, Pandya D: Corticothalamic connections of the posterior parietal cortex in the rhesus monkey. *J Comp Neurol* 1985; 237:408–426.

Chapter 13

# Audiologic Management of Central Auditory Processing Disorders

Daniel Schneider, M.A.

The preceding chapters have discussed the underlying neurophysiological bases for central auditory processing disorders (CAPDs) as well as the techniques used to diagnose these disorders. Progress in these areas is truly impressive but also of little consequence unless it can be translated into effective management strategies for the child with CAPD. It is therefore incumbent upon the examining audiologist to be able to interpret test results and recommend appropriate management strategies.

This chapter will discuss useful auditory training approaches as well as FM amplification and classroom sound reinforcement. The techniques recommended for a particular child will be determined by the CAP test battery and the category or categories of CAPD identified by the basic test battery (see Chapter 4). The two major categories are "decoding" (poor auditory processing at the phonemic level) and "tolerance–fading memory" (associated with difficulty in listening in the presence of noise and poor short-term memory). Phonemic training is recommended for subjects in the "decoding" category; noise desensitization training and FM amplication are recommended for those in the "tolerance–fading memory" classification. The principles of classroom acoustic management and classroom sound reinforcement are discussed. These techniques reduce classroom noise and reverberation while electronically reinforcing the teacher's voice. It is hard to imagine a child who would not benefit from this approach. Since it is more expensive than a personal FM system, this approach becomes more cost effective when several CAPD children are in the same classroom.

These management strategies are not all inclusive; they represent management approaches that correspond to the categories of CAPDs specifically discussed: that is, decoding problems and tolerance-fading memory. The auditory training approach assumes that weaknesses can be improved with systematic and sustained training. There are certainly many equally effective language-mediated or cognitively mediated approaches to management of CAPD. These approaches fall more within the domain of speech-language pathology; some of them will be discussed in Chapter 14.

## PHONEMIC TRAINING

Two approaches to phonemic training will be discussed here: phonemic synthesis and phonemic analysis. Both Lindamood and Lindamood[10] and Katz[35] report that phonemic ability is not dependent on intelligence. Lindamood and Lindamood reported that instead of a normal distribution of this ability, there tends to be a bimodal distribution of "haves" and "have-nots." They describe phonemic analysis as an auditory ability that is predictive of reading and spelling success in kindergarten through seventh grade.[10] Katz[5] concurs that skill in phonemic synthesis is more related to verbal measures than performance measures of intelligence. He suggests that phonemic synthesis is an auditory ability that is frequently underdeveloped in CAPD children. He notes that improvements in phonemic synthesis can result in improvement in reading and spelling, as well as articulation.[5]

Both Katz and Harmon[6] and Lindamood and Lindamood[10] used isolated phonemes presented in neutral contexts to minimize the effects of coarticulation. Although this eliminates the natural acoustic transitions between phonemes that occur in coarticulated speech, it does not interfere with the success of these programs. Further, it is possible that this enhances the carryover to reading and spelling success because phonic approaches to reading also use discrete phonemic elements, as does the orthographic code. This carryover is maximized if auditory training occurs when the child is at the reading-readiness or early-reading stage.

## Phonemic Synthesis

Phonemic synthesis is simply the blending of discrete phonemes into a coarticulated syllable. Use of the Phonemic Synthesis program[6] is an excellent training program for decoding problems because it is effective, yet simple to administer. The program uses a tape-recorded format, which requires a quiet room and a high quality tape recorder. High-fidelity headphones are also necessary. The entire program consists of 15 lessons; however, since mastery is required, the program will call for repetition of lessons that are not mastered. This requires a sequence of 20 to 30 lessons for most students to complete the program.

### *Essential Elements of Phonemic Synthesis Program*

- Auditory only/unisensory approach.—The child is allowed to listen without visual or orthographic interference.
- Phonemes presented in isolation.—Phonemes are presented in their most neutral/medial form, minimizing unnecessary coarticulation.
- Slow rate of presentation.—Phonemes are presented slowly at a rate of one per second, giving the child adequate time to listen.
- Sequential/hierarchial program organization.—The program introduces short, easier blends first and builds on learned behaviors. This usually allows students to move through the program smoothly with success at each level.
- Discovery learning.—Children are never told whether a blended response is correct or incorrect. They must discover the correct answer through auditory learning. They are praised for appropriate attending behavior, not correct answers.
- Mastery learning.—The mastery level for each phonemic synthesis lesson is defined as is the requirement for completing that lesson. Mastery of this skill is required for accurate auditory phonemic decoding as well as success in phonics.
- Training stops at syllable length.—Four- and five-phoneme, one-syllable blends are the longest required in the latter training stages.
- Control of stimulus.—The tape-recorded format allows for complete stimulus control as well as ensuring an auditory-only presentation.

## Phonemic Analysis

If the CAP evaluation identifies a decoding problem, it is actually a phonemic analysis problem, not a phonemic synthesis problem. The Lindamood Auditory Conceptualization (LAC) test by Lindamood and Lindamood[10] is a test of phonemic analysis ability that begins at a level appropriate for most kindergarten students. The most difficult items can be completed by most sixth- and seventh-grade students. The LAC test is a part of the Auditory Discrimination in Depth training program also developed by the Lindamoods.[10a] This program contains training exercises based on the LAC test as well as many aspects that go beyond auditory phonemic analysis training. Only the LAC test will be discussed here. Phonemic analysis training uses the same techniques as the test.

The precheck on the LAC requires the child to understand four basic concepts: same-different, number concepts to 4, left-to-right progression, and first-last. Category I test items are isolated phonemes presented in groups of two or three. On the easier items the child must use colored blocks to demonstrate whether the phonemes were all the same or all different. The blocks are arranged left to right with spaces separating them to represent the discrete, separated presentation of the phonemes. On more difficult items in this category, the child must be able to detect the sequence of three discrete phonemes. Category II items use coarticulated nonsense syllables consisting of two to four phonemes. The child must detect subtle phonemic changes between two nonsense syllables and represent those changes with the colored blocks. In this category, the blocks are ordered left to right without spaces. This visually represents the coarticulation of the nonsense syllable. This task is easy enough that even kindergarteners learn the response format quickly and enjoy arranging the colored blocks.

The program offers a training tape to prospective examiners to demonstrate the live-voice technique. Since an auditory-only approach is preferred, children can be asked to close their eyes when listening. For therapy using discrete phonemes, the rate of presentation can be slowed to one phoneme per second from the recommended rate of two per second to give the child adequate listening time.

Occasionally a child will have difficulty on a phonemic synthesis lesson. It may be helpful to break away and utilize a different technique (e.g., phonemic analysis) to work on the same phonemes that were a problem in the phonemic synthesis program.

## NOISE-DESENSITIZATION TRAINING

Noise-desensitization therapy does not have the same degree of research support as phonemic training. Speech-in-noise training is a drill-type training. Extra effort will be required to make this activity enjoyable. Since noise desensitization is similar to other skills that must be drilled, it should occupy only a short portion of the therapy period. When drilling speech production in the hearing-impaired child, Ling[11] recommends frequent, short training intervals (5 to 7 minutes in length) since such intense concentration is required. Similar high levels of concentration are required in training speech-in-noise skill. Short training intervals are appropriate.

Katz and co-workers[8] recommend that monosyllables be used in a background of increasingly noxious and increasingly intense noise. Monosyllables are selected because of their low predictability. This allows the therapist to more accurately measure the benefit of the therapy. Care is taken throughout therapy to maintain success and avoid frustration. Higher-interest sentences or stories can also be used for therapy but progress checks should utilize monosyllables.[8]

Katz et al[8] recommend presenting the speech and the noise via tape recorders. The speech is kept at a constant comfortable listening level throughout therapy. Therapy begins in a quiet background followed by a minimally distracting noise such as fan noise or audiometric speech spectrum noise at a very quiet level. Relaxation exercises are helpful at this stage in the training. As training progresses noise levels are increased (the volume control on the tape playback equipment should be carefully marked with about 15 levels so that the volume of the noise can be increased in measurable steps). As the child progresses, the noxiousness of the noise is also increased (e.g., fan noise to cafeteria noise to single-talker discourse). When the noise produces an adverse effect (e.g., poor discrimination of the words), the background noise is eliminated for about ten items. Following this drill in quiet, the noise should again be raised in small steps with approximately ten items presented at each noise level.[8]

Katz et al[8] report speech-in-noise skills tend to deteriorate following the termination of therapy unless they are periodically reinforced. Once-a-week reinforcement by the parent at home is suggested.

FM amplification systems are often recommended when the CAP evaluation indicates a speech-in-noise problem.[7, 8, 14] These systems can minimize the distracting effects of background noise but they do not address the heart of the problem, intolerance for background noise. Training may improve this intolerance by systematic and sustained practice functioning with reduced acoustic cues. Emotional desensitization should also occur as the child learns that she or he can function in noise with minimal auditory information.

## FM AMPLIFICATION

FM amplification fits very nicely into the management program for children with CAP disorders who are intolerant of poor signal-to-noise ratios. FM systems improve the signal-to-noise ratio at the user's ears. The face validity and construct validity of this approach are obvious and strong. This may be the very reason that there is little published research into the effectiveness of this treatment option. Still, research support and anecdotal clinical support are required, especially if school systems are going to be asked to purchase FM systems for "normal-hearing" CAP-disordered children.

Stach and co-workers[14] published an article on their clinical experience with FM systems in four patient groups: (1) mainstreamed hearing-impaired students; (2) hearing-impaired adults with heavy communication demands; (3) elderly patients with speech-in-noise problems; and (4) children with normal hearing and a CAPD. If their CAP evaluation indicated an FM system might be of benefit, the authors performed a clinical FM evaluation to verify clinically that an FM system could increase speech intelligibility. This evaluation, performed in the sound room, utilized a message-in-competition task (using sentences from the Synthetic Sentence Inventory or Pediatric Speech Intelligibility test presented through the front loudspeaker and single-talker discourse competion presented through the rear speaker). Message-to-competition ratios were varied and then repeat measurements were made with an FM microphone-transmitter positioned 8 inches from the front loudspeaker. These authors found this "clinical verification" to be necessary because they have found CAP patients who do not benefit clinically from an FM system owing to the "degree of their central auditory deficit."[14]

When these authors recommend an FM system for a CAP child they find a trial use period to be essential so that parents and teachers can monitor the benefit of the device. Following the trial period, 8 of 20 potential candidates found the FM system to be of enough benefit to warrant personal purchase of the equipment.[14]

Katz et al[7] in a recently completed (unpublished) study evaluated the clinical benefit of FM amplification. Fifteen students with confirmed CAP disorder and speech-in-noise difficulty were tested in the sound field with and without the FM microphone-transmitter suspended from the front speaker. Noise was delivered through two separate speakers at horizontal azimuths of +45 and −45 degrees. As would be expected, these students scored significantly more poorly in noise as compared to quiet. However when using the FM system, their performance improved to the point that the FM vs. quiet scores were not significantly different. Also of interest is the finding that all of the children performed better in FM condition than in the noise condition.

There is also research support for the use of FM systems with unilaterally hearing-impaired children. Children with unilateral hearing loss share some auditory characteristics with CAPD children; therefore, some of the information that has been obtained with this group may also apply in CAPD cases. Speech-in-noise difficulty and localization ability are often cited as problem areas for unilaterally impaired students.[1] As is the case for children with CAP disorders, unilaterally hearing-impaired students are also at marked risk for academic difficulties.[1, 3, 4]

Studies on unilaterally hearing-impaired children have found contralateral-routing-of-signal amplification to be of limited benefit, while FM amplification directed to the student's good ear has been shown to be beneficial.[1, 9] These studies utilized FM systems that were coupled to mild-gain behind-the-ear hearing aids either by teleloop/induction or direct audio input. The Kenworthy et al.[9,11] study (utilizing direct audio input coupling) provided frequency response data on their FM-hearing aid system that revealed significant rolloff in the frequency response starting at approximately 4 KHz. FM systems utilizing headsets with wider frequency responses may help to enhance the FM benefit noted in future research efforts.

### Benefits of FM Amplification for CAP Child

#### *Improved Signal-to-Noise Ratio*

This is the most often cited and most important benefit of FM systems. The signal-to-noise ratio will be affected by the signal enhancement of the FM system and the noise reduction at the child's ear due to the headset or earmold.

***More Uniform Intensity Level of Teacher's Voice***

The proximity of the transmitting microphone to the teacher's mouth assures a more uniform intensity of the teacher's voice that is relatively immune to the teacher's physical orientation in the classroom (e.g., where he or she is relative to the student and the direction that the teacher is facing).

***Wideband Frequency Response***

The proximity of the transmitting microphone to the teacher's mouth also allows the high-frequency spectral information in the teacher's voice to be preserved in the transmitted signal. The bandwidth of FM receiver-headset systems allows frequency responses to extend to 8 KHz and beyond.

## Fitting Considerations

There is no established fitting protocol for FM systems with CAPD children. The FM systems currently being manufactured for this group of children are mild-gain systems with safe maximum power outputs. The FM receivers are typically used with Walkman-style headsets or earbuds that can provide flat wideband responses from 250 to 8,000 Hz and beyond. Since CAPD children perform poorly with distorted (filtered) or low-redundancy speech signals, our fitting goal is to provide students with high-fidelity, broad-frequency-response, low-distortion amplification.

Flat wideband frequency responses are easily obtained with modern FM equipment. The real ear insertion response (REIR) of an FM system can be measured quickly and easily to reveal the frequency response delivered to the child's ear. Accurate real ear insertion response measurements require that the FM transmitter-microphone be positioned close to the reference microphone at the student's ear. Kenworthy et al[9] chose a high-frequency emphasis response (1 to 4 KHz) for their clinical FM study with unilaterally hearing-impaired children. While appropriate in their study, this degree of low-frequency attenuation, typical in hearing aid fittings, is not required in FM fittings. Flat FM frequency responses should not amplify low-frequency background noise to any significant extent owing to the very favorable signal-to-noise ratio at the FM transmitter microphone.

This is not to minimize the importance of the high-frequency response. In striving for a flat wideband response we desire to preserve the frequency-intensity relationships in the speaker's voice. The wideband frequency responses of "stereo-quality" headphones suit this purpose well. Walkman-style headphones or earbuds perform extremely well. They are lightweight and comfortable for extended use periods.

The noise rejection properties of Walkman-style headphones and earbuds, as measured by negative real ear insertion gain, are very slight. If greater noise rejection is required a larger headset or a circumaural muff may be required. Earbuds can be inserted into commercially available noise-protection muffs (circumaural muffs) for excellent noise rejection. These muffs will not be as comfortable or as cosmetically acceptable as the lightweight headsets, but they remain a viable option for children with more severe speech-in-noise problems.

The Stetoclip "stethoscope type" headset (Phonic Ear, Inc., Mill Valley, Calif.) has impressive noise-rejection properties but it is designed to be used with a button-style transducer typical of some FM systems and body-style hearing aids. The frequency responses of these output transducers (earphones) do not meet the wideband frequency response criterion. Figure 13–1 shows several undesirable real ear insertion responses with a button-style transducer at midline and at the ear. The transducer coupled at ear level

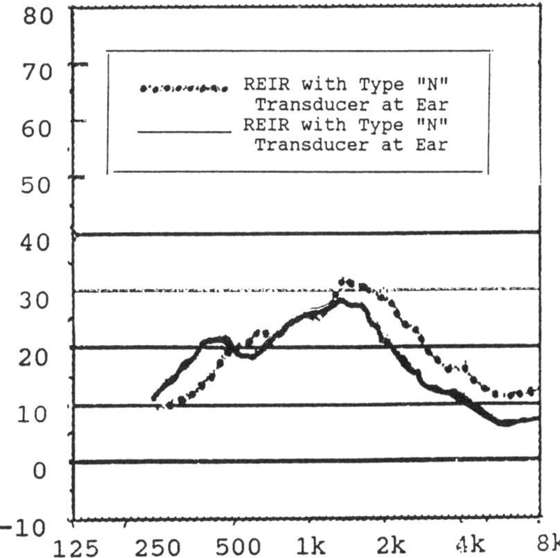


**FIG 13–1.**
Undesirable real ear insertion responses for FM system with button-style transducer.

avoids the acoustic transmission of sound through the Stetoclip tubing but does not improve the response enough to meet our wideband criterion.

The choice of microphone for the FM transmitter also affects the frequency response of the system. Figure 13–2 simulates the differences in frequency response between a boom-style microphone and a lapel microphone. The boom microphone's placement (approximately 2 inches in front of the side of the mouth) captures more of the speaker's high-frequency vocal spectrum. The lapel microphone (placed approximately 6 to 8 inches below the speaker's mouth) loses some of the highs as well as receiving a weaker input signal overall (a less favorable signal-to-noise ratio is captured at the FM microphone). The lapel microphone is also somewhat susceptible to intensity variations because of changes in the teacher's head position. The disadvantages of the boom microphone are: (1) teachers may not like to wear them, (2) a loud-spoken teacher can drive a mild gain system into saturation, and (3) the boom microphone can visually obscure the teacher's mouth from some angles.

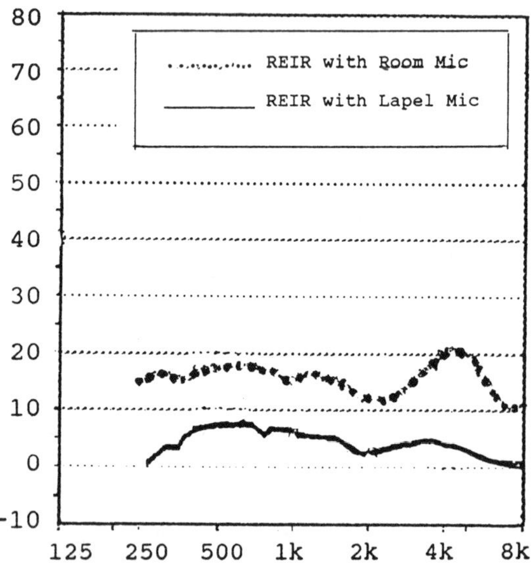


**FIG 13–2.**
Real ear insertion response of phonic ear FM system utilizing directional lapel microphone placed in boom position (3 inches in front of speaker at side of speaker cone) and in lapel position (6 inches below and 1 inch back from front edge of speaker). Note: reference microphone is at standard position with subject approximately 1 m from speaker.

**Recommended Fitting Protocol**

Until future research studies define the optimal FM fitting for the CAPD child, it is recommended that flat wideband FM systems with safe saturation sound-pressure levels (not exceeding 105 dB SPL) be fitted on a trial basis when the CAPD evaluation indicates the potential for FM benefit. If possible the response of the FM system should be clinically checked using real ear measurements to verify the appropriateness of the response.

The student, parents, and teachers should be counseled as to the rationale for using the FM system, appropriate use of the equipment, and the emotional impact of wearing an adaptive device. The trial fitting should be judged successful if the student shows willingness to continue wearing the equipment. It is helpful, but not necessary, that the teacher notices an improvement in listening ability and attendant behaviors.

## CLASSROOM SOUND REINFORCEMENT SYSTEMS

When several CAPD students are placed in the same classroom it can be cost effective to provide a classroom sound reinforcement system. Our experience with these systems indicates that the enhanced audibility of the teacher's voice benefits all students in the classroom.

Classroom sound reinforcement systems are utilized for the same reasons as personal FM systems. It is the opinion of this author that they can be more effective than personal FM systems if the sound reinforcement system is properly installed and equalized and if classroom noise and reverberation are reduced.

Success with a classroom amplification project was reported by Sarff.[12] A sound-field amplification project was established in three southern Illinois public schools after a school psychologist noted that students being referred for learning disabilities services typically demonstrated deficitsin auditory areas. Learning-disabled students were mainstreamed into regular classrooms that provided amplification for the teacher's voice. In addition, they received individual or small-group instruction in an amplified resource room.

Three general conclusions were drawn from this study:

1. Significant gains in academic achievement were realized in the first year of the project for those students in the amplified classrooms.
2. The gains of the children in the amplified classrooms were greater than the gains made by students only receiving regular resource room assistance.
3. Reading and language arts scores increased more than math scores.

Additionally, the impressions of the teachers and students were generally very favorable. Easier and more accurate listening was often cited by students. Teachers reported less vocal strain during teaching. The project led to greater awareness of "the problem of ambient noise and has led to suggestions for sound treating classrooms."[12]

Several sound-reinforcement systems have been installed in suburban Buffalo, New York, in self-contained classrooms for language-delayed and CAPD children. Although we do not have controlled experimental data to support the benefit of these systems, anecdotal data from the teachers will be presented.

The first classroom to be treated was quite typical of modern elementary school classrooms, measuring approximately 20×30×20 feet. All surfaces were hard and reflective with the exception of the porous, tiled ceiling of unknown acoustic properties. Noise levels in the occupied classroom were in the 50 to 65 dBA range. Reverberation was determined empirically to be approximately 0.9 seconds, which is considered to be typical of a modern classroom.[2]

Before installing a sound-reinforcement system we reduced the classroom noise and reverberation by installing a wall-to-wall carpet. Carpeting is the most efficient acoustic modification since it reduces reverberation at the same time it damps chair noise, foot noise, and desk noise. We went one step further and reduced reverberation by covering the rear wall of the classroom with absorptive foam baffles (Illbrook, Inc., Minneapolis, Minn.). Blackboard space was maintained behind the teacher. This is appropriate for teaching as well as for maximizing short-latency reverberation that enhances intelligibility.[13] These acoustic modifications reduced classroom noise to the 40 to 45 dBA range and reverberation to approximately 0.4 seconds.

The new classroom acoustic environment had a soft, absorptive feel, which was quickly sensed by anyone entering the room. The reverberation was reduced to the point that the teacher's voice seemed quite weak without considerable vocal effort. A mild-gain sound system was installed to electronically reinforce the teacher's voice. The system consisted of an FM microphone-receiver and an amplifier-equalizer. The loudspeaker was positioned centrally and near the ceiling in the front of the classroom near the point where the teacher would normally stand to address the entire class.

With wideband electronic enhancement from the amplifier/speaker the teacher's voice was reinforced in a natural manner. Both signals emerged from the same direction and were perceived as coming from one source. The FM microphone gave the teacher complete mobility in the classroom and the ability to continually monitor the performance of the system. If a malfunction occurred, the teacher would hear it immediately.

The classroom teacher observed that reducing the noise made the students less distracted and actually seemed to have a calming effect on the students. She felt the sound reinforcement system was particularly helpful for presentations to the entire class and that it seemed to make each spoken sound clearer and more precise. She noted that the children were able to listen with greater ease yet with increased comprehension.

A resource teacher (who tutored two hearing-impaired students in this classroom) who herself has a severe bilateral hearing impairment noted that the classroom was the best listening environment she had ever experienced. She felt it was acoustically better than any personally worn FM system that she had used with her bilateral behind-the-ear hearing aids not to mention freeing her from wearing the FM receiver (and depending on the person speaking to turn the FM transmitter on). She noted that concentrating was easier and that even the children's voices seemed clearer. She also noted improved classroom comprehension in both of the hearing-impaired students with whom she worked.

The success of this project is totally anecdotal but would seem to be of sufficient merit to justify similar projects. The acoustic modifications to the classroom are judged by the author to be just as important as the sound reinforcement. Although installations of foam baffles would go beyond the resources of many programs, carpeting is still the most efficient way to reduce both noise and reverberation. Newer acoustic ceiling tiles also offer greater noise-absorbing properties. Sound reinforcement systems should include a central speaker (or speaker cluster), an FM microphone for the teacher, and an amplifier-equalizer. Equalization allows the frequency response of the system to be shaped for the most pleasing and effective response. Although classroom sound-field systems are now commercially available it is also possible to cost-effectively assemble a system with an appropriate FM system and locally available stereo components, as was done in this project.

**Acknowledgments**

The classroom sound reinforcement project would not have been possible without cooperation and assistance from Thomas Wolff, Rita Clarey, and Jayne Lehsten from the Erie #1 BOCES Special Education Program. Their contributions are gratefully acknowledged.

## REFERENCES

1. Bess F, Klee T, Culbertson J: Identification assessment and management of children with unilateral sensorineural hearing loss. *Ear Hear* 1986; 7:43–51.
2. Bess F, Sinclair S: Amplification systems used in education, in Katz J (ed): *Handbook of Clinical Audiology,* ed 3. Baltimore, Williams and Wilkins, 1985.
3. Bess F, Tharpe A: An introduction to unilateral sensorineural hearing loss in children and case history data on unilaterally hearing impaired children. *Ear Hear* 1986; 7:3–19.
4. Culbertson J, Gilbert L: Children with unilateral sensorineural hearing loss: Cognitive, academic, and social development. *Ear Hear* 1986; 7:38–42.
5. Katz J: Phonemic synthesis, in Lasky E, Katz J (eds): *Central Auditory Processing Disorders.* Austin, Tex, Pro-Ed, 1983.
6. Katz J, Harmon C: *Phonemic Synthesis.* Allen, Tex, Developmental Learning Materials, 1982.
7. Katz J, Nast K, Oleksy K: The effect of an assistive listening device on speech recognition in a background of speech babble in children with speech-in-noise difficulties. Unpublished observation, 1991.
8. Katz J, Yeung E, Metwetsky L: SSW C-I-R *Manual for Calculations, Interpretation, Recommendation of SSW Test Results.* Amherst, NY, Jimm Co, 1988.
9. Kenworthy O, Klee T, Tharpe A: Speech recognition ability of children with unilateral sensorineural hearing loss as a function of amplification, speech stimuli, and listening condition. *Ear Hear* 1990; 11:264–270.
10. Lindamood C, Lindamood P: *Lindamood Auditory Conceptualization Test.* Allen, Texas, Developmental Learning Materials, 1971.

10a. Lindamood C, Lindamood P: *Auditory Discrimination in Depth.* Allen, Texas, Developmental Learning Materials, 1975.

11. Ling D: *Speech and the Hearing Impaired Child.* Washington DC, Alexander Graham Bell Association for the Deaf, 1976.
12. Sarff L: An innovative use of free field amplication in regular classrooms, in Ross R, Downs M (eds): *Auditory Disorders in School Children.* New York, Thieme-Stratton, 1981.
13. Nabelek A, Nabelek I: Room acoustics and speech perception, in Katz J (ed): *Handbook of Clinical Audiology,* ed 3. Baltimore, Williams and Wilkins, 1985.
14. Stach B, Loiselle L, Jerger J, et al: Clinical experience with personal FM assistive listening devices. *Hear J* 1987; 40:24–30.

*Chapter* **14**

# Speech and Speech Disorders: Implications for Central Auditory Processing

**Mary Ellen Tekieli Koay, Ph.D.**

The relationship between auditory perception or the "ability to process information obtained through the auditory modality"[1] and speech disorders (articulation disorders specifically) has been studied extensively during the past 35 years. A great deal has been written about the role of auditory skills in speech and language development. Although there seems to be agreement that complex relationships exist between audition and speech and language, specific details are lacking or at best are controversial. The reasons for the lack of a solid foundation in this area include the following:

1. Confusion in terms and definitions used to describe the auditory phenomenon often referred to as "auditory perception" or "auditory processing."[2–5]
2. Differences in approach to the evaluation of auditory skills using formal and informal tests.
3. Variations among authors in what they consider to be the essential perceptual "subskills"[2] of auditory processing. Moreover, the same term or subskill may be used differently by different authors.
4. Variations in test stimuli used to tax the auditory system (e.g., dichotic presentation of syllables, words, digits; binaural fusion tests; filtered speech).

The questions that still remain include which auditory deficiencies are found with certain disabilities. This has prompted us to continue our search to delineate and define parameters of central auditory processing and evaluate these processes in individuals with speech and language disorders.

This chapter focuses on (1) central auditory processing from a speech-language (vs. audiological) viewpoint, (2) developmental auditory skills in normal children, and (3) central auditory processing in children with speech disorders.

## SPEECH-LANGUAGE APPROACH TO CENTRAL AUDITORY PROCESSING

### Variations in Terminology

The speech-language pathologist and audiologist may have a similar clinical profile in mind when they use terms such as auditory perceptual disorder (a speech-language pathology term) or central auditory processing disorder (an audiological term). These and a host of other synonymous terms have been used to describe specific communication deficiencies in certain children and adults. For example, one author uses "auditory perception" and "auditory processing" synonymously[5]; whereas other writers may differentiate these terms based on areas of the brain that may subserve these functions. These authors caution us to distinguish between a perceptual dysfunction and a processing disorder.[6]

### Variations in Clinical Profile

About a decade ago, Rampp[5] suggested that speech-language pathologists had become "sophisticated enough" to diagnose auditory perceptual disorders. At approximately the same time, at West Virginia University, a clinical profile of children with auditory perceptual disorders was being compiled for the use of speech-language pathologists (Table 14–1). It is not surprising that the list of behaviors included in Table 14–1 resemble, more or less, the behavior constellations discussed by others over the years.[2, 5, 7, 8] However, at the time, my co-workers and I felt as though we were breaking new ground in suggesting such an exhaustive list of behaviors. We cautioned our colleagues that many of the behaviors resembled characteristics of those with hearing loss and possibly other disorders. Therefore, differential diagnosis may be an issue with an individual patient.

Although the speech-language pathologist recognizes and uses a group of behaviors to diagnose auditory perceptual disorders, he or she must also be aware of variations in constellations of communication behaviors associated with central auditory processing disorders. For example, a point of confusion lies in whether or not the child with an auditory perceptual disorder (or central auditory processing disorder) always demonstrates speech or language problems. That is, do language and/or articulation problems always exist in children with central auditory processing disorders? The answer is no. For example, Willeford and Burleigh[2] state that many of the children they evaluate do not have obvious speech or language problems. However, these authors further state that subtle speech or language difficulties may have existed when the children were younger.

The speech-language pathologist may see children with mild, moderate, or severe articulation problems who also have central auditory processing disorders. In fact, speech-language pathologists often view the central auditory processing disorder as an etiological factor for some children with articulation or language problems.[3] Whether central auditory processing provides the foundation for language or whether its function is dependent on language has been debated.

The central auditory processing disorder itself may be mild, moderate, or severe.[9] Furthermore, in its most severe form, the central auditory processing disorder may manifest itself first and foremost as a speech and language problem in the preschool years. That is, the preschool child with a severe central auditory processing disorder is initially brought to the clinic for evaluation because his or her speech and language problems are extremely noticeable to the parents, not because someone suspects difficulty with auditory skills.

During the preschool years, the child is usually in favorable listening conditions since most interactions are one-to-one. Therefore, mild central auditory processing disorders may not be detected. However, more severe problems may be confusing to the parent since the child displays inconsistent responses in communication. Many times a hearing loss is suspected.

Although there are variations in the clinical profile of central auditory processing disorders, there have been attempts to sort the characteristics. Katz and Smith[10] organized the communication behaviors manifested in central auditory processing disorders into three groups which "encompass most auditory processing difficulties."[10]

**TABLE 14–1.**
Central Auditory Processing: Implications in Those With Speech Disorders

| Frequent characteristics of children with auditory perceptual disorders |
|---|
| Reduced attention behaviors |
| Discrimination problems |
| Localization problems |
| Memory problems |
| Inconsistent responses |
| Prolonged therapy with little progress |
| Strong visual channel |
| Unexpectedly high performance on language comprehension tasks |
| Academic failures |
| Hyperactivity or hypoactivity |

1. The auditory decoding group has a central auditory processing disorder that is reflected in an early childhood articulation problem, many times affecting the /r/ and /l/ phonemes. Poor phonic skills in these children are believed to contribute to the spelling and reading problems later.
2. The auditory tolerance-fading memory group includes persons who are very much distracted by background noise and demonstrate poor auditory memory skills.
3. The auditory integration group includes one subgroup that exhibits severe reading and spelling problems and one group that demonstrates less severe learning problems. Both groups demonstrate poor integration and delays in responding.

The Katz and Smith[10] data appear to be a good first step to a better understanding of different subgroups of central auditory processing disorders, especially since the authors related the behaviors to neurological sites. Speech-language pathologists will be interested in learning more about constellations of behaviors, severity levels, and any possible interrelationships.

## Philosophies of Evaluation and Management

Assessment techniques employed to evaluate central auditory function by speech-language pathologists and audiologists are quite different both in construction and in presentation. However, it has been my experience that what a speech-language pathologist calls an auditory perceptual ability is referred to as central auditory processing by the audiologist. The speech-language pathologist assesses "auditory perceptual abilities" with formal tests, such as the Goldman-Fristoe-Woodcock Auditory Skills Test Battery, whereas the audiologist employs a battery of perceptual tests to assess central auditory processing disorders. Of course, the two disciplines may be testing completely different skills or subskills, since the speech-language pathologist usually evaluates auditory perceptual skills from a language processing or cognitive view.[11, 12]

Proponents of the language processing view use auditory language tests to study cognitive and linguistic competencies. Such tests require higher-level language processing and use stimuli and responses across the modalities.[12, 13] For example, when a child is asked to point to a line drawing, it is difficult to know whether visual perception or auditory perception is the problem in an incorrect response. Auditory language tests and remediation programs are generally based on a top-down model of central auditory processing with little emphasis on the acoustic signal and its analysis.[11, 12] Conversely, a bottom-up view is the auditory processing view usually held by the audiologist (though not to the exclusion of cognitive and linguistic factors) who assesses the integrity of the central auditory system by evaluating basic auditory processes.[11, 12]

Pure dichotomies, such as a speech-language vs. auditory approach,[2] a language processing vs. an auditory processing view,[11] or a top-down vs. a bottom-up view of central auditory processing[11, 12] will surely result in the loss of valuable diagnostic information and subsequent remediation recommendations. I very much agree with the more contemporary views that combine the models by asserting that central auditory processing tasks involve both signal analysis and higher-order processes.[11, 12, 14] These views are discussed in Chapter 1.

## Joint Approach to Management

This volume, with its transdisciplinary view, addresses the issues that various professionals face in dealing with the complex area of central auditory processing. This task is further complicated, since auditory skills relate to a variety of speech disorders or other communication problems from developmental disabilities in children to brain lesions in the elderly.

A better understanding of different subgroups of central auditory processing disorders is essential, especially in children.[15] For example, it is necessary to understand the implications of early brain lesions on cognition. Moreover, we should be aware of the different outcomes of brain lesions on a developing brain due to its plasticity vs. the outcome in an adult brain with a similar lesion.[15] We must go beyond a speech-language approach, or an audiological approach, or a neuropsychological approach and use the knowledge and talents of various disciplines in dealing with central auditory processing in those with speech disorders.

## CENTRAL AUDITORY PROCESSING IN NORMAL CHILDREN: DEVELOPMENTAL TRENDS

If we are expected to evaluate and manage central auditory processing in articulation- or language-disordered children, it is necessary to know more about how both normal children and children with disabilities develop auditory processing skills.

Limited data are available relative to the perception of spoken speech by children. There is evidence, however, that several aspects of speech perception follow a developmental sequence. For example, investigators have observed improvement in subject performance with an increase in chronological age on immediate memory span,[16] auditory comprehension,[17] dichotic listening ability,[18, 19] discrimination of stop consonants,[20] and performance in temporal segmentation.[21]

Several colleages and I have carried out a series of research projects designed to investigate central auditory processing skills in children using both commercially available tests with different formats (e.g., Illinois Test of Psycholinguistic Abilities[22] and the Goldman-Fristoe-Woodcock Auditory Skills Test Battery[1]) and tests that tax or "uniquely stress"[2] the central auditory system (e.g., identification of brief consonant-vowel [CV] syllables, also known as a temporal segmentation task, and dichotic CV syllables).

The following is a brief description of the research protocol used in the series of studies. In both the temporal segmentation and dichotic tasks, six CV syllables (three voiced stops and three unvoiced stops followed by the vowel /a/) were employed. The verbal stimuli for the temporal segmentation task were available from an earlier study. An adult male speaker had recorded the verbal stimuli in an acoustically isolated room with a low ambient noise level. Intensity of the productions and fundamental frequency of the vowel portions of the CV syllables were carefully controlled. The CV syllables were segmented temporally by means of electronic gating equipment to yield stimuli that included the onset characteristics of each stimulus and that ranged in duration from 10 msec to 150 msec in 10-msec steps. Since each of the six CV syllables was segmented into 15 different durations, there were 90 stimuli available for the study with children.

The dichotic task was prepared by Charles I. Berlin. The six CV syllables were presented in pairs, with each syllable competing with each other syllable an equal number of times. The tape-recorded stimuli were presented at 75 dB SPL via a Sony TC-377 two-channel tape recorder coupled to a set of acoustically balanced headphones. The customary switching of headphones was carried out following the first 30 presentations as a precaution against instrumental channel effects. The dichotic task was administered on two different occasions for purposes of test-retest reliability.

During both the temporal segmentation and dichotic listening tasks, each child listened to stimuli and pointed to the appropriate stimulus/stimuli, which was printed on a chart in front of him. The responses were recorded by the experimenter. For the temporal segmentation task, a recognition threshold duration was determined for each consonant in each CV and was designated as the minimum duration necessary for at least 50% of the subjects to identify the consonants in the CV syllable. In the dichotic task several possible responses could be obtained to the stimulus pair: double correct, single correct, and double error.[24]

## DEVELOPMENTAL TRENDS IN NORMAL CHILDREN'S PERCEPTION OF SPEECH STIMULI

Young children, ages 5, 7, and 9 years, with normal speech and language skills served as subjects in our studies designed to investigate developmental trends in children's perception of speech stimuli. The children's performance was assessed on a temporal segmentation task,[21,25] a CV dichotic listening task[26] (both of which were discussed in the preceding section), and four subtests of the Illinois Test of Psycholinguistic Abilities: Auditory Reception, Auditory Association, Auditory Sequential Memory, and Auditory Closure.[22]

On the temporal segmentation task we found a significant decrease ($P < .05$) in the mean recognition threshold segment duration needed for recognition of consonants in CV syllables as chronological age increased. That is, 5-, 7-, and 9-year-old children showed significant improvement identifying brief durations of consonants as they got older.[21] As expected, the children's performance also improved with an increase in chronological age on the four subtests of the ITPA.

On the dichotic task, the 7- and 9-year-old children with normal speech, language, and hearing ability demonstrated the significant right ear advantage that is typically found in normal listeners.[19, 24, 25] Moreover, the children demonstrated a significant increase in double correct responses with an increase in chronological age from 5 to 9 years.[25] Berlin and McNeil[27] noted earlier that the number of double correct responses on a dichotic task increased with age from 5 to 13 years, and thus may be correlated with improved language skills throughout that age range.

A developmental sequence in children's perception of speech stimuli is supported by the results obtained from our dichotic and temporal segmentation studies. Moreover, our results are consistent with those of other investigators who have reported improvement in subject performance with an increase in chronological age on a variety of speech perception tasks.[16–21]

### Relationships Among Auditory Perceptual and Auditory Processing Tasks in Normal Listeners

Using correlational studies we investigated relationships among auditory "subskills" as tested basically by the Illinois Test of Psycholinguistic Abilities[22] and the Goldman-Fristoe-Woodcock Auditory Skills Test Battery.[1] We found significant correlations among the Auditory Sequential Memory (a digit sequential memory task) and Auditory Association (e.g., "A dog has hair; a fish has________.") Subtests of the Illinois Test of Psycholinguistic Abilities and the recognition of brief syllables and dichotic listening ability.[25] Although our initial evidence provides insights into the specific relationships found between auditory skills, recognition thresholds for brief syllables, and dichotic listening ability, we have yet to understand the specific relationships between patterns of auditory test performance and functional auditory disorders. We have noted, however, that these difficult auditory tests place stress on the auditory system in ways that demonstrate variations in performance according to age and function.

## CENTRAL AUDITORY PROCESSING IN CHILDREN WITH SPEECH DISORDERS

### Audiological Assessment Procedures

Audiological central auditory tests (that is, those that follow a bottom-up model) include such tasks as dichotic listening, temporal segmentation, binaural fusion, and filtered speech. Although we have used all of the abovementioned procedures, my colleagues and I have used the dichotic consonant-vowel (CV) task most often in our research projects. When replicating the dichotic syllables study with children who had articulation disorders, we found that although 7-year-old articulation-disordered children demonstrated more single correct responses in the right ear than the left ear, they did not show the significant right ear advantage[24] seen in our children of similar age or in Berlin's normal children of the same age.[19] In an earlier study we found that children with cleft palate also did not show a significant right ear advantage.[26] Pinheiro and Musiek[6] discuss the popularity of dichotic CV tests for research but suggest that the task is not used as often for clinical purposes. Although we obtained good group data, we probably could not make use of the information clinically for a particular child. However, this assessment information may be helpful to others.

Clinically, audiological central auditory tests have been used with adults to help determine the site of the lesion in central auditory nervous system disorders and with children to assess the function and efficiency of the central auditory nervous system. The goal is to use tests that will tax the auditory system at different levels of the nervous system with the objective of identifying deficiencies.[2] A variety of central auditory tests have been used successfully with children, most of which fall into four classifications: (1) monotic tests, (2) dichotic tests, (3) binaural interaction tests, and (4) electrophysical tests.[2] Specific tests and procedures are discussed elsewhere in this volume. Information is sparse, however, regarding the use of audiological central auditory tests with articulation- and/or language-disordered children who are suspected of having auditory processing problems.

## Tests That Measure Auditory Perceptual Skills

Numerous commercially available, nonaudiological tests have been developed in attempts to measure the various functions of auditiory perception.[2] Since the authors of these tests seem to vary in their concepts of what is entailed in auditory processing, the tests are very different in design and format.

Two of these nonaudiological tests, the Illinois Test of Psycholinguistic Abilities[22] and Goldman-Fristoe-Woodcock Auditory Skills Test Battery[1] have been used extensively in our own research projects. In fact, we have attempted to categorize these tests and their subtests, as well as several other nonaudiological procedures, along a continuum of auditory events necessary for central auditory and language processing (Fig 14–1). Figure 14–1, which is modified continually over time, provides at least a working model for us to

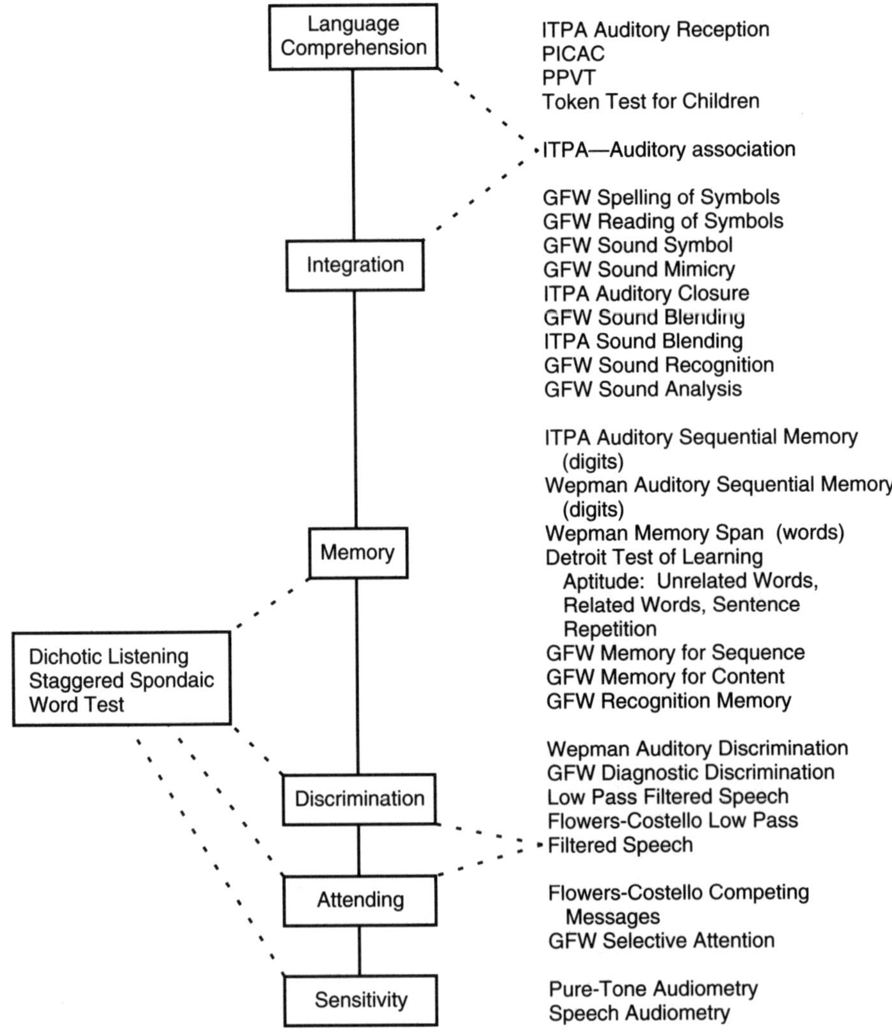


**FIG 14–1.**
Suggested categorization of tests for a continuum of auditory events necessary for central auditory and language processing. GFW = Goldman-Fristoe-Woodcock; ITPA = Illinois Test of Psycholinguistic Abilities; PICAC = Porch Index of Communicative Ability in Children; PPVT = Peabody Picture Vocabulary Test.

organize our procedures and is by no means conclusive.

We have been able to demonstrate relationships between performance on some of the "subskills" of the commercially available tests and single right ear, single left ear, and total correct dichotic scores.[24] For example, the single left ear dichotic performance of articulation-disordered children correlated significantly with the Goldman-Fristoe-Woodcock Reading of Symbols subtest. What is tested by the Reading of Symbols subtest? The client is supposed to read nonsense words. How does the reading of symbols relate to reading skills? The Goldman-Fristoe-Woodcock Test's authors include the sound-symbol test to "measure several basic abilities [that] are prerequisite to advanced language skills, including reading and spelling." Furthermore, "the [Goldman-Fristoe-Woodcock] Sound-Symbol Test has been designed to identify subjects who are deficient in certain sound-symbol skills, and further, to describe this deficiency."

To follow up, we designed investigations of the relationships between dichotic tasks and temporal segmentation tasks and several measures of reading. Although inconclusive, the results[28–30] warrant further research on the relationships between reading and auditory skills. It may be that common skills are required to perform both of these tasks, as is suggested in the literature.

## SUMMARY

Central auditory processing plays a role in the development and use of normal speech and language and contributes in some complex manner to certain communication deficits. Because of the variety of tests, approaches, and populations that have been studied by a variety of disciplines, we are often at a loss to derive a clear-cut understanding of the problem. To understand the problem, it is important that we strive to use operational definitions of our procedures. Furthermore, we must work together in our approaches to central auditory processing in the speech-disordered population. A combined approach (top-down and bottom-up[11, 12] or speech-language and audiologic[2]) should be common in the routine clinical evaluations of the speech-disordered population with suspected central auditory processing disorders.

## REFERENCES

1. Goldman R, Fristoe M, Woodcock R: *Goldman-Fristoe-Woodcock Auditory Skills Test Battery.* Circle Pines, Minn, American Guidance Service, 1974.
2. Willeford JA, Burleigh JM: *Handbook of Central Auditory Processing Disorders in Children.* Orlando, Fla, Grune & Stratton, 1985.
3. Lasky EZ, Katz J: Perspectives on central auditory processing, in Lasky E, Katz J (eds): *Central Auditory Processing Disorders: Problems of Speech, Language, and Learning.* Austin, Texas, Pro-Ed, 1983, pp 3–9.
4. Katz J, Wilde L: Auditory perceptual disorders in children, in Katz J (ed): *Handbook of Clinical Audiology.* Baltimore, Williams & Wilkins, 1985, pp 664–688.
5. Rampp DL: Auditory perceptual disorders: Speech and language considerations. *Semin Speech-Language Hearing* 1980; 1:117–126.
6. Pinheiro M, Musiek FE (eds): *Assessment of Central Auditory Dysfunction: Foundations and Clinical Correlates.* Baltimore, Williams & Wilkins, 1985.
7. Keith RW, Pensak ML: Central auditory function. *Otolaryngol Clin North Am* 1991; 24:371–379.
8. Sanger DD, Keith RW, Maher BA: An assessment technique for children with auditory-language processing problems. *J Commun Disord* 1987; 20:265–279.
9. Keith RW (ed): *Central Auditory Dysfunction.* New York, Grune & Stratton, 1977.
10. Katz J, Smith PS: The staggered spondaic word test: A ten-minute look at the central nervous system through the ears. *Ann NY Acad Sci* 1991; 620:233–251.
11. Duchan JF, Katz J: Language and auditory processing: Top down plus bottom up, in Lasky E, Katz J (eds): *Central Auditory Processing Disorders: Problems of Speech, Language, and Learning.* Austin, Texas, Pro-Ed, 1983, pp 31–45.
12. Young ML, Protti-Patterson E: Management perspectives of central auditory problems in children: Top-down and bottom-up considerations. *Semin Hearing* 1984; 5:251–261.
13. Keith RW: Audiological and auditory language tests of central auditory function, in Keith R (ed): *Central Auditory and Language Disorders in Children.* Houston, College-Hill Press, 1981, pp 61–76.

14. Butler K: Language processing disorders: Factors in diagnosis and remediation, in Keith R (ed): *Central Auditory and Language Disorders in Children*. Houston, College-Hill Press, 1981, pp 160–174.
15. Keith RW, Jerger S: Central auditory disorders, in Jacobson J, Northern J (eds): *Diagnostic Audiology*. Austin, Pro-Ed, 1991, pp 235–248.
16. Boswell SL, Sanders B, Young SJ: The effects of exposure duration and practice on the immediate memory spans of children and adults. *J Exp Child Psychol* 1974; 17:167–176.
17. Carrow MA: The development of auditory comprehension of language structure in children. *J Speech Hearing Disord* 1968; 33:99–111.
18. Nagafuchi M: Development of dichotic and monaural hearing abilities in young children. *Acta Otolaryngol* 1970; 6:409–414.
19. Berlin CI, Hughes LE, Lowe-Bell SS: Dichotic right ear advantage in children 5–13. *Cortex* 1973; 9:394–402.
20. Wolf C: The perception of stop consonants by children. *J Exp Child Psychol* 1973; 16:318–331.
21. Farris ME, Tekieli Koay ME, Cullinan WL: Children's perception of temporally segmented spoken consonant-vowel syllables. Paper presented at the Annual Convention of the American-Speech-Language-Hearing Association, San Francisco, Nov 1978.
22. Kirk S, McCarthy J, Kirk W: *Illinois Test of Psycholinguistic Abilities* (revised edition). Urbana, University of Illinois Press, 1968.
23. Tekieli Koay M, Cullinan W: The perception of temporally segmented vowels and consonant-vowel syllables. *J Speech Hearing Res* 1979; 22:103–121.
24. Tekieli Koay M. Curl B: Dichotic listening abilities of mild and severe articulation disordered children. Paper presented at the Annual Convention of the American Speech-Language-Hearing Association, Los Angeles, Nov 19–23, 1981.
25. Tekieli Koay ME, Alderson TL, Cullinan WL, et al: Developmental trends in children's perception of speech stimuli. Paper presented at the Annual Convention of the American Speech-Language-Hearing Association, Cincinnati, Nov 18–22, 1983.
26. Tekieli Koay M, Leeper H: Dichotic listening abilities of cleft palate children and adults. Paper presented at the Annual Convention of the American Speech-Language-Hearing Association, San Francisco, Nov 1978.
27. Berlin C, McNeil M: Dichotic listening, in Lass N (ed): *Contemporary Issues in Experimental Phonetics*. New York, Academic Press, 1976, pp 327–387.
28. Tekieli Koay ME, Prichard CL, Koh N, et al: Children's speech perception and reading skills: Developmental trends and relationships. Paper presented at the Annual Convention of the American Speech-Language-Hearing Association, Washington, DC, Nov 21–25, 1985.
29. Tekieli Koay ME, Koh N, Kesecker H, et al: Temporal recognition thresholds, visual perception, and reading performance in children. Paper presented at the Annual Convention of the American Speech-Language-Hearing Association, New Orleans, Nov 13–15, 1987.
30. Tekieli Koay ME: Dichotic performance and reading in adults and articulation disordered children. Paper presented at the Annual Convention of the American Speech-Language-Hearing Association, Boston, Nov 18–20, 1988.

*PART* 5

# SPEECH-LANGUAGE CONSIDERATIONS AND APPROACHES

*Chapter* **15**

# Language, Language Learning, and Language Disorder: Implications for Central Auditory Processing

**Christine Sloan, Ph.D.**

The purpose of this chapter is to look at some examples of research in language, language learning, and language disorder to see what issues might be relevant to the topic of central auditory processing. In this way I hope to show how auditory processing and language processing might be related and also why it is important to consider a disorder of auditory processing as one possible factor in disorders of language and communication.

## ISSUES IN LANGUAGE

Language can be defined quite simply as a system of sound-meaning correspondences. This definition points to the two levels or representations of spoken language that must be processed when language is comprehended and expressed. In learning to speak and understand language, the child learns how to relate sound and meaning.

At first glance one might think that at least one task involved in learning language is learning the words themselves and their different meanings. Surely this is one very important aspect of language development. However, in looking at how this learning might be accomplished, one begins to see that it is not a simple matter. Understanding the relationship between the spoken sounds of the language and their meaning requires going beyond the individual words themselves to consider the context in which these words are expressed.

An example from Pinker[15] on the meaning of verbs illustrates this point. First it must be recognized that we typically speak in utterances—words put together in sentences and phrases. To do this, it is not enough just to select the appropriate words and string them together in a particular order. As Pinker says, verbs are choosy; not all verbs can appear in all sentence orders, even when the combinations make perfect sense. Look at the following examples from Pinker[15]:

John *fell*.
John *fell* the floor.

John *devoured* something.
John *devoured*.

John *put* something somewhere.
John *put* something.
John *put* somewhere.
John *put*.

John *became* sick.
John *became*.

As these examples illustrate, different verbs make different demands on how they can be expressed. Specifically, one must know which other linguistic forms need to accompany each verb to express its meaning. Notice that the verb *fell* requires only a subject (John); the verb *devour* requires a subject and an object to fulfill its meaning (you cannot just devour; you have to devour something); the verb *put* requires a subject, an object, and a location to accompany its meaningful use; and so on. These different structures that individual verbs require are called *predicate-argument structures* or simply, *argument structures.*[15] As illustrated above, there are different kinds of argument structures associated with different kinds of verbs.

These illustrations raise interesting questions for those involved in facilitating language learning, particularly with language-disordered children. Any attempt to explain how the meaning of a verb is acquired must necessarily take these argument structures into account. Language learning, then, involves more than simply learning the meaning of individual words. Entire phrases, or in some cases utterances, need to be processed as a whole. In the same way, language use, that is, language expression and comprehension also goes beyond the individual word.

Pinker[15] says that each argument structure expresses a combination of thematic relationships plus information about the particular semantic field in which these relationships are interpreted. In other words, meaning comes from the relationships expressed by the verb and its argument structure as well as by the more general semantic context in which these relationships occur (e.g., a *man talks,* a *dog barks; rings* are put on *fingers, shoes* are put on *feet*). Sometimes these grammatical rules are violated, as when a verb is combined with an inappropriate argument structure, and the meaning of the utterance is altered. There are two common situations in which this occurs. One is from poetry and constitutes part of what we call poetic license. To express something beyond our conventional logic and understanding, the poet often combines linguistic forms that would be ungrammatical in everyday speech. These lines from e.e. cummings[4] illustrate:

> someones married their everyones
> laughed their cryings and did their
> dance (sleep wake hope and then) they
> said their nevers they slept their dream
>
> *e.e. cummings*
> "anyone lived in a pretty how town"

The poet uses the verbs "laughed," "said," and "slept" in new argument structures (you do not sleep your dreams or laugh your cryings). But in doing so he has evoked new meanings.

Another example of how meaning changes when verbs are used with new or inappropriate argument structures can be found in the grammatical errors of young children. These are examples from accounts of children's spontaneous speech:[15]

> Don't giggle me.
>
> I poured you with water.
>
> I'll brush him his hair.
>
> Pick me up all these things.
>
> Mommy, fix me my tiger.
>
> How come you're putting me that
> kind of juice?
>
> I wish the war had peace.

The last line in this example was spoken by an adolescent boy with acquired aphasia who was being treated many years ago during the Vietnam war.

The point of all this is to illustrate that learning the sound-meaning correspondences of a language is a complicated process and is likely to involve much more than simply associating a string of sounds (a word) with a specific meaning. The examples from Pinker[15] suggest that several things must be involved. First, children must be able, or become able, to deal with spoken inputs of some length, not just with individual words. This is because it is necessary to learn not only the words themselves but also their permissible contexts (both syntactic and semantic). To do this, some kind of working memory is required that can store in a relatively exact form (i.e., phonetic code) an entire phrase or utterance. Second, because it is unlikely that children learning language are told in any consistent way which of their utterances have the right linguistic forms and which do not, children must engage in some kind of internal comparison between the adult language forms presented to them on the one hand and their own early grammatical forms on the other. In the case of learning verbs, this comparison process goes on until the child has learned the particular argument structures that can accompany each verb to express its meaning appropriately. This process of comparison also requires memory, both a long-term store of the child's existing linguistic forms and a short-term store to hold new input. Finally, for the child to compare old and new forms there must be a mechanism that enables the child to scan the new input and identify the relevant features that are different from her or his own existing forms. To make matters more difficult, these critical features may not be the most perceptually salient (e.g., be the more intense or stressed sound units) in the spoken input. Further, distractions in the environment can be present that vie for the child's attention. These distractions have to be ignored while the child directs attention to the critical features in the new language data.[1]

What is important in all of this for auditory processing is that these memory, retrieval, and comparison mechanisms rely on accurate phonological coding of the spoken input. Potentially, any error in auditory processing of the input can interfere with this phonological coding and subsequently with accurate storage, retrieval, and comparison of language forms.

## ISSUES IN LANGUAGE LEARNING

Research in language learning also has implications for understanding the importance and potential contribution of central auditory processing to language. Bowerman[1] studied the emergence of spatial forms in children from two language groups—English and Korean. She wanted to know what influences the child's early use of these spatial words—the child's cognitive understanding of space or the specific sound-meaning relationships of the language being learned. She chose to study English and Korean children because spatial relationships are expressed differently in these two languages. For example, English-speaking children express early spatial relationships with words like *on, off, in,* and *out*. These terms together express the path of motion or static location of an object in relation to another object. Bowerman calls this, loosely, the geometry of spatial relationships. So in English, *in* and *on* are differentiated in a very particular way: if one object is seen as moving toward another object, usually larger, such that it ends up contained by that object, then *in* is used, as in *Put the apple in the bowl* or *Put your finger in this ring* . But if the object ends up on a flat surface or partially covering or encircling the other object, then *on* is used, as in *Put the apple on the table* and *Put the ring on the finger*.

In Korean the words used to express actions such as "putting in" or "putting on" do not express the same spatial relationships as *in* and *on* do in English. For example, the Korean word *kki-ta* expresses both *put in* and *put on,* as well as *put together*. However, *kki-ta* has another meaning that restricts its use to only those actions in which objects are brought into a relationship of tight fit or attachment. *Kki-ta* is used for both putting a ring on a finger and a finger in a ring, a screw on a jar and a cassette in a tape recorder; but it is also used for buttoning a button, snapping a snap, and wedging a book between other books. (Incidently, there is another Korean word for describing a "loose fit" arrangement.)[1]

There are more differences between these two languages in their expression of spatial relationships; however, the point of this comparison related to what Bowerman discovered. Recall that she was trying to understand how much of early language development is directed by nonlinguistic cognitive understanding and how much is determined by how the input language codes spatial relationships. If sensorimotor concepts rather than experience with the language guide children's acquisition of early relational words, then there should be similarities between the situations in which English children say *in* and those in which the Korean children say some Korean word, for example, *kki-ta*. In other words, this hypothesis would suggest that the meanings expressed by the children's early spatial forms (either *in* for English or *kki-ta* for Korean) would be the same, although the words themselves are different, because language acquisition is driven by the child's cognitive understanding. Only after some experience with the language would children begin to use these terms to express those spatial relationships peculiar to their own language.[1]

But Bowerman[1] found that by as early as 20 months, and perhaps earlier, English and Korean children's expressions of spatial relationships were diverging in ways consistent with the unique categories of each language. Although the cognitive understanding of space might be considered similar for children from both language groups, at a very early age the input language began to determine how and what spatial relationships were expressed.

Bowerman's findings suggest that very early on in development the input language is influencing and guiding language development. Perhaps this is not surprising. But when we consider what must be involved in this process and just how early in development the language of the environment exerts its influence, it becomes apparent that accurate and efficient auditory processing must play a significant role. The child must be able to construct a stable phonetic representation for these early words (e.g., *in, on*) to be able to associate them with the relevant semantic features of the environment. Further, the child must be able to distinguish among referents (e.g., *in* versus *on*) even when these may not be in the most salient words or stress positions within an utterance. Finally, it appears that much of this early learning may be "incidental"; that is, not formally taught but learned as the young child goes about interacting with the environment.

This notion of incidental learning has been the focus of more recent research on the processes of language learning. Rice[18] has studied this process with both normal and language-disordered children using a procedure called *quick incidental learning* or QUIL. The QUIL procedure presents children with an opportunity to learn new words and then measures their ability to do so. Children view animated television programs that have been dubbed experimentally so that the narration tells a simple story featuring a selected set of new words. Children watch the program individually and are instructed simply to "watch carefully." No further instruction is given and no interaction with adults is allowed so that whatever learning occurs takes place spontaneously, while the child observes the program.

Using this research procedure, Rice[18] has shown that normally developing 3- and 5-year-old children can learn new words after only two viewings of a 12-minute video. Three-year-olds learn about two new words out of 20 and 5-year-olds about five new words. However, this effect is limited to object names and attribute words, such as *gramophone* and *malicious*. Verbs and affective state words are not learned in this way. As might be expected, under conditions of QUIL, language-disordered children learn significantly fewer words (about 1.5 of out 20) than members of control groups matched for either mean length of utterance (MLU) or for age. Although the finding that language-disordered children are slow word learners is not new, the results obtained with the QUIL technique suggest that at least part of the problem lies in on-line processing mechanisms—mechanisms that appear to be independent of standard indices of language development, such as general vocabulary development (as indexed by the Peabody Picture Vocabulary Test) and general linguistic development (as indexed by MLU).[18]

Rice's research is particularly interesting and relevant to auditory processing for several reasons. First, it is an attempt to evaluate and measure language-learning processes, as they occur naturally. Second, it suggests that language-disordered children are not just delayed language learners; they are different language learners. Finally, these differences appear to be related to processing mechanisms, which may very likely include auditory processing abilities. Rice's language-impaired subjects were inefficient language processors.[18] Tallal's research (briefly discussed later) has shown that language-impaired children also are inefficient auditory processors.[23, 24] It is to be hoped that further research of this kind will help us understand more about these processing difficulties.

## ISSUES IN LANGUAGE DISORDERS

The notion that problems in auditory processing or auditory perception underlie some language disorders in children is not new and in fact dates at least to the 1950s, when children were first identified who seemed normal in every way except for their development of language.[7, 14, 23] Somewhere around the time of the psycholinguistic revolution in the 1960s and 1970s interest in the auditory basis of language disorders fell away; later, developments in pragmatics and the social correlates of language became the focus of attention. At the same time, however, research in speech perception was advancing.[10, 11, 16] The results of speech perception research forced us to look once again at the speech signal, which is the language input, and how it is processed by the auditory system, and to reconsider how problems in speech processing might contribute to difficulties in speech and language development.[22]

Added to these developments was the slow accumulation of clinical reports of adults and some children with brain lesions in the central auditory pathways that affected speech processing but did not produce aphasia or a general language disorder.[2, 8,14a, 17] These reports of central auditory disorders that affected language comprehension in the absence of any general language impairment challenged our understanding of language processing once again and rekindled the interest in auditory processing and its relationship to language disorders. They suggested that at least some persons, including language-disordered children, could be language-impaired because of a primary difficulty in auditory processing.[22]

Researchers who have been studying the linguistic, cognitive, or pragmatic underpinnings of language disorder now are asking new questions and positing new mechanisms for understanding these problems in children. Leonard and colleagues[13, 19] have been engaged in cross-language comparisons of language-disordered children as a means of discovering the basis for one of the prominent features of children with specific language impairment—their deficits in grammatical morphology. Leonard and others[9, 12, 24] have reviewed the literature on language impairment in children and have noted that morphology appears to be an especially weak area for these children. Language-disordered children, when compared with their language-age-matched peers, are more likely to omit grammatical inflections (like plural *-s* or past tense *-ed*) and function words (like *the* and *is*).[19] Leonard et al[13] postulated two hypotheses to explain this difficulty. The one that is relevant here is called the *perceptual salience* hypothesis. This hypothesis takes note of the fact that grammatical morphemes in English are nonsyllabic consonant affixes and unstressed syllables that in fluent speech are shorter in duration than adjacent morphemes in the sentence. Hence, these grammatical forms are less salient perceptually (i.e., shorter, less stressed, relatively less intense). Indeed, this saliency argument is the one often taken to explain the telegraphic nature of the early sentences of young children.[19] The following sentence illustrates these less salient segments of the sentence.

*The* cat*s* *are* play*ing* on *the* table.

Telegraphic: "Cat play table" or "Cat play on table"

Leonard[12] cites the work of Tallal and colleagues as a source of evidence that language-disordered children have difficulties in auditory processing—specifically, that they cannot distinguish auditory segments of brief duration (i.e., a sound or syllable in a word) when these occur in the context of other segments (i.e., within a word or phrase), as occurs naturally in speech. To test this hypothesis, Leonard and colleagues[12] studied language disordered-children from other language backgrounds in which morphological features, such as plurality or gender, are marked differently; in particular, in cases in which these elements are more salient than in English. They hypothesized that if saliency was the critical factor, and not the morphological structure per se, then morphology, which is difficult for English language-disordered children, would not be as difficult for language-disordered children learning languages in which morphological information is represented in a perceptually salient form, such as a stressed syllable.

Leonard and colleagues[12, 19] have reported on studies of Italian- and Hebrew-speaking children, and the results lend support to the perceptual salience hypothesis. Italian language-disordered children, although behind in morphological development when compared with their age peers, had a morphology that was considerably more developed than that of their English-speaking counterparts.[12] Italian is a language rich in morphological features and these are marked in the language by word-final monosyllabic vowels or word-final multisyllables that end in vowels, or in some cases they receive primary stress or else benefit from vowel lengthening.[19]

The Hebrew language contains morphological information with both highly salient and less salient features. Rom and Leonard[19] found that the Hebrew-speaking language-disordered children were less impaired in their acquisition of the highly salient morphological features and more impaired with those less salient. In fact, the type of errors children made on these salient and non-salient features differed as well. Errors on highly salient markers were substitutions, but errors on less-salient markers were omissions. English language–disordered children resembled Hebrew language–disordered children in their acquisition of the less salient markers, but as a group they were more impaired.

Connell[5] incorporates the notion of saliency in his approach to language disorders and in particular to the objectives of treatment. Connell proposes that all languages emerge out of a universal grammar that sets certain limits and provides certain operations.[5] This is the innate part of the language-learning mechanism. But as we have seen, the language that is to be learned begins to exert its influence very early in development. Connell suggests that children begin to modify this universal grammar and reset its parameters by responding to specific triggers in the input language. A trigger refers to a specific instance of a unique parameter of the language such as a specific word order. In English, for example, the verb in a verb phrase precedes the rest of the phrase; this is called the head parameter.[5] Children learning English must learn this word order. Children learning Japanese, on the other hand, must learn that the verb comes after the rest of the phrase. The only way to learn which option corresponds to the language the child is learning is to receive sufficient evidence from exposure to the language. Such exposure triggers the appropriate setting of the head parameter.

Because these triggers will differ for different languages, they cannot be included in the universal grammar itself but must be identified by the child as she/he correlates the units in the speech stream with meaning; that is, as the child identifies the components of the verb phrase thereby triggering the verb-first or verb-last syntactic option. Connell suggests that this process of identifying the triggers in the input language may involve some perceptual and cognitive processes that are not language specific as well as some that are.[5]

Connell[5] advocates a teaching approach that makes triggers more salient to the learner. In this approach, saliency is obtained by having the learner understand and say contrasting sentences in which trigger material is highlighted. Connell states that children need to say as well as to understand the contrasting sentences for learning to occur. He suggests that this may indicate that language-disordered children cannot identify triggers because of an inability to hold in memory a mental representation (I would say phonetic representation as well) of the structure of a sentence long enough for analyzing the critical parts. Because the evidence available suggests that language-disordered children take the same circuitous route to the adult language that normal children take, although over a longer period of time, Connell concludes that the differences between these groups may be in how able they are to readily identify triggers in the input language.[5]

Some research in language disorders has sought to investigate directly the relationship between language measures and auditory processing. The work of Tallal is most notable, but others have validated her findings.[21, 22, 25] These studies demonstrate that children with language disorders experience difficulty with certain types of auditory tasks, in particular tasks involving temporal resolution of auditory patterns, phoneme identification and discrimination, auditory memory, and categorical perception. Research also has shown that certain auditory processing variables are highly correlated with or predictive of oral language measures.[25]

Again we see the mainstream of research in language disorders looking to factors related to auditory processing, auditory perception, attention, and memory as potential explanations for the difficulties in learning language observed in language-disordered children. It must be made clear, however, that not all language disorders are the result of deficits in these areas. In a recent 25-year retrospective of the area of child language disorders, Chapman[3] writes:

> A problem in all the foregoing research is that language disordered children are more variable in their language skills than the accounts suggest.

> Children can be identified who are delayed in comprehension and production; but other children appear delayed only in production, yet others seem to have poorer comprehension than their (productive) syntax would warrant. Some of these children have associated phonological problems; others do not. All these children have been included, usually to unknown degrees, in the groups studied. . . .
>
> Despite the limitations in our subject identification, studies suggest a number of potential causes of language disorder. Associated problems in cognition are well-documented . . . Associated etiologies . . . including genetic factors, inborn errors of metabolism, . . . postnatal infections (prominently, otitis media), and brain damage . . . (and) problems linked to the processing of temporally brief auditory events. . . .
>
> If we can more fully describe our subjects and the many potential associated causes of language disorder, our next decade of work may yield new insights.

Researchers must recognize the heterogeneity of the language-disordered population and formulate specific criteria for selecting groups of subjects. In addition, children must be observed over time to identify how patterns of impairment change as children grow and mature. Perhaps more thorough single-subject studies, particularly long-term studies of individual children, would reveal more clinically useful information than studies of groups of children observed only at one point in time. This type of longitudinal case study research has already documented that some preschool-age language-delayed children, who seem to have recovered from their language delay by age 6, become reading- and learning-disabled school-age children in later years.[20] We must improve our precision in describing and defining our subject groups, not only because of the heterogeneity of language disorder, but also because of the considerable individual differences among children. Children differ not only in their disabilities but also in their abilities and talents, in their experiences, and in their styles of learning—a subject that would take another paper to discuss (see Ferguson[6] for a discussion of individual differences in language learning). Finally, we must develop more precise and valid measures of central auditory functions, tests that are free of linguistic bias and tests that can be linked directly to problems in processing the acoustic speech signal.

Clinicians also can and must contribute to our understanding of auditory processing and language disorders. It is the clinician who sees these children in all their many colors and patterns and can observe their behavior over time. Please be thorough; try not to be biased toward only one version of language disorder; and use your skills, intuition, and knowledge of language, language learning and development, and of auditory and speech processing to home in on the basis of the problem for each child individually. Then tell us about them by publishing or presenting these case studies. The best understanding will come about when clinicians and researchers work together and share their understanding.

## REFERENCES

1. Bowerman M: Learning a semantic system: What role do cognitive predispositions play? in Rice ML, Schiefelbusch RL (eds): *The Teachability of Language*. Baltimore, Paul H Brookes Publishing Co, 1989, pp 133–170.
2. Breedin SD, Martin RC, Jerger S: Distinguishing auditory and speech-specific perceptual deficits. *Ear Hear* 1989; 10:311–317.
3. Chapman R: Child language disorders: A twenty-five year retrospective. *Speech Lang Pathol Audiol* 1991; 15:5–10.
4. cummings e.e.: *e.e. cummings, poems 1923–1954, first complete edition*. New York, Harcourt, Brace & World, 1954.
5. Connell PJ: Linguistic foundations of clinical language teaching: Grammar. *J Speech Lang Pathol Audiol* 1990; 14:25–36.
6. Ferguson CA: Individual differences in language learning, in Rice ML, Schiefelbusch RL (eds): *The Teachability of Language*. Baltimore, Paul H Brookes Publishing Co, 1989, pp 187–198.
7. Harris C: Language disorders: Some unanswered questions. *Communicative Disorders: An Audio Journal for Continuing Education,* vol 2. New York, Grune Stratton, March 1977.
8. Jerger S, Martin RC, Jerger J: Specific auditory perceptual dysfunction in a learning disabled child. *Ear Hear* 1987; 8:78–86.
9. Johnston J: Specific language disorders in the child, in Lass N, McReynolds L, Northern J, et al (eds): *Handbook of Speech-Language Pathology and Audiology*. Toronto, BC, Decker, 1988, pp 685–715.
10. Kuhl PK: Speech perception: An overview of

current issues, in Lass N, McReynolds LV, Northern JL, et al (eds): *Speech, Language, and Hearing. Normal Processes,* vol 1. Philadelphia, WB Saunders, 1982, pp 286–322.

11. Kuhl PK: Auditory perception and the ontogeny and phylogeny of human speech. *Semin Speech Lang* 1990; 11:77–91.
12. Leonard L: Language learnability and specific language impairment in children. *Appl Psycholinguist* 1989; 10:179–202.
13. Leonard L, Sabbadini L, Volterra V, et al: Some influences on the grammar of English- and Italian-speaking children with specific language impairment. *Appl Psycholinguist* 1988; 9:39–57.
14. Lubert N: Auditory perceptual impairments in children with specific language disorders: A review of the literature. *J Speech Hear Disord* 1981; 46:3–9.

14a. Mendez MF, Geeham GR Jr: Cortical auditory disorders: Clinical and psychoacoustic features. *J Neurol Neurosurg Psychiatry* 1988; 51:1–9.

15. Pinker S: Resolving a learnability paradox in the acquisition of the verb lexicon, in Rice ML, Schiefelbusch RL (eds): *The Teachability of Language.* Baltimore, Paul H Brookes Publishing Co, 1989, pp 13–62.
16. Pisoni D: Speech perception: Some new directions in research and theory. *J Acoust Soc Am* 1985; 78:381–388.
17. Rapin I: Cortical deafness, auditory agnosia, and word deafness: How distinct are they? *Hum Commun Can* 1985; 9:29–37.
18. Rice ML: Children with specific language impairment: Toward a model of teachability, in Krasnegor NA, Rumbaugh DM, Schiefelbusch RL, et al (eds): *Biological and Behavioral Determinants of Language Development.* NJ, Lawrence Erlbaum Associates, 1991, pp 447–480.
19. Rom A, Leonard L: Interpreting deficits in grammatical morphology in specifically language-impaired children: Preliminary evidence from Hebrew. *Clin Linguist Phonet* 1990; 4:93–105.
20. Scarborough HS, Dobrich W: Development of children with early language delay. *J Speech Hearing Res* 1990; 33:70–83.
21. Sloan C: Auditory processing disorders and language development, in Levinson P, Sloan C (eds): *Auditory Processing and Language: Clinical and Research Perspectives.* New York, Grune and Stratton, 1980, pp 101–116.
22. Sloan C: *Treating Auditory Processing Disorders in Children.* San Diego, Singular Publications, 1986.
23. Tallal P: Auditory processing disorders in children, in Levinson P, Sloan C (eds): *Auditory Processing and Language: Clinical and Research Perspectives.* New York, Grune and Stratton, 1980, pp 81–100.
24. Tallal P: Developmental language disorders. I. Definition. *J Speech Lang Pathol Audiol* 1988; 12:7–21.
25. Whites M: Temporal auditory processing abilities in learning disabled children. Unpublished doctoral dissertation. University of Kansas, 1988.

Chapter 16

# Relationship of Otitis Media to Speech Processing and Language Development

Paula Menyuk, D.Ed.

The theme of this chapter is the relationship between fluctuating peripheral hearing loss caused by persistent otitis media and the development of speech processing. The theme of the other papers in this book is the relationship between central auditory processing difficulties and speech processing. However, the argument that will be made is that peripheral and fluctuating loss can also have a profound effect on the development of speech-processing abilities of children, and, in this way, on their language development. It might be expected that a great deal of research examines the effect of fluctuating hearing loss on the ability of the infant and young child to perceive speech and to develop language. Unfortunately, this is not the case. The facts about otitis media make studying the effect a difficult task.

Although large numbers of infants have episodes of otitis media over the first 3 years of life (some estimate over 90% of all infants[6]), the frequency with which episodes occur and the amount of hearing loss suffered during the episodes vary widely from infant to infant. The hearing losses suffered during the episodes are usually mild, but the amount of time that the infant suffers a hearing loss varies from episode to episode. Further, infants who have frequent episodes of otitis media frequently feel ill or are in pain. This may affect the communicative interaction of infants with persistent otitis media and their caregivers. It is difficult to partial out additional complicating factors, outside of hearing loss, that might affect speech processing.

Perhaps because of these factors, the effect of early otitis media on the course of language development has been a matter of great controversy over the past two decades, one that as of this date has not been resolved. The controversy is concerned with whether frequent occurrence of the disease in the early years of life has *long-lasting or only short-term* detrimental effects on the speech and language-processing abilities of children. Further, because physicians will continue to treat the disease in the best manner possible and attempt to find a vaccine or vaccines to prevent the disease it is not clear to some why there appears to be so much passion generated by those on both sides of the controversy. However, finding the answer to the question of whether the disease has long-term detrimental effects is an important matter for the children concerned. If the results of research indicate that any children are at risk for language problems at school age (and therefore at risk for academic problems) as a result of episodes of otitis, then more vigorous educational as well as medical interventions might be contemplated.

This chapter will briefly review some of the research results that have led to the controversy. The studies that will be reviewed were deliberately chosen to represent what I think are the important aspects of the arguments. Then the results of some recent studies that my colleagues and I have carried out will be discussed. Finally, I will attempt to interpret the results of our own and others' research findings to see what conclusions about the issue best fit the data.

## REVIEW OF SOME RESEARCH RESULTS

Many early studies of the relationship between early and persistent otitis media and later language problems were retrospective studies; that is, the incidence of otitis media episodes was retrieved from the medical records of children who were having speech and language problems during the preschool and school years.[7, 22] Most of these studies did find a significant relation between early frequent episodes and later speech and language problems. Although these studies played the important role of bringing the possible developmental effects of persistent otitis media to our attention, they raised many more questions than they answered. The principal problem was that these studies were not able to document the occurrence and duration of early otitis episodes. Therefore, it was difficult to use data from them to help resolve the controversy. For that reason only the data from some prospective studies will be reviewed, and they present a very mixed picture. The studies to be discussed fall into two categories: those that are concerned with language development and academic achievement broadly, and those focused on the speech processing of infants and children with otitis.

Two prospective studies of two socioculturally different populations have found no relation between number of early otitis episodes and later language and academic performance. In one study 3-year-old children who resided in a Danish municipality were invited to take part in an otological study.[8] Some 435 children participated and underwent pneumatic otoscopy, tympanometry, and, as far as possible, pure-tone audiometry four times over a period of approximately 1 year. Among these were 40 children who had constant signs of secretory otitis media. At age 8 the entire group, including 28 children with long-lasting otitis media, was given a silent-reading word test. Six months later 26 of the children with persistent otitis media and 26 control children were given the revised Peabody Picture Vocabulary Test and a standard intelligence test. There were no significant differences between the scores of the target children and the other children on any of the tests. There was, however, greater variability in scores in the target group as compared with the control group on the latter two tests. The researchers suggested that more comprehensive and varied studies seem needed to elucidate the relationship between language development and persistent otitis media.

Roberts et al.[16] studied 61 children who could be classified as coming from families of low socioeconomic status (SES) and were attending a day-care program in the United States when they were enrolled in the study. The numbers of episodes of otitis and the duration of the episodes were documented from the time the children were 2 months of age. When signs of illness were reported or observed nurse practitioners did pneumatic otoscopic examinations. The children were followed up from age 2 months until they completed the first 3 years of elementary school.

These children's scores on standard tests of intelligence and academic achievement were used to examine the question of a relation between early otitis and later language performance. The intelligence and achievement tests were administered when the children were 42 to 60 months. This study revealed no relationship between number of days with otitis media in infancy and later performance on verbal components of standardized intelligence tests or later academic achievement. As the researchers point out, this was a prospective study in which the occurrence and duration of otitis was documented. Thus, many of the problems with retrospective studies were eliminated. However, the researchers also point out that perhaps the language domains affected by otitis media were not assessed in this study despite the fact that the measures used are predictive of later academic performance.

A study using subjects from the study population described above examined language function in a group of 44 children, selected at birth, who had varying histories of otitis over the first 3 years of life.[2] A regression model was used to examine the effect of a number of variables on the ability of the children to retell or paraphrase a story at 5 and 7 years. The frequency and duration of episodes of otitis media during the first 3 years, as well as other selected variables, were used in the regression model. These other variables included mother's measured IQ, mother's education, the home environment, and a standard IQ measure at 5 years. Frequency and duration of otitis media were not predictive of mean length of utterance, a measure used by many researchers who study early language development. However, the significant predictors of narrative skills were both the standard intelligence test and frequency and duration of otitis media. Thus it might be the case that the ability to *recall and regenerate connected discourse* are affected by early histories of otitis media. If they were, then the measures of language and academic achievement used in the two studies described earlier would not be adequate assessments of these children's oral and written language problems.

The above study found that children with nine or more episodes of otitis over the first three years were more inattentive and distractible. It is possible that suffering a fluctuating hearing loss might lead to difficulties in attending to the stream of speech. A further study[1] indicated that children aged 12 and 18 months who suffer from otitis media more than 20% of the time over this age period attended less during a book reading session. They were also more often off-task, even during the times they were well, than infants who had diagnosed otitis media less than 20% of the time. Thus, the negative effects of frequent episodes of otitis on attention appeared to carry over to different types of tasks.

It is also possible that suffering a fluctuating hearing loss renders infants less capable of using the hearing capacities that they do have. Finitzo and Friel-Patti[3] made just such a suggestion at the early stages of their study. In their study 400 infants were followed from age 6 months to age 30 to 36 months. They were to be evaluated every 6 months by immittance screening, an otoscopic examination, and some form of hearing assessment. At 6 months auditory brain-stem response (ABR) audiometry was undertaken and repeated at 12 months if the ABR was abnormal. Behavioral audiometric measures began at 12 months. Measures were taken to detect silent episodes of otitis. In the 1987 report[3] it was found that the mean minimal response level for 500 Hz at 12 months was 26 dB for children with pressure equalization tubes and 32 dB for children with otitis media. The same pattern of response was observed at 2,000 Hz. Further, some infants in the study could hear the pure tones but could not localize them. This problem was accentuated in infants with ventilation tubes and active otitis media. The researchers hypothesized that even when long-standing otitis media resolves, the affected infant may have difficulty in responding to and localizing sounds in the environment. As stated initially, this may be the cause of attention difficulties in infants who suffer frequent episodes of otitis.

In a later publication of this same study,[5] the researchers report that the correlation between days of effusion and average hearing thresholds for children over time is significant and consistent for the periods 6 to 12 months and 6 to 18 months of age. Further, it was found that within this population hearing thresholds for infants from 6 to 12 months of age were significantly related to receptive scores on an inventory of language development at 12 months. At 18 and 24 months both receptive and expressive scores were significantly related to hearing at 6 to 18 months of age. Hearing, in turn, was related to frequency and duration of otitis media. The children in this study were much younger than those tested in the studies described above. Therefore, the effects of persistent otitis media may only be seen at early ages.

Infants with frequent early episodes of otitis might suffer a permanent hearing threshold shift. Fria et al[4] examined speech reception thresholds and pure-tone thresholds (500, 1,000 and 2,000 Hz) in infants and children aged 7 months to 11 years who were experiencing otitis media. They found that the average speech reception threshold was 22.7 dB and the pure-tone average was 24.5 dB for the 540 children in the study over 2 years of age. For the 222 infants below 2 years, the average speech reception threshold was 24.6 dB. Although the means for all these measures were within what is considered the normal range, the wide standard deviations from the mean indicated to these researchers that many of these children have elevated thresholds. This will be discussed further in the next section of the paper.

Children with otitis media have particular difficulty in processing speech sound categories that have little energy such as the voiced stop consonants (/p/, /t/, and /k/) and strident sounds (/s/,

/sh/, and /th/) since threshold shifts from 0 to 20 or 30 dB can affect perception of these sounds. Two recent studies have examined speech sound production in infants with varying histories of otitis media. In one study[14] 40 children between the ages of 18 and 35 months, who were scheduled for tympanostomy and ventilation tube placement, were assessed one day before the procedure took place. They were given an otological and audiological examination, and a phonological screening test. Twenty words were elicited by asking the children to name objects or in some instances to repeat the names. The words in the list were selected to examine the production of phonological patterns that are in the process of being acquired during the age range of the children tested. In addition, the children's medical histories were examined and their parents' education and occupational status determined.

The children were given the phonological screening every 3 to 4 months until they reached their third birthday or until they mastered the patterns being assessed in the screening. It was found that a combination of factors were good predictors of later delays in phonological development. Children who did not catch up to their peers in phonological production at age 3 had inadequate-for-age production of velars (for example /g/, /k/), liquids (for example /l/, /r/), consonant clusters (for example /pr/, /st/, and /skr/) and postvocalic singleton obstruents (syllable final or word final consonants), elevated thresholds at 500 Hz, and a history of early onset and late remission of otitis media.

A continuation of the above study was carried out.[13] All the children who were delayed in phonological production (except five whose parents had selected to put them into speech therapy) plus additional children who had completed the test protocol were reassessed at age 4. There were 36 children who were in the study group, and all had had ventilation tubes. Of these children 22 caught up with their peers in phonological production at age 4, but 14 had not. Those who did and did not catch up differed significantly in scores on initial phonological testing of certain patterns. These children exhibited postvocalic singleton obstruent omission (deletion of medial and final consonants), velar deviation (primarily fronting back sounds), and stridency deletion (omission of such sounds as /s/, /sh/, etc.). These are sounds in positions in words where the energy is reduced. However, it was a combination of factors that was most predictive of phonological performance at 4 years. Discriminant analysis revealed that over 97% of the subjects who had and had not caught up to their age peers on phonological production could be correctly classified by a set of four variables: velar deviation, cluster reduction, retest adequacy score (phonological test score 4 months after tube placement), and elapsed time between initial diagnosis of otitis media and age of first significant remission. Although only 24% of the original subject group were delayed in phonological development at age 4 this is still a sizeable number. Further, sex differences and hearing threshold differences between the groups both before tube placement and after remission of otitis media did not account for phonological differences between the group that caught up and the one that did not.

A study of the relation between early otitis media and the language and phonological development of 55 children from low-SES families indicated that there was no significant relation between otitis media and a number of speech and language measures.[15] There was a relation between the total number of developmental phonological processes used by the children between the ages of 4½ and 8 years. These children continued to use phonological realizations rules such as weak syllable deletion, consonant cluster reduction, and metathesis ("goggie" for "doggie") for a longer period of time than children with no or few episodes of otitis. Such indications of delayed phonological development dropped out more slowly for children with early persistent otitis media, but no consistent patterns were observed in phonological processes or in the particular speech sounds with which they had difficulty.

In summary, this brief review of the literature indicates that the relation between early and persistent otitis media and language development is far from a simple one. The data collected thus far seem to indicate a number of different possible conclusions about the relationship. First, the studies that have used standard tests and measures of language development after 3 years of age have found that number of episodes and duration of otitis media are not significantly related to measured intelligence, word recognition on an oral or written test, or mean length of utterances. There appears to be a relationship between number of episodes and duration of otitis media and hearing at 6, 12, and 18 months, and a relationship between average hearing levels for these months and a measure of receptive language at 12 months, as well as measures of both reception and production of language at 18 and 24 months.

Number of episodes and duration of otitis media, together with measured intelligence, are related to the ability of preschool children to recall and act out stories. Their degree of distractability can be related to early and persistent otitis media. An episode of otitis media can cause a shift in the speech reception threshold of children and in the threshold of pure-tone detection. Their ability to localize sound and their speech reception and pure-tone detection thresholds may be minimally (in the range of 20 to 30 dB) but permanently affected. Phonological development is delayed at age 4 in some children. The children who exhibit phonological delay are those who have the general early phonological problems outlined above and those who suffer early and continuous episodes of otitis media. Table 16–1 presents a summary of these findings.

**TABLE 16–1.**

Summary of Research on Effects of Early Otitis Media on Speech, Language, and Hearing

| Age | Behavior |
|---|---|
| 6 to 18 months | Elevates pure-tone response[3] |
| 12 months | Depresses receptive language[3] |
| 18 months | Depresses receptive and expressive language[3] |
| 24 months | Negatively affects attention[1] |
| 24 months to 11 years | Elevates pure-tone and SRT[4] |
| 36 months | Delays phonological processes[14] |
| 48 months | Delays phonological processes[13] |
| 54 to 60 months | No effect on IQ[16] |
| | No effect on achievement[16] |
| | No effect on MLU[16] |
| 5 to 7 years | No effect on MLU[1] |
| | No effect on IQ[1] |
| | Depresses story recall[1] |
| | Negatively affects attention[1] |
| 8 years | No effect on word comprehension[8] |
| | No effect on silent word reading[8] |
| | No effect on IQ[8] |
| | Delays phonological processes[15] |

## RESULTS OF OUR RESEARCH

This part of the chapter discusses three studies. The first is a study of 205 children selected from a large cohort (N=2,568 children) followed from birth to 3 years.[19] Pediatricians in an urban health center and in two suburban practices began enrolling children into a study group. For 27 continuous months they enrolled each child who made a first visit before 3 months of age. Demographic data, family medical histories, and each member's history of ear disease were obtained initially and updated when the children were 2 years old. At each visit, regardless of its purpose, a physician examined the children's ears and a form was completed that included the purpose of the visit, interval history, and information relevant to middle-ear disease.

Each participating pediatrician was trained in the use of the otoscope. Each time a diagnosis of acute otitis media was made, the child was considered to have had 29 days of effusion unless the period of effusion was observed to be shorter. At three years children were randomly selected for testing from lists prepared by computer that displayed age, sex, race, number of episodes of otitis media, and number of siblings. The sample of 205 children selected at 3 years was divided into three groups: those who had experienced 32 days of effusion, those who had experienced 32 to 108 days of effusion, and those who had experienced more than 108 days of effusion during each of the first 3 years of life. Given the data on hearing losses suffered during days of effusion, it is clear that the children in the latter group were not hearing normally for a large number of days in each year of their first 3 years of life.

The children were given standard tests of speech and language that examined their ability to perceive words, comprehend and produce relations among words in utterances, and to articulate sounds. Their mean length of utterances and the structural complexity of their spontaneous utterances were also determined. These children's hearing was assessed before testing and if any child had an average pure-tone threshold greater than 25 dB for the speech frequencies in either ear, their assessment was postponed until the ear or ears had cleared. It was found that for the entire population the only significant differences between effusion groups was on the assessment of word comprehension. When the performance of urban and suburban children (or children from primarily low-SES and middle-SES families) was examined separately, significant differences among effusion groups were found only in the middle-SES group of children. For this group significant differences in language comprehension and production as well as word comprehension were observed. No differences were found in mean length of utterances or complexity of utterances. The important findings are presented in Table 16–2.

The explanation for finding only differences among effusion groups in the middle-SES population could be the very narrow range of scores obtained by the low-SES children, as a group, on all the tests given.[10] The finding that there was a significant difference among the scores of the middle-class children on reception and production of language at 3 years of age that was related to amount of effusion in the first year of life is in agreement with the studies reviewed. The finding that there was no significant difference in MLU among effusion groups is also in agreement with the studies reviewed, which indicate no general delay in language development at 3 years in relation to amount of effusion during the early years of life. The finding that there was no difference among effusion groups in articulation disagrees with the studies reviewed above, which indicate that there is some phonological delay in children who have early and particularly persistent effusion during the early years of life. The group in this study with most days of effusion could theoretically fall into this category of children.

**TABLE 16–2.**

Effects of Duration of Otitis Media in Year 1 on Language at 3 Years in Middle-Class Children*

| Variable | Effusion Groups | | |
|---|---|---|---|
| | <30 days | >130 days | *P* Value |
| Zimmerman Preschool Scale | | | |
| Comprehension quotient | 135.0 | 120.4 | .003 |
| Production quotient | 130.0 | 112.4 | .004 |
| Peabody Picture Vocabulary Test (mean) | 113.5 | 104.2 | .01 |

*Data from Teele et al[19] and Menyuk.[10]

The second study to be reported here was a continuation of the first one.[18] Of the originally enrolled cohort of 1,067 children, 498 were seen through their seventh birthday. From this group children were randomly selected in each of the clinical settings for additional testing as they became 7. Of those selected 207 agreed to participate. Again, time spent with effusion over the first 3 years and in subsequent years was recorded. Using parental occupation, the children could also be categorized as belonging to the low or the high SES group in the population. All the subjects received a hearing screen just before they received other testing. Children with bilateral thresholds of 20 dB and above at 500, 1,000, 2,000, and 4,000 Hz were deferred for later testing. The average hearing thresholds were recorded when the children were tested.

Cognitive, academic, and linguistic assessments were carried out. All the children were given a standard intelligence test (the WISC-R, Wechsler, 1974) and a standard measure of reading and mathematics skills (the Metropolitan Achievement Test, Primer level, form JS). The linguistic measures included analyses of spontaneously generated speech, performance on experimenter-generated tasks, and performance on standard tests of language abilities (Goldman-Fristoe and Goldman-Fristoe Woodcock Test, the "WUG" test [Berko-Gleason], the Peabody Picture Vocabulary Test, and the Boston Naming Test). Stepwise multiple regression was used to investigate the association between amount of effusion calculated from hypothesized days with effusion, and the scores the children achieved on all measures while controlling for other predictor variables such as gender and SES.

Amount of effusion during the first year of life and over the first 3 years was significantly related to measured intelligence, both verbal and nonverbal. A significant relation was found with amount of effusion and performance on a test of mathematical knowledge. Although the relation between the reading scores and amount of effusion was not significant there was a tendency for scores to be lower in children with greatest amounts of effusion. These findings are in direct conflict with those of other studies that have been reviewed. In these other studies both measured intelligence and academic achievement were not significantly different in relation to amount of

OME. The test of intelligence used in these other studies was the same; therefore differences in tests used cannot account for the conflicting results obtained in testing intelligence. Variation in the children who participated in the respective studies might account for conflicting results, but the exact kind of variation that is the cause of the conflict is unclear. It may be the SES of the children, the age at which the children were assessed, or the criteria for estimating days of effusion.

The analyses of the relations between amount of OME in the first 3 years of life and language measures yielded very few significant results. This was the case despite the fact that there was a significant relation between duration of otitis media during the first year of life and average hearing threshold for the children at 7 years. The areas in which significant effects were found were all in morphophonology: articulation of speech sounds and production of morphological markers. There was a tendency for amount of effusion to be associated with word production. These results and the results for cognitive and academic assessments are shown in Table 16–3.

The findings concerning phonology and morphology are in agreement with several other studies. There were particular sounds that caused the greatest difficulty on the articulation test for children with greater amounts of effusion. They were primarily strident and stop sounds. This is also in agreement with other studies of phonological production in children with lots of effusion early in life referred to earlier. The morphological task was an experimenter-designed task that required the children to repeat sentences that contained lexical items that had final consonants and consonant clusters that were a part of the stem (*fuzz* and *friend*) or were bound morphemes (*he's* and *planned*). It was the latter repetitions that caused the greatest difficulty. Both sets of findings suggest that the children paid the greatest attention to the most meaningful aspect of a lexical item and were letting other aspects go. It should also be noted in Table 16–3 that this particular task was

**TABLE 16–3.**

Effect of Duration of Otitis Media Over First 3 Years on IQ, Achievement, Speech, and Language*,†

| Variable | Regression | SE | t ratio | *P* | $R^2$ |
|---|---|---|---|---|---|
| IQ | | | | | |
| SES | −0.183 | .035 | −5.19 | <.001 | .137 |
| Male | 1.263 | .482 | 0.76 | NS | .196 |
| Otitis media | −1.78 | .482 | −3.69 | <.001 | .193 |
| Mathematics | | | | | |
| SES | −1.19 | 0.20 | −5.85 | <.001 | .156 |
| Male | −13.81 | 9.58 | −1.44 | NS | .194 |
| Otitis media | −6.51 | 2.79 | −2.33 | <.001 | .185 |
| Reading | | | | | |
| SES | −1.53 | 0.33 | −4.68 | <.001 | .099 |
| Male | −40.84 | 15.40 | −2.65 | <.009 | .139 |
| Otitis media | −8.32 | 4.48 | −1.85 | <.065 | .155 |
| Articulation | | | | | |
| SES | 0.001 | .005 | −0.17 | NS | .053 |
| Male | −0.220 | .219 | −1.00 | NS | .053 |
| Otitis media | −0.186 | .066 | −2.81 | <.005 | .048 |
| Morphologic markers | | | | | |
| SES | −0.010 | .002 | −2.45 | <.001 | .067 |
| Male | −0.263 | .128 | −2.06 | <.041 | .121 |
| Otitis Media | −0.086 | .039 | −2.21 | <.028 | .101 |
| Confrontation naming | | | | | |
| SES | −0.148 | .025 | −5.85 | <.001 | .163 |
| Male | 1.805 | 1.21 | 1.49 | NS | .183 |
| Otitis Media | −0.651 | 0.37 | −1.78 | <.077 | .174 |

*From Teele D, Klein J, Chase C, et al: *J Infect Dis* 1990; 162:685–694. Used by permission.
† SES = socioeconomic status; NS = not significant.

significantly more difficult for boys than for girls.

The last study to be discussed is still in progress (the data that were collected are still being analyzed). The children in this study range in age from 1 to 3 years and were randomly selected for testing from pediatric practices in middle- or upper-middle-class suburban communities. Samples of mother-child communicative interaction were recorded when the children were approximately 12 months old. Such samples were also collected at approximately 24 months; in addition, the children were given a sentence repetition task and a standard test of vocabulary knowledge that has been standardized on children aged 30 months and more. At approximately 36 months the children were given a number of tests to examine articulation, word comprehension, and morphosyntactic knowledge. We have collected data on 138 subjects at 1 year, 105 subjects at 2 years, and approximately 60 at 3 years. These differences in numbers are due not to attrition but rather to the fact that the time we had for testing children limited the number that could be entered into the study each year. In addition, the term "approximate" is used for the number of children at 3 years because at this point we have not weeded out the subjects for whom there may be incomplete data.

The findings that will be reported on here should be considered tentative since the data analysis is still not complete. The language samples of the infants at year 1 have been transcribed, coded, and analyzed; therefore, data from this analysis will be discussed. Only some of the data from the language sample at year 2 have been analyzed, although the language sample has been completely transcribed and coded. The sentence repetition data have been coded and analyzed for the morphophonological rules used. Despite the fact that the picture is far from complete, our findings thus far are quite interesting and shed some light on the issues that have been discussed thus far.

At year 1 there is significant effect of frequency of otitis media episodes on the phonological repertoires of the infants.[9] The greater the frequency of episodes, the fewer the consonant phones used in the utterances of these infants. The frequency of episodes also has a negative effect on the proportion of consonant phones to vowel phones used and on the total number of consonant tokens to vowel tokens in the entire language samples obtained from each child. Distinctions among consonants are harder to hear than those among vowels so the results are in the expected direction. There is a tendency for frequency of episodes to have a negative effect on the number of different places (labial, alveolar, and velar) used to differentiate among the consonants produced. Such differences have been found between normally hearing infants and those with sensorineural hearing losses.[17] There is no effect on the number of words produced (as reported by the mother). One could argue that the differences observed in proportion of consonants to vowels in babbling are probably representative of a delay in the development of canonical or true babbling, which is composed of clear consonant-vowel (CV) patterns, and therefore a subsequent delay in word acquisition. However, there was a tendency for the frequency of otitis episodes to have a positive effect on the amount of variegated (different CV sequences) over repetitive (same CV sequences) babble the infants produced, and apparently no effect on the acquisition of lexical items at 1 year. Thus the hypothesized delay in lexical development was not evident in our data.

The measures of language development at 2 years that are available at present are measures of the development of grammatical morphemes (markers of plural, tense, and possession), the performance of the children on a test of word comprehension, MLU,[21] and the syllabic structure of their words.[20] If one controls for the influence of sex, frequency of otitis media at year 1 for boys only is significantly negatively correlated with word comprehension, MLU, maximum sentence length, the number of different words used, and the number of different bound morphemes (markers of tense, plural, etc., that appear at the ends of words) produced. There is a significant negative effect of frequency of episodes in year 1 *and year 2* on the girls' production of plural and possessive markers ($P<.03$).

Finally, the analysis of syllable production at year 2 produced very mixed results. Subjects were classified into two otitis media groups: those with one or no episodes in the first year and those with two or more episodes. Lexical productions that were longer than one syllable were analyzed. The parameters looked at were syllable reduction as a function of position and stress and accuracy of production of phones in various positions in the syllables. In both groups the patterns of syllable reduction as a function of stress and position were very similar. Both groups were more likely to preserve stressed syllables regardless of position. There were differences, however, in the correctness with which phones in syllables were produced as a function of the frequency of episodes of otitis media. There was a significant negative effect of frequency of otitis media on correct production of syllables ($P<.001$), and although the girls had significantly more correct production than the boys ($P<.001$), episodes of otitis media had a negative effect on their correct production as well.

The patterns of errors were interesting. Infants with the more frequent episodes of otitis media produced such syllables with more frequent consonant cluster reduction (*banket* for *blanket*), postvocalic obstruent deletion (*puppe* for *puppet*), stridency deviation (*Kati* for *Kathy*) and liquid deviation (*daion* for *lion*). These, again, are phonological errors that one might expect to result from hearing loss.

The results of this preliminary analysis of the relation between duration of otitis media early in life and speech production indicates that there is a relation between otitis media during the first year of life and morphophonological development during the first 2 years. It is especially marked in boys' acquisition of morphological markers and in how correctly multisyllabic words are produced. Boys may be more affected by otitis media than girls in the second year of life because boys are slower than girls in language development and otitis media may add a factor that slows development even further. The data from other studies that we have reviewed seem to indicate that this may also be true of other factors such as measured IQ and how long over the early life span otitis media episodes frequently occur. These data on morphophonological development seem to reflect what might occur if the hearing losses suffered because of episodes of otitis affect how clearly children can hear the more difficult-to-hear sounds in linguistic contexts that complicate the task. Table 16–4 summarizes the results obtained in the study thus far.

In summary, the results of the studies carried out by my colleagues and me indicate that during the first 2 years of life there is a relation between duration of otitis media experienced, the resultant hearing losses suffered, and the infants' morphophonological production at year 1 and 2. At year 3 there is a significant relation between otitis media and the child's comprehension of words and language and the production of language. At 7, there is a significant relation between amount of otitis media over the first 3 years of life and verbal and nonverbal intelligence, early mathematical skills, and morphophonological production. As indicated, these results are in agreement with some studies and in disagreement with others.

**TABLE 16–4.**
Effects of Frequency of Otitis Media in First Year on Morphophonological Development

| Morphophonological Variable | *t* Ratio | r Value | *P* Value |
|---|---|---|---|
| During year 1 (N=138)* | | | |
| Number of consonants | −2.17 | | <.03 |
| Proportion of consonant/vowel phones | −3.29 | | <.001 |
| Proportion of C/V tokens | −2.41 | | <.02 |
| Number of consonant places | −1.66 | | <.09 |
| Proportion variegated babble | 1.73 | | <.08 |
| During year 2 (N=105, boys only)† | | | |
| PPVT raw score | | .40 | <.01 |
| MLU | | .33 | <.05 |
| Maximum sentence length | | .28 | <.04 |
| Number different words | | .27 | <.05 |
| All bound morphemes | | .30 | <.03 |
| /s/ only | | .34 | <.01 |

*Data from Luloff, Menyuk, and Teele.[9]
†Data from Wendler-Shaw, Menyuk, and Teele.[21]

## SUMMARY AND CONCLUSIONS

It should be clear from the data reviewed that a discussion of the relationship between duration of otitis media and speech processing and language development cannot be a simple one. The expected relationship is: otitis media can lead to hearing losses of approximately 40 dB in the affected ear. Such losses should raise the speech reception threshold for that ear. This should affect the perception of speech sounds that have low intensities and all speech sounds in linguistically complex contexts such as the morphological ends of words and in multisyllabic words, as well as in noisy environments. Such differences should lead to delays in lexical acquisition because lexical development is dependent on the ability to store a phonological sequence and relate that sequence to a semantic category. Lexical acquisition plays a crucial role in language development. This theoretical relation is depicted in Figure 16–1.

The data from our own and others' studies do not indicate that such a clear developmental relationship exists between early and persistent otitis media with effusion, and language development. Two outstanding questions arise about the findings of research thus far. They are: What relationships between otitis media and language development are consistent across studies? and, Why isn't there a clear-cut significant relationship between otitis media and language development?

The answer to the first question appears to be that otitis media leads to differences in language development of different kinds during different periods of development. A consistent finding is that otitis media leads to across-the-board delays in language development between 2 and 3 years of age. This is the period when there is rapid acquisition of lexicon and acquisition of basic syntactic structures.[11] Most studies, but not all, indicate that those aspects of language "catch up" as measured by MLU, analysis of spontaneous speech samples, and standard intelligence tests. However, there is more variability in the performance of children with early histories of otitis media than those without such histories. Speech development, as measured by diversity in phonological repertoire and phonological realization rules, is delayed throughout the entire period of development from 0 to 8 years. The development of the morphological system of the language, which involves particular phonological realizations such as final stridents or /t/ and /d/ as in past tense markers, is delayed.

The answer to the second question is a complex one and requires much more research. If there is a consistent finding that phonological development is delayed in children with persistent early otitis media, it is not clear why there is not a consistent finding that there is a delay in language development. This should be a consequence of delayed morphophonological development for the reasons outlined above. The reason for the finding that there is no significant relation may lie in the variability in language knowledge within the populations studied. That is, there may be some children who do suffer language delay, and others who do not. Not enough children with early persistent otitis media suffer sufficient language delay for statistical significance. Those who do suffer delay may do so for a number of environmental reasons as well as otitis media.

HEARING PROBLEM
SPEECH PROCESSING PROBLEM
LEXICAL PROBLEM??
LANGUAGE PROBLEM??
METAPROCESSING PROBLEM??
READING PROBLEM??

**FIG 16–1.**
Theoretical sequence of difficulties caused by early otitis media with effusion.

Another and more theoretically satisfactory reason may be that the measures of language knowledge that have been used to assess older children with early histories of otitis have not as yet addressed their particular problems. Complex aspects of language processing may be those areas of language performance in these children that still have to be examined. There are hints in the data that this may be the case. For example, it has been found that children with frequent episodes of otitis have attention problems and are easily distractible both early and late. This should affect their ability to process narratives, and it does. Variation in the narrative abilities of children can be significantly accounted for by early histories of otitis media. The ability to retrieve morphological endings as distinct from word stems is significantly related to amount of days spent with otitis media during the first year of life. Confrontation naming, or rapid retrieval of lexical items, tends to be related to otitis media. Given these findings it is possible that measures that look at these children's abilities to bring to conscious awareness (metaprocess) what they know about the morphophonological structure of lexical items, or derivation rules, or the meaning of complex sentences, or the intentional meanings of stories may be those aspects of later language processing that are related to early histories of persistent otitis media. They also are measures that are signifi-

:antly related to reading success.[12] Children who nave reading disabilities or learning problems are often children without any familial histories of reading disorder who do have histories of early persistent otitis media. It is findings such as these that first set researchers on the track of looking for relations between early otitis media and language development, and it is these possibilities that keep us on the track.

## REFERENCES


1. Feagans L, Blood I: Attention to language in day care attending children: A mediating factor in the developmental effects of otitis media. Poster presented at the First International Congress of Behavioral Medicine, Uppsala, Sweden, June 1990.
2. Feagans L, Sanyal M, Henderson F, et al: Relationship of middle ear disease in early childhood to later narrative and attentional skills. *J Pediatr Psychol* 1987; 12:581–594.
3. Finitzo T, Friel-Patti S: Assessment of hearing in infants and young children: The otitis media quandry. Paper presented at Biennial Meeting of the Society for Research in Child Development, Baltimore, April 1987.
4. Fria T, Cantekin E, Eichler J: Hearing acuity of children with otitis media with effusion. *Arch Otolaryngol* 1985; 111:10–16.
5. Friel-Patti S, Finitzo T: Language learning in a prospective study of otitis media with effusion in the first two years of life. *J Speech Hear Res* 1990; 33:188–194.
6. Howie V: Acute and recurrent otitis media, in Jaffe B (ed): *Hearing Loss in Children*. Baltimore, University Park Press, 1977, pp 421–430.
7. Jerger S, Jerger J, Alford B, et al: Development of speech intelligibility in children with recurrent otitis media. *Ear Hear* 1983; 4:138–145.
8. Lous J, Fiellau-Nikolajsen M, Jeppesen A: Secretory otitis media and language development: A six-year follow-up study with case control. *Int J Pediatr Otorhinolaryngol* 1988; 15:185–203.
9. Luloff A, Menyuk P, Teele D: Effect of persistent otitis media on the speech sound repertoire of infants. *Abstracts of the Fifth International Symposium on Recent Advances in Otitis Media, Ft. Lauderdale, Fla,* 1991, p 178.
10. Menyuk P: Predicting speech and language problems with persistent otitis media, in Kavanaugh J (ed): *Otitis Media and Child Development*. Parkton, Md, York Press, 1986, pp 83–98.
11. Menyuk P: *Language Development: Knowledge and Use*. Glenview, Ill, Scott, Foresman/Little, Brown College Div, 1988.
12. Menyuk P, Chesnick M, Liebergott J, et al: Predicting reading problems in at risk children. *J Speech Hear Res* 1991; 34:893–903.
13. Paden E, Matthies M, Novak M: Recovery from OME-related phonologic delay following tube placement. *J Speech Hear Disord* 1989; 54:94–100.
14. Paden E, Novak M, Beiter A: Predictors of phonologic inadequacy in young children prone to otitis media. *J Speech Hear Disord* 1987; 52:232–242.
15. Roberts J, Burchinal M, Koch M, et al: Otitis media in early childhood and its relationship to later phonological development. *J Speech Hear Disord* 1988; 53:416–424.
16. Roberts J, Sanyal M, Burchinal M, et al: Otitis media in early childhood and its relationship to later verbal and academic performance. *Pediatrics* 1986; 78:423–430.
17. Stoel-Gammon C: Prelinguistic vocalizations of hearing-impaired and normally hearing subjects: A comparison of consonantal inventories. *J Speech Hear Disord* 1988; 53:302–315.
18. Teele D, Klein J, Chase C, et al: Otitis media in infancy and intellectual ability, school achievement, speech and language at age 7 years. *J Infect Dis* 1990; 162:685–694.
19. Teele D, Klein J, Rosner B: Otitis media with effusion during the first three years of life and development of speech and language. *Pediatrics* 1984; 74:282–287.
20. Tsushima T, Menyuk P, Teele D: The effects of otitis media on syllable realization in the speech of children. *Abstracts of the Fifth International Symposium on Recent Advances in Otitis Media,* Columbus, Ohio, Ohio State University, College of Medicine, Department of Otolaryngology and The Deafness Research Foundation, 1991, p 191.
21. Wendler-Shaw P, Menyuk P, Teele D: Effects of otitis media in the first year of life on language production in the second year of life. *Abstracts of the Fifth International Symposium on Recent Advances in Otitis Media,* Columbus, Ohio, Ohio State University, College of Medicine, Department of Otolaryngology and The Deafness Research Foundation, 1991, p 179.
22. Zinkus P, Gottlieb M: Pattern of perceptual and academic deficits related to early chronic otitis media. *Pediatrics* 1980; 66:246–253.

*Chapter* **17**

# Speech-Language Management of Central Auditory Processing Disorders

**SusanEllen Bacon, Ph.D.**

As you have read and absorbed the information from this book, you may have had two thoughts: how exciting, and how do I assimilate this information and apply it to my clinical setting? The excitement will be reinforced as you modify your diagnostic procedures or your interactions with a client because of the information you have read, but the clinical challenge remains.

It is possible in this concluding chapter to provide a single approach to the speech-language management of central auditory processing disorders (CAPDs) only if we would all reach consensus on the definition and etiology of central auditory processing problems, if each of our clients would exhibit the same behavioral abnormalities, if parents and educators would share the same concerns, and if the utopian remedial strategy (with a universal theoretical foundation) could be purchased from one educational supply house. I wish that were the case.

But there would be some downsides to my wish. In order to make my wish come true it would be necessary to clone one client and one therapist to remove any individual differences. The twinkle in the eye of the child who mischievously poked the teacher's aide and the confusion on the face of the child who looks at you plaintively after hearing your directions would be gone. Clients would loose their individual personalities and your unique treatment style, once mixed with enthusiasm and compassion, could not be differentiated from the session being conducted in the next room.

Since there would be such obvious downsides to my wish coming true, we are going instead to need to develop strategies to deal with our differences in philosophy, clients, and treatment methodology so that we can develop effective protocols for the speech-language management of CAPDs.

## NEW GESTALT

Before we become immersed in the technical aspects of our fields, I would like to suggest that we interject a more global intervention schema. Many speech-language pathologists place auditory processing problems in children under the category of receptive speech disorders. While this categorical placement is correct, I believe that we need to step back further to provide a more comprehensive viewpoint.

In that regard, I propose a new gestalt. We must determine the student's ability to process auditory information by asking the question: "How well does he or she listen? Students are required to listen an average of 42% of the school day and yet even the most optimistic findings indicate classroom teachers spend only 8% of the available instructional time teaching students how to listen.[2, 7]

What researchers have also found is that as students advance through the educational system the amount of time they are required to listen increases and their listening ability decreases.[6, 12]

Students who exhibit auditory perceptual problems are not only struggling with the diagnosed receptive language disorder but are caught in the same listening syndrome as their educational counterparts. If we are to do these students a service, it is important to infuse information about general listening strategies into their daily curriculum. One of the most effective ways to impact the language arts curriculum (where listening is already placed) is for speech-language pathologists to share information about listening with the regular classroom teacher.

We not only have instant credibility because of our past practices as resources for receptive language strategies, but many of the materials we have on hand include general listening lessons. However, to teach this new gestalt, it is vital that we be able to define listening using a clear, workable model.

The SIER model[11] provides an easily understandable description of activities performed by effective listeners. This model depicts listening as a four-stage sequential process: sensing, interpreting, evaluating, and then responding to information. Helping students to improve their ability to listen in a classroom environment provides us with a more comprehensive strategy to address auditory process problems.

Once we have adopted a more global viewpoint, we can add additional management strategies such as: classroom management techniques, implementation of the consultative model, a systematic hierarchy of auditory skills, and creative uses of existing therapy materials. While each of these strategies will be discussed as unique treatment components, no strategy is effective in isolation and each technique will require modification according to the practitioner's personality and the individual needs of the client.

## CLASSROOM MANAGEMENT STRATEGIES

Classroom management techniques should be used as our first intervention strategy and we should begin by stressing to the classroom teacher the significance of CAPD as a handicapping condition. Not only do educators need to realize that the behaviors exhibited by a child with auditory process problems are symptoms rather than indices of a disorder, but educators need to be aware that the implementation of appropriate classroom techniques will reap rewards not only for the targeted student, but for the teacher and each of the other students in the class.

A variety of authors[4, 8] have suggested schemas that impact classroom management. As you review their treatment protocols—or any treatment protocol—you should be struck by the similarity between the classroom management of students with auditory perceptual deficits and of students who are hard of hearing. This fact should prove reinforcing on two levels: first, it reemphasizes the concept that these strategies generalize to other students; and second, it adds credence to the general management of students who have difficulty processing auditory signals.

Because of the similarity between classroom management of students who are hard of hearing and students who exhibit auditory perceptual problems, we already have in our repertoire a series of strategies that can be provided to teachers as they deal with students in their classroom. These strategies facilitate the student's ability to process language in the classroom environment and provide modeling of ideal language behaviors. It is important that we consider the following:

1. *Delivery style.*—Educators should speak in a clear, animated, and audible tone of voice. Gestures that enhance the message are effective tools, but extraneous gestures are detracting. Teachers should be aware of their speaking rate; if increased comprehension is noted at a slower than average rate of speech (about 150 words per minute), instruction should be provided at the reduced rate.

2. *Preferential seating.*—Students with auditory processing problems should be provided optimal seating in regard to both auditory and visual stimuli. Ideally the student should be away from noise (e.g., windows, heater) and placed so that the visual field contains the instructional material. The concept of preferential seating should be flexible and the student should be involved in the seating decision.

3. *Visual aids.*—Teachers should be encour-

aged to use visual aids, especially when new concepts are introduced. Strategies such as cognitive mapping (student-created pictorial representations and interactions of auditory information), graphic organizers (teacher-provided illustrations/statements which help students "track" the lecture), and pictures in the mind (imagination strategies) are all effective reinforcements for auditory information.

4. *Unambiguous directions/instructions.*—Students benefit from clear, concise, and succinct instructions. They equally benefit by clearly understanding the purpose of the activity. A clearly stated purpose provides a preparatory attitude that allows the student to focus on the appropriate information.

5. *Effective teaching strategies.*—This statement is not included to pass judgment on educators but to reinforce the concept that educational practices such as instructional transitions, organized presentations, and clearly delineated concepts do improve the ability of students to comprehend and retain information.

6. *Facilitate cueing strategies.*—Many students with auditory process deficits exhibit difficulty with word-retrieval strategies. It is our responsibility to determine the most effective retrieval strategy, provide the student success in retrieval exercises, encourage self-awareness of effective strategies, and gradually withdraw the external cue so that the student can achieve independent success.

7. *Maintain records.*—Regardless of which classroom management strategy is implemented, it is important to maintain records. These records should include which strategies are most successful and under what circumstances other techniques failed. The success stories need to be shared with all of the resource personnel working with the student so that a consistent reinforcing plan can be implemented. The student deserves to achieve success in as many arenas as possible.

8. *Auditory exhaustion.*—Educators need to be aware that even when the most successful strategies are implemented there will be days, and especially afternoons, students with the best of intentions struggle to process information. One effective way of dealing with this phenomenon is to instruct in segments no longer than 20 minutes and vary instructional strategies.

9. *Monitor the message.*—Regardless of how effective teachers are in implementing all of the strategies we have discussed so far, it is important that they realize that sometimes the information just isn't processed. From recognizing the "blank" or "puzzled" look on students' faces to stopping and asking, "Lets see if I said everything I thought I did," teachers need to use strategies other than tests to make sure the message is received. The *least* effective way to ensure message reception is repetition. Let me repeat . . .

10. *Compassion.*—Most of us went through training programs that used the phrase "establish rapport." What I mean here is a step beyond that: it is truly connecting with the child by letting him or her know you understand his or her struggles and are willing to listen and to brainstorm about strategies that will help the student perform in the classroom.

If we realize that for most of the students who exhibit auditory process deficits the regular teacher provides the majority of language stimulation, we must agree that by providing strategies to improve the student's ability to process information in the classroom, we have taken a vital first intervention step.

## IMPLEMENTATION OF THE CONSULTATIVE MODEL

The next intervention step builds on the new gestalt. It is important to change the specific treatment philosophy. The pull-out model of therapy, the one that says that we remove the student from the classroom for 20 minutes three times a week, may be viable for remediating some speech and language disorders. It may even be helpful for introducing new concepts, reviewing, and providing individual strategies, but I do not believe that it is the appropriate single model for the speech-language management of students with auditory processing disorders.

So the challenge is, how do we make the transition from the pull-out model to a more integrated, consultative approach? And the answer is, you have already begun if you have shared with your regular education teachers the information on listening and classroom-management strategies. The advantages of using the consultative model as an intervention strategy are numerous. We can coordinate intervention programs with the student's primary teacher. There is an opportunity for "our" students to be "stimulated" by the performance of the "regular" education student. And we can meet the speech-language needs of more students (especially those students who are exhibiting auditory problems but have not been referred for evaluation). Incidentally, therapists report a reduction in referrals for auditory process diagnosis and treatment when the consultative model is implemented!

There are also disadvantages. These include practitioners' lack of training in the implementation of consultative service delivery, the need to acquire a clear understanding of curricular issues, and the problem of needing to learn "classroom" teaching styles.[5]

However, when we look at success stories in implementing the consultative model, the advantages outweigh the disadvantages. And the success comes because we are implementing our intervention strategies where the students spend the majority of their school day: the classroom.

One technique for designing auditory remediation programs for the classroom is to look at the language arts skills that are stressed at each grade. Another strategy is to develop "tip" sheets or short newsletters and share ideas on a monthly basis. Or be creative and do demonstration teaching. By drawing from your materials on receptive language remediation an exciting in-class auditory program can be developed. Such a program will be one *all* of the students learn from and enjoy.

## SCOPE AND SEQUENCE OF AUDITORY SKILLS

Regardless of whether pull-out or in-class remediation is deemed most appropriate, a systematic hierarchical management strategy *must* be implemented. There exists in our field an argument over whether or not it is possible to view auditory processing as a series of individual components that must be mastered to achieve the whole, or if it is necessary to view the process as a whole. Although this argument is not settled, many authors have presented a systematic series of skills that require mastery before information can be efficiently processed. I do not purport to settle that argument at this time: what I do want to share is that learners crave structure and organization. Without some conceptual framework to begin intervention, there is no way we can manage the speech-language remediation of students who exhibit auditory problems. Using concepts from both the communication literature as well as theory from speech-language pathology and audiology, I propose as a minimum the following strategies be included in a scope and sequence of remediation:

1. *Attending behavior.*—The student must be alert to the stimuli for an adequate amount of time.
2. *Awareness.*—Once alert to the stimuli, the student must appropriately direct his or her focus.
3. *Identification.*—This component includes sound recognition and labeling. (It is hard to differentiate here between the auditory skill and the language activity.)
4. *Discrimination or fine-tuning the identification skills.*—Included here is the ability to tune out distractions.
5. *Memory.*—The discrimination process involves using this process for pattern comparison, but here we are stressing the improvement of both short- and long-term storage capacity.
6. *Sequencing.*—There are variable components to the memory process; the order and length of recall are addressed here.
7. *Directions.*—Building on the memory and sequencing components, this skill is directly related to classroom success and is considered one of the major indicators of auditory processing problems.
8. *Context.*—The student who is able to identify an isolated linguistic event needs to be able to address the arena in which the stimuli are presented. The same sound pattern could take on different meaning.
9. *Relevance.*—Continuing the concept of context, appropriate and inappropriate information must be identified.
10. *Purpose.*—Here one begins to address fulfilling auditory goals and implementing auditory strategies. The listener is given specific concepts to recall and discuss.
11. *Conceptualization.*—Here the message

has been heard, internalized, sorted, and retained using a "to me" value.

12. *Critical analysis.*—The focus here is whether the message has been understood and whether the understanding is accurate, relevant, and appropriate. This step adds a "judgment" component.
13. *Feedback.*—It is important that one of the strategies we teach is the ability to appropriately respond to information.
14. *Appreciate.*—It is also important to provide some auditory stimuli that are just for "pure" enjoyment.

This scope and sequence should not be viewed as a series of isolated, individual tasks, but as interdependent strategies that can be individually stressed during speech-language therapy. In order to conduct traditional therapy procedures, such as treatments for articulation, syntax, or semantic disorders, students need to have strategies to process the auditory stimuli. It should also be remembered that the typical student exhibiting auditory processing problems is not easily identified on one of our "standard" language assessment instruments. In order to "fine tune" these children's speech-language skills, it is necessary to improve their ability to process the nuances of our language.

## TAP INTO YOUR CREATIVITY

The amount of structure necessary in the session/lesson is also a debated topic. Some therapists firmly believe that structured sessions are necessary to elicit change and suggest taped programs and message redundancy. Other therapists stand firmly on the other side of this issue and hold that a variety of situational contexts must be contrived in order to prepare the student to deal with the "real world."

Programs are available that can provide structured therapy sessions. A few of these programs that have been used effectively in therapy procedures include:

- Auditory Discrimination in Depth (1969)
  C. Lindamood and P Lindamood
  Teaching Resources Corporation
  Boston, Massachusetts
- Language Processing Remediation (1987)
  Gail Richard and Mary Anne Hanner
  Linguisystems
  Moline, Illinois
- Semel Auditory Processing Program (1976)
  Elizabeth Semel
  Follett Publishing Co.
  Chicago, Illinois

The repetoire of strategies available to the creative therapist appears limitless.

Of all of the types of speech-language therapy sessions we conduct, therapy for the management of children exhibiting auditory processing problems can and should be our most creative. We are given an opportunity to provide innovative strategies for students who usually are struggling in the typical classroom environment. That struggle often lessens the student's self-esteem. Yet student after student, when provided creative, energetic therapy sessions addressing their auditory processing deficit, not only will show significant growth in ability to use appropriate strategies, but will leave each session with a smile.

## CHOOSING THE APPROPRIATE THERAPY

The questions we need to ask to help us choose the optimal remedial procedure are, "How is the child functioning in his or her environment?" and "How should that child be performing?" And the answer for improving speech-language and auditory proficiency is not cloning our clients but determining how best to implement a strategy that provides the same answer to both questions. That process necessitates choosing a new gestalt, working with the classroom teacher, using an organized systematic therapy approach, providing students with individualized coping strategies, and providing opportunities for students to succeed by utilizing their strongest learning modality when presenting new information. When implementing the program you deem appropriate based on those criteria you have the opportunity to make a real difference in the speech-language status of students exhibiting central auditory processing disorders.

## REFERENCES


1. Bacon S: Listening and the consultative model. *Clin Connect* 1990; 4:12–13.
2. Barker L: *Listening Behavior*. Englewood Cliffs, NJ, Prentice-Hall, 1971.
3. Butler K: Language processing disorders: Factors in diagnosis and remediation, in Keith R (ed): *Central Auditory and Language Disorders in Children*. San Diego, College-Hill Press, 1981.
4. Clark J: Central auditory dysfunction in children: A compilation of management suggestions. *Long Speech Hear Serv Schools* 1980; 11:208–213.
5. Miller L: Remediation of Children With Auditory Language Learning Disorders, in Roeser R, Downs M (eds): *Auditory Disorders in School Children*. New York, Thieme Medical Publishers, 1988.
6. Nichols RG, Stevens L: *Are You Listening?* New York, McGraw-Hill, 1957.
7. Rankin PT: The measurement of the ability to understand spoken language, in Duker S (ed): *Listening Bibliography*. Metuchen, NJ, Scarecrow Press, 1926, pp 219–279.
8. Rampp D: *Auditory Processing and Learning Disabilities*. Omaha, Cliff Notes, 1980.
9. Richard G, Hanner MA: *Language Processing Remediation*. Moline, Ill, LinguiSystems, Inc, 1989.
10. Sloan C: Auditory processing disorders in children: Diagnosis and treatment, in Levinson P, Sloan C (eds): *Auditory Processing and Language*. New York, Grune and Stratton, 1980.
11. Steil L, Watson KW, Barker LL: *Effective Listening: Key to Your Success*. Reading, Mass, Addison-Wesley Publishing, 1983.
12. Swanson C: Teachers as listeners: An Exploration. Paper presented at the International Listening Association, San Diego, March 1986.
13. Willeford J, Burleigh J: *Handbook of Central Auditory Processing Disorders in Children*. Orlando, Fla, Grune and Stratton, 1985.

# Index